Lymphedema Caregiver's Guide

arranging and providing home care

Mary Kathleen Kearse, PT, CLT-LANA
Elizabeth McMahon, PhD
Ann Ehrlich, MA

Lymph Notes
San Francisco

Lymphedema Caregiver's Guide: arranging and providing home care
© 2009 by Lymph Notes

Lymph Notes
2929 Webster Street
San Francisco, CA 94123 USA
www.LymphNotes.com   sales@lymphnotes.com

Notice of Rights
All rights reserved. No part of this book may be reproduced in any form or by any means without prior permission of the publisher.

Notice of Liability
The information in this book is provided on an "as is" basis without warranty. It is sold with the understanding that the publisher and authors are not engaged in providing medical or other professional services. Neither the authors, nor Lymph Notes, shall have any liability to any person or entity for any loss or damage caused or alleged to be caused, indirectly or directly by the instructions contained in this book.

Trademarks
Lymph Notes and the Lymph Notes logo are registered trademarks, and LymphNotes.com is a trademark, of Lymph Notes. All product names and services identified throughout this book are used in editorial fashion only; usage does not imply an endorsement or affiliation.

ISBN 978-0-9764806-7-9
Library of Congress Control Number: 2008938315
Publishing history—first edition, printing 1-01

Cover is based on an original quilt by Sue Andrus of Andrus Gardens, www.AndrusGardensQuilts.com.

Dedication

This book is dedicated to Bob Weiss, a very special caregiver, in recognition of his efforts to help everyone with lymphedema treatment access and insurance obstacles.

Bob became a lymphedema caregiver when his wife, Pearl, developed lymphedema. Soon Bob found an additional calling as a Lymphedema Activist, using the knowledge he acquired advocating for Pearl, and his analytical skills, to guide patients through the quagmire of healthcare laws and reimbursement policies.

Bob developed a legal and medical argument that compression garments for lymphedema treatment should be covered by Medicare because they fall within the definition of prosthetic devices given in the law that created Medicare—and has received favorable rulings in several coverage appeals.

He continues to lobby for lymphedema legislation at the state and national levels, and works with Medicare and other organizations to establish the administrative policies and codes needed to facilitate payment for lymphedema treatment and devices. Bob educates patients and professionals through his column in the NLN newsletter, conference presentations, and via online communities and e-mail lists.

On behalf of the lymphedema community, we say *"Thank you Bob (and Pearl), your efforts are greatly appreciated."*

Acknowledgements

I sincerely thank my mother for her inspiration and strength through the years, and my family and friends for their many words of encouragement. I greatly appreciate Mary Jo Marino and my colleagues at Marino Therapy Centers for your faith and support of my work, and my patients and their caregivers for allowing me to know, love, and serve you. I am indebted to the lymphedema community for their expertise, my coauthors Ann and Liz for the special honor of writing with you, and Lymph Notes for the wonderful opportunity to expand my work through this book. My humble gratitude extends to Saints Therese and Faustina for their prayers of love and mercy. Most especially, I thank my husband Kelly for the wisdom, laughter, and music you share with me every day; you are my all. *This work is dedicated to my father for his love beyond measure.*
—Kathy

I would like to acknowledge my coauthors who inspire me by the breadth of their lymphedema knowledge and their dedication to empowering patients and caregivers. It was a pleasure to work with you. I also wish to acknowledge my patients who are inspiring examples of courage in the face of adversity. Thanks are due to my wonderful extended family for their love and support. And, lastly, thank you to my husband and my daughter who have been extraordinary caregivers, when needed, and whose love means more to me than I can say.
—Liz

It is an honor to be part of the team that brought to life a book with the potential to improve the health and quality of life for lymphedema patients, especially those who are unable to manage home care on their own. It has been a pleasure working with my coauthors as they graciously shared their extensive knowledge and experience and willingly putting in the effort required to "*Get it just right*" throughout. Also special thanks to the Lymph Notes team who put in even more hours to create a book that meets so many needs. I want to thank my lymphedema therapists for the excellent care they have provided that has made my participation in this project possible. They have generously, and very patiently, answered my endless questions—and often provided additional ideas. Special thanks to my loving family for their support and patience, especially during endless conversations about lymphedema care.
—Ann

The authors and publisher would like to thank our reviewers for their attention to detail and thoughtful comments.

Jane Armer, PhD, RN
Carole Bentley
Linda Boyle, PT, DPT,
    CLT-LANA
Jillian Bracha, B.Sc., PT, CLT, CI
Laura Ehrlich
Wade Farrow, MD, CWS
Alison Humble Golla, MA,
    OTR/L, CLT
Tina Hammond, PTA,
    CLT-LANA
Liliya V. Jones, MD, PT, CLT
Anna Kellogg, OTR/L, CLT
Bonnie Lasinski, PT, MA, CI,
    CLT-LANA

Ruthi Peleg, PT
Bonnie Pike
Barbara Kate Repa
Sheila Ridner, PhD, RN
Nate Rinehart
Mary Sommers
DeCourcey Squire, PT,
    CLT-LANA
Debi Stowers
Kathryn Thrift, CLT-LANA
Bob Weiss
Kathleen Westbrook, PT,
    CLT-LANA
Chris Whiteaker
Barbara Zanzig

We would also like to thank the caregivers and patients who appear in the photo illustrations for their time and cooperation.

Figure 1-3 and Figure 12-3 are reproduced from **Living Well With Lymphedema** by permission of the publisher. All other photos were provided by Mary Kathleen Kearse. Illustrations in Figure 1-1, Figure 2-1 and Appendix A are based on artwork licensed from Giunti International, www.giunti.it. Cover design is based on an original quilt by Sue Andrus of Andrus Gardens, www.AndrusGardensQuilts.com.

Foreword

This book has changed my thinking about lymphedema care. Since 1998, when my colleagues and I founded the Lymphology Association of North America (LANA), my focus has been on improving the competency of lymphedema therapists who provide treatment proven to reduce disability and pain related to lymphedema.

In reviewing this book, I found myself forced to think beyond the demands of delivering excellent treatment. This book so clearly and simply states the obvious: failure of treatment these days is not due to a lack of competent therapists; but, more often, to a lack of supportive care in the home. So often, patients are unable to provide self-care for maintaining compression on the affected limb, which is the key aspect of lymphedema management.

This book clearly argues the need for competent caregivers and then sets about to bridge the gap that exists in lymphedema home care. Ms. Kearse has carefully researched her subject and gives concise and clear explanations as to why a caregiver shortage exists. She then provides ways in which concerned family and friends can pick up the burden of care, with excellent text, diagrams, and pictures. In an effort to better train family members to provide care for their loved one at home, our lymphedema treatment program will be using this book as part of our curriculum for patients and family.

Many unmet needs remain within the field of lymphedema, including insurance coverage for compression garments and aids; adequate medical school education and the availability of trained physicians; research into cause and treatment of lymphedema; and training dollars for therapists to receive an excellent education. This book so competently and completely addresses the need for caregivers within the field of lymphedema that at least one of the unmet needs has been addressed.

It is deeply pleasing to me that I have been asked to write a foreword for such an important book within the field of lymphedema.

Paula J. B. Stewart, MD, MS, CLT-LANA
Medical Director
HealthSouth Lakeshore Rehabilitation Hospital

Table of Contents

Contents in Brief

Contents in Detail

Introduction

We extend a warm welcome whether you are reading this book because you provide or receive lymphedema care, arrange for care, or educate, supervise, or collaborate on care. Home care can seem overwhelming at first, but it gets easier with time and practice.

Home care is an essential part of lymphedema treatment. Caregivers play an important—and under-recognized—role in providing this care. A knowledgeable caregiver can improve the effectiveness of home care, adherence to the home care routine, and the quality of life for a patient with lymphedema. Many patients cannot perform home care on their own; for them, home care does not happen without a caregiver.

We wrote this book to give you, in one easily accessible place, practical information you can use every day including step-by-step instructions with photographs and explanations, forms to make care organized and easier, problem-solving support, help arranging care, and answers to frequently asked questions. You will find information you might need on a daily basis: from routine care to identifying emergencies, from providing physical care to providing emotional support, from communication skills to body mechanics. In addition, you will find lists of resources and sources of further information.

The book is addressed to caregivers, but we recognize that a successful treatment team includes patients, caregivers, and lymphedema therapists working together and we hope that all team members will find this book useful.

We respect and honor the work you do and want to offer a helping hand to those providing or arranging care, to those with lymphedema, and to therapists.

What do we mean by home care?

By home care we mean the daily lymphedema regimen that includes skin care, compression wrapping and garments, lymphatic drainage, and exercise or other activities prescribed by the patient's healthcare provider and explained here. Home care also includes a number of important support activities—such as managing supplies and equipment—which are also covered in this book.

What does a caregiver do?

Very few people are able to manage all of the activities of daily lymphedema care on their own due to limitations in reaching, grasping, flexibility and mobility. Individual needs vary, but most patients need some assistance with the physical aspects of lymphedema care—such as skin care, lymph drainage, putting on and removing compression bandages or garments, and exercise. Many patients also need emotional care and support.

Some patients—especially the very young and very old—may need assistance organizing and remembering care routines. A caregiver provides structure to help these patients complete their care routine.

Depending on the patient's medical condition, the need for caregiver assistance may be short-term—to help someone learn the home care routine initially or during recovery—or long-term. For more information see "Types of Care" on page 39 and "Care Goals" on page 39.

Are caregivers therapists?

Caregivers are not therapists; they are persons who can assist in carrying out a daily care routine prescribed by a therapist or healthcare professional. Caregivers are expected to monitor the patient's health, identify changes in the condition of the affected area, and alert the patient's medical team if there are significant changes. Caregivers are not expected to make treatment decisions.

To avoid confusion with Manual Lymph Drainage (MLD) performed by professional therapists, we use the term Simple Lymph Drainage (SLD) to describe the techniques a caregiver uses to activate the lymphatic system (see "Lymphatic Drainage" on page 32). SLD has been used to describe home care massage for some time, primarily in the United Kingdom.[1]

Why a caregiver shortage?

In the next few years we will need many more lymphedema caregivers while the number of potential family caregivers drops sharply, as explained below. In order to close this care gap, the lymphedema community must create ways to provide trained caregivers.

As the baby boomers age, we are experiencing a major demographic shift in the United States (and other countries). Between 2011 and 2031 the 'Over 65' population is expected to double from 10% of the total population to nearly 20%.

As the 'Over 65' population increases, so will the number of people with lymphedema. Despite changes in certain cancer treatments to lower the risk of lymphedema, the increase in the older population, and improvements in cancer survivorship, will result in a larger number of people with lymphedema as a consequence of cancer treatment.

Our current obesity epidemic will also result in more people with lymphedema, some of whom will be over 65 but many will be younger. In general, people with obesity-related lymphedema are more likely to need assistance. Training is especially important to minimize the risk of lifting injuries in caregivers working with the obese.

Historically both family and paid caregivers have been women between the ages of 25 and 54. As the population ages, predictions show many fewer women in this age range relative to the number of people needing care. In 2000 there were approximately two women in this age bracket for every person 'Over 65,' by 2030 there will be less than one.

The lymphedema caregiver shortage is part of a larger shortfall in medical professionals including lymphedema therapists, direct-care workers, and informal caregivers that the Institute of Medicine describes as "an impending health care crisis as the number of older patients with more complex health needs increasingly outpaces the number of health care providers with the knowledge and skills to adequately care for them." [2]

Who is this book for?

This book is a guide to providing daily care for people with lymphedema and is intended for two audiences:

- **Care providers** including partners, children, parents or other family members, friends, home health aides, visiting nurses, hospice workers, and other professional caregivers.

- **Care arrangers** including people arranging care for themselves, friends or family, or as part of a healthcare service or facility.

In order to simplify the text, we use the terms caregiver, care arranger, and patient. These terms were selected to cover all possible relationships.

Patients with lymphedema may use this book to learn more about lymphedema care and may be capable of providing some, or all, of their own care. Please note that **Living Well With Lymphedema**[3] focuses on self care (including self-massage) while this book provides instructions for a caregiver.

We assume that the patient has been diagnosed with lymphedema and that their treatment is being coordinated by a physician (or other health care provider) and a qualified lymphedema therapist who can provide advice as needed. If this is not the case, or if you need information on how lymphedema is diagnosed or finding treatment, please start with the relevant chapters in **Living Well With Lymphedema**.

Goals of this Book

Our goals for this book include:

- Giving the reader a basic understanding of lymphedema, lymphedema treatment with Complete Decongestive Therapy (CDT), and the importance of home care.

- Enabling the caregiver to identify conditions, or changes in condition, that should be brought to the attention of the patient's medical team.

- Making it easier for a caregiver to learn the hands-on aspects of lymphedema home care, in cooperation with the patient's therapist.

- Providing a process and tools for managing supplies and equipment and arranging and coordinating care, especially when multiple caregivers are involved.

- Offering the caregiver guidance on how to provide emotional care and support, and how to protect themselves from injury and burnout.

We have tried to make this a practical book with:

- Clear explanations in plain English. We have included some medical terminology to make it easier to communicate with health professionals.

- Just enough anatomy and physiology to help you understand what you are doing and why.

- Proven tips from therapists and caregivers with years of experience.

This Book Does Not Provide

Please understand what this book is not:

- **It is not a substitute for lymphedema therapy**. Daily care is an essential part of lymphedema treatment in combination with the care of a professional therapist.

- **It is not therapist training**. Lymphedema therapists are medical professionals with specialized training. For information on how to become a lymphedema therapist see "Therapist Training" in **Living Well With Lymphedema**[4] or the Resources section of www.LymphNotes.com.

- **It is not a comprehensive home care manual**. Although we discuss care planning that includes care for other medical conditions, we only provide instruction for lymphedema care.

- **It is not a directory of home care providers or eldercare facilities.**

How to Use this Book

We have organized this book to meet the needs of readers in different situations:

- If you are new to lymphedema, especially if you or someone you care about has just been diagnosed, start at the beginning and read the entire book roughly in order. There are some areas that you can skip over; these are noted in the text.

- If you will be a lymphedema caregiver, read the sections on "Understanding Lymphedema Care," "Daily Care Skills," and "Caring for the Caregiver." Depending on your situation and your responsibilities, you may also want to read the sections on "Activities of Daily Living," "Managing Supplies and Equipment," and "Arranging and Managing Care."

- If you are arranging or coordinating lymphedema care, read the section on "Understanding Lymphedema Care," skim "Daily Care Skills," and skip to "Managing Supplies and Equipment" and "Arranging and Managing Care." Read other sections as needed.

Like many specialties, lymphedema care has its own language. We introduce terms you may hear from therapists or other professionals but we also explain them and pair them with common terms. Explanations are usually given the first time a term appears, check the index if you encounter an unfamiliar term.

Book Website

Supplementary materials and additional information will be available on the book website (www.Lymphedema-Caregiver.com) including:

- Forms that you can download and print on letter size paper.

- Color versions of selected images.

- Ability to submit questions or corrections online.

- Clarifications and corrections based on reader feedback.

We look forward to hearing from you.

Notes

1   "Guidelines for the use of MLD and SLD" by the
    British Lymphology Society, 2001. Available from
    www.lymphoedema.org/bls/membership/guidelines.htm.

2   **Retooling for an Aging America: Building the Health Care
    Workforce** by the Institute of Medicine, National Academies Press,
    2008. Available from www.nap.edu.

3   **Living Well With Lymphedema** by Ann Ehrlich, Alma Vinjé-
    Harrewijn, and Elizabeth McMahon. Lymph Notes, 2005.

4   **Living Well With Lymphedema** by Ann Ehrlich, Alma Vinjé-
    Harrewijn, and Elizabeth McMahon. Lymph Notes, 2005.

Understanding Lymphedema Care

The goal of this section is to help the caregiver or care arranger understand lymphedema and the lymphatic system, lymphedema treatment, and the importance of daily care in lymphedema treatment.

We begin with an overview of the lymphatic system, the causes of lymphedema, the progression or stages of lymphedema, and possible complications. Since many lymphedema patients also have other medical conditions, we discuss some common conditions and how these conditions relate to lymphedema and lymphedema treatment.

The chapter on "How is Lymphedema Treated" explains the principles of lymphedema treatment and treatment options. The actual practice of daily care is explained in Section II, "Daily Care Skills."

Caregivers who are not familiar with the lymphatic system should also read Appendix A. Understanding the anatomy and physiology of the lymphatic system makes it easier to provide lymphedema care, especially lymphatic drainage.

Chapter 1

What is Lymphedema?

This chapter explains lymphedema including:

* What is the lymphatic system and why is it important?

* Classification and causes of lymphedema.

* Progression of lymphedema, including degenerative skin changes, and techniques for monitoring and staging lymphedema.

* Complications that may develop as a result of lymphedema. Lymphedema treatment focuses on reducing the likelihood of these complications and their impact on the patient's health and quality of life.

* Other medical conditions that may cause, or complicate, lymphedema.

Readers who are familiar with lymphedema may skim or skip this chapter. Readers who are not interested in the medical details may want to skip or skim the subsection on progression (starting on page 16) but they should read about complications of lymphedema and any of the 'other medical conditions' that apply to their patient or situation.

Lymphedema Defined

Lymphedema (or lymphoedema) is abnormal swelling (*edema*) that occurs when the lymphatic system does not develop properly, is damaged, or is overloaded. Lymphedema is a chronic and degenerative condition that currently cannot be cured. Lymphedema can be managed through prompt and ongoing treatment that helps reduce swelling in the affected area, minimize the risk of infections, and slow adverse tissue changes.

The fluid that builds up in the tissues and causes swelling is described as being "protein-rich" because it contains more protein molecules than normal. Bacteria thrive in this stagnant protein-rich fluid. Any break in the skin allows bacteria to enter and can result in a serious infection.

Swelling can be disfiguring, it can cause functional impairment, and in severe cases it can be disabling. The swelling, infections, and other complications of lymphedema can have a negative impact on the patient's quality of life including work, home, and social relationships. Patients can develop reduced self esteem, distorted body image, depression, and anxiety.

Lymphedema, and related medical conditions, can be painful. The swollen area may feel uncomfortable, achy, heavy or tight. Patients can have background pain at rest, incident pain caused by daily activities, or procedural pain related to treatment. When pain is involved, pain management becomes an essential part of lymphedema treatment. Swelling related pain can often be relieved through lymphedema care techniques including simple lymph drainage, compression, and decongestive exercise. Severe pain is usually not associated with lymphedema; seek medical help if the patient has severe pain. Specific pain management techniques are not addressed in this book.

What is the Lymphatic System?

The lymphatic system is part of the immune system that keeps us healthy by destroying cancer cells and other pathogens. The lymphatic system also:

- Removes waste and excess fluid from tissues and returns proteins and fluid to the cardiovascular system.

- Circulates *lymphocytes*, which are specialized white blood cells that help destroy harmful organisms.

- Absorbs fats and fat-soluble vitamins in the digestive system.

The lymphatic system has several parts (see also the diagrams in Appendix A):

- *Lymphatic capillaries* are tiny tubes where tissue fluid enters the lymphatic system and becomes lymphatic fluid or lymph. About 70% of the lymphatic capillaries are located in, or just under, the skin and the other 30% are located around internal organs.

- *Pre-collectors, collectors, trunks,* and *ducts* are progressively larger lymphatic vessels that collect lymph, process it through the lymph nodes, and return the filtered lymph to the cardiovascular system.

- *Lymph nodes* are bean-shaped nodules connected to the lymphatic trunks and ducts where lymph is filtered and processed. Lymph nodes may become enlarged while fighting an infection; what people call 'swollen glands' are actually enlarged lymph nodes.

Tissue fluid, or interstitial fluid, is a watery liquid found between the cells in the body that carries fats, large blood proteins, and waste products that are too large to be removed by the blood capillaries. Excess tissue fluid flows into the lymphatic capillaries and becomes lymph.

The small initial lymphatic capillaries flow into progressively larger vessels (pre-collectors and collectors) that flow into lymph nodes. The lymph nodes filter the lymph, remove most of the water, and contain lymphocytes which destroy harmful substances like bacteria or cancer cells. The lymphatic trunks carry the fluid out of the lymph nodes and into larger lymphatic ducts which return the purified lymph to the cardiovascular system.

Hundreds of lymph nodes are located throughout the body. The larger lymph nodes are located in clusters as shown in Figure 1-1 on page 14. These include the cervical nodes along either side of the neck, axillary nodes in each armpit, and inguinal nodes at the upper thigh near the groin.

Lymph is propelled through the lymphatic vessels by pulsed contractions of the smooth muscles in the vessel walls that create pressure differences within the lymph vessel, and one-way valves that prevent the lymph from flowing backward within the vessel. Lymph flow is aided by body movements, including nearby skeletal muscles and joints, and by breathing—especially deep, or diaphragmatic, breathing. Without a strong pump like the heart, lymph flow can be disrupted easily by obstructions or inactivity. Swelling initially stretches the vessels and causes the one-way valves to leak; chronic swelling eventually causes these valves to stop working (see Figure A-1 on page 401).

Lymph from the body flows upward (towards the heart) and reenters the cardiovascular system at the base of the neck, in an area known as the *terminus* (end point) or *venous angle.* The *right lymphatic duct* drains lymph from the upper right quadrant of the body, the right arm, and the right side of the

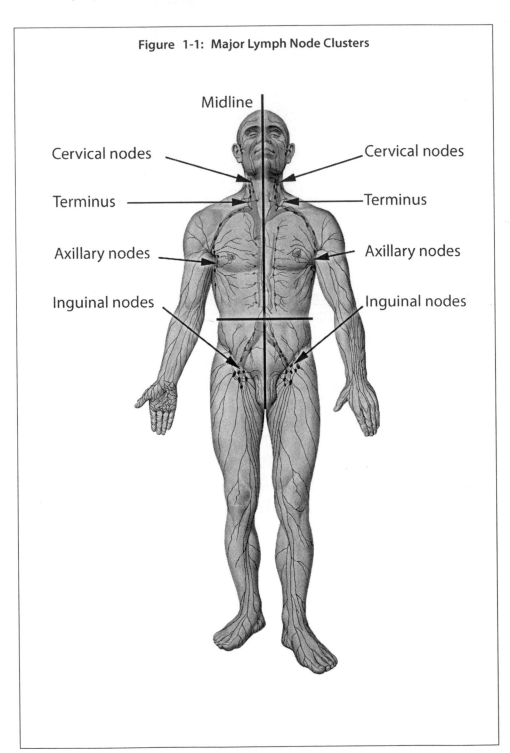

Figure 1-1: Major Lymph Node Clusters

neck and head into the right subclavian vein. Lymph from all other areas of the body, including both legs, is drained primarily by the *thoracic duct* that flows into the left subclavian vein.[1]

For more detail on the anatomy of the lymphatic system, see Appendix A starting on page 399.

Classification and Causes of Lymphedema

There are two classifications of lymphedema that are distinguished based on the origin of the condition:

- *Primary lymphedema* (PLE) is caused by abnormal development of lymphatic vessels and nodes. Swelling can occur at any age but is most commonly observed during puberty, and less commonly seen at birth or after age 35; primary lymphedema affects both sexes and may affect upper and lower extremities; it is seen most frequently in females with swelling in one or both legs that begins at the foot and progresses up toward the trunk.

- *Secondary lymphedema* (SLE) is an acquired disorder caused by obstruction, interruption, or functional impairment of the lymphatic system. Circulatory problems and cancer treatment are the most common causes of secondary lymphedema in North America; other causes include injuries, burns, surgical scars, and tropical parasites. Swelling in secondary lymphedema most commonly affects one or both arms or legs but it can develop anywhere on the body; swelling frequently starts near the damaged lymphatic structures and extends out.

Primary lymphedema is usually diagnosed after ruling out other causes of swelling, including secondary lymphedema. Both classifications of lymphedema are managed using the same treatment methods.

Lymphedema is sometimes described in terms of the affected area(s):

- *Upper Extremity Lymphedema* affects the arm and sometimes the hand and may be caused by damage to the axillary lymph nodes in the armpit.

- *Lower Extremity Lymphedema* affects the leg and sometimes the foot and may be caused by damage to the inguinal or pelvic lymph nodes or other medical conditions (see page 25).

- *Breast Lymphedema* affects the breast and the surrounding tissues and may be caused by damage to axillary lymph nodes or the lymphatic structures in the breast.

- *Truncal Lymphedema* affects the upper or lower body and may be caused by damage to the axillary, inguinal, or pelvic lymph nodes.

- *Head and Neck Lymphedema* affects the head, neck, mouth, and may extend to the upper chest. It may be caused by damage to the cervical lymph nodes in the neck or the lymph nodes in the head.

- *Genital Lymphedema* affects the pubic area, as well as the penis and scrotum in males or the vulva in females, and may be caused by damage to the inguinal, pelvic, or abdominal lymph nodes.

Lymphedema of the extremities may be described as *bilateral* when it affects both arms or legs or *unilateral* if only one arm or leg is affected.

Lymphedema Progression

Lymphedema is a degenerative condition and this section describes the natural progression of changes caused by lymphedema. Effective treatment is important to slow or halt this progression and treatment may be able to reverse some tissue changes.

Readers who are not interested in medical details may want to continue reading with "Complications of Lymphedema" on page 22.

During the *latent phase* or *subclinical stage* before lymphedema is visible or swelling is measurable, lymph transport capacity is reduced but is still sufficient to manage the normal load. The patient may report a feeling of heaviness, fullness, tingling, or aches and pains in the limb, or notice that jewelry, clothing, or shoes no longer fit easily. There are subtle changes in the affected tissues which may include an increase in the level of extra-cellular fluid and a buildup of fibrous tissues.

In the early stages of lymphedema, the accumulated fluid stretches the lymphatic capillaries and collectors, disabling the valves that normally prevent backflow and inhibiting the normal lymph pumping mechanisms. The walls of the lymphatic collectors and capillaries can harden and fibrous clots may block the lymph channels.

Lymph nodes can harden or shrink and lose their ability to fight infection. These lymph nodes also stop concentrating lymphatic fluid by separating out water and returning excess water to the blood circulatory system. The net result is an increase in the amount of fluid to be removed at the same time as the ability to remove fluid is diminished.

The immune system response in the affected area is compromised and the risk of infection increases significantly. An infection may lead to the first clinically observable swelling. Frequently, an infection (or a series of infections) is the event that leads to lymphedema being diagnosed.

Lymphedema becomes visible when the size and circumference of the affected limb is obviously larger than the normal limb. At this point there may be 200 ml (7 ounces) or more of extra fluid and other substances in the affected limb and the difference in circumference between the affected and unaffected limbs may be 2 cm (0.8 inch) or more.

Protein and fluid buildup in the swollen area triggers an inflammatory response with increased macrophage activity that destroys elastic fibers and may result in abnormal fibrous growths. Fibroblast cells migrate into the area and synthesize scar tissue (collagen). Abnormally large amounts of subcutaneous fat may form and treatment may not completely reduce the swelling or restore the area to its previous state.

This inflammatory response results in a change from soft pitting edema (see "Pitting" on page 18) seen in early stage lymphedema to brawny non-pitting edema with hard, leathery, skin known as fibrosis or fibrotic tissues found in later stage lymphedema. Recurrent infections are common.

The overlying skin becomes thicker and may develop an orange peel appearance (*peau d'orange)* from the congested lymphatic vessels. Scaly deposits of debris may form on the skin and warty growths (*papillomas*) may develop, especially in the legs. Excess fluid may leak onto the surface of the skin (*lymphorrhea* or *weeping lymphedema*) or the skin may develop cracks or folds that are prone to infection.

Elephantiasis is lymphedema characterized by severe swelling, hard, thickened tissue, deep skin folds, and warty growths. See, for example, Figure 1-2.

Chronic swelling from untreated lymphedema can cause tissues to degenerate into malignant lymphangiosarcoma, a rare but serious cancer (see page 25).

Pitting

Pitting is a test for edema and the status of the tissues. Pitting can be tested by pressing on the swollen area with a finger or thumb for 10 seconds. If an indentation remains after the examiner ceases pressing, pitting is present. The depth of the indentation reflects the severity of the edema. See Figure 1-3 on page 19.

Edema is described as being "non-pitting" when pressure is applied but little or no indentation occurs. Excess fluid that cannot be displaced with mere pressure indicates advanced subcutaneous tissue changes or fibrosis.[2]

Figure 1-2

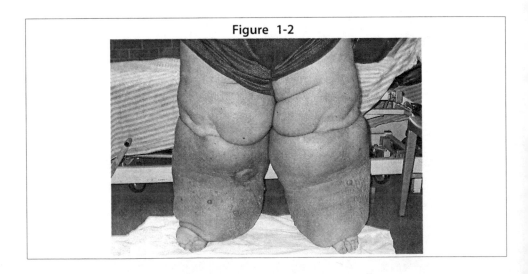

Figure 1-3

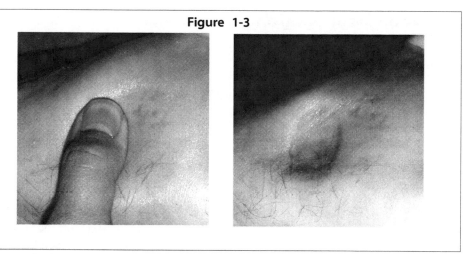

Skin Changes in the Affected Area

Swelling interferes with the flow of nutrients from the blood vessels to the skin and with the oil producing glands that lubricate the skin, resulting in skin that is malnourished, dry, and fragile. These changes also disrupt the natural acid barrier or acid mantle on the surface of the skin that protects the skin and body from infection.

In patients experiencing uncontrolled swelling, the skin becomes red and inflamed as it stretches to accommodate extra fluid. In severe cases, the skin may blister and open as fluid continues to build up in the tissue spaces. In uncontrolled swelling, these blisters may eventually burst. Typically, a clear watery fluid exudes from openings in the skin and the area may feel wet, a condition known as "weeping lymphedema" or *lymphorrhea.*

Breaks in the skin can lead to chronic open wounds, resulting in a greater susceptibility to infections. Unless the swelling is properly controlled, these wounds may never fully heal.

Swollen skin that initially feels soft or watery with pitting edema gradually begins to feel stiffer, like a gel, and lumpy due to protein build-up and the start of fibrosis. As fibrosis progresses, the skin will become hard and leathery from continued protein build-up and scar tissue formation. Some patients also accumulate fatty deposits under the skin so the fibrosis feels spongy. See also, "Fibrosis" on page 24.

Condition Monitoring and Measurement

Patient condition and treatment effectiveness are monitored based on changes in the:

- Amount of swelling as measured by limb circumference or volume.

- Skin condition including pitting (see "Pitting" on page 18), fibrosis, and the presence of open wounds or weeping lymphedema (see "Weeping Lymphedema" on page 238).

Swelling may be determined by comparing the involved and uninvolved limbs or by measuring the same limb over time to track any increase or decrease in size. Most therapists measure limb circumference at multiple locations and track changes in circumference measurements or the limb volume calculated from the circumference measurements. Research institutions may use a device that measures limb volume based on water displacement (volumeter) or an electromechanical device that measures limb cross section (perometer) and calculates limb volume. Bioimpedance is a new and more sensitive way of evaluating lymphedema-related tissue changes.

A caregiver typically monitors swelling, skin condition, and other indicators of the patient's health on a daily basis as part of skin care (see page 45) and measures limb circumference once a week as explained in the chapter on "Taking Measurements" (page 59). More frequent monitoring may be required if there are signs of infection.

Stages of Lymphedema

Medical personnel may describe the condition of an area with lymphedema in terms of stages that relate to the progression of the condition. There are several different staging systems that use the similar terms with slightly different meanings. The International Society of Lymphology (ISL) system and the newer American Society of Lymphology (ASL) system are summarized in "Lymphedema Staging Systems" on page 21.

Lymphedema Staging Systems

ISL Lymphedema Staging[3]

- *ISL Stage 0*: subclinical state where the lymph transport capacity is impaired but still sufficient for the normal lymph load, there is no evident swelling.

- *ISL Stage I*: early onset, swelling subsides with limb elevation, edema may be pitting.

- *ISL Stage II*: pitting edema, limb elevation rarely reduces swelling.

- *ISL Late Stage II*: fibrosis is more evident, edema may or may not be pitting.

- *ISL Stage III*: tissue is hard or fibrotic and edema is not pitting, skin changes may include thickening, hyperpigmentation, increased skin folds, fat deposits, and warty overgrowths.

ASL Clinical Lymphedema Staging is based on a composite of three or more findings[4]

- *ASL Stage I*: mild or reversible edema, no skin changes, no infections, no functional limitations, no limits on activities.

- *ASL Stage II*: moderate edema, none to minimal skin changes, none to occasional infections, mild to moderate functional limitations, occasional limits on activities.

- *ASL Stage III*: moderate to severe edema, moderate skin changes with significant fibrosis, less than four infections per year, moderate to significant functional limitations, frequent and significant limits on activities.

- *ASL Stage IV*: severe edema, severe skin changes with advanced fibrosis, more than four infections per year, moderate to severe functional limitations, constant and severe limits on activities.

Complications of Lymphedema

Although lymphedema is not fatal, patients with lymphedema are at risk for serious complications. Some of these complications can be fatal or disabling and all of them diminish the patient's overall health and quality of life. Treating complications such as infection—that can require hospitalization and intravenous antibiotics—can be much more expensive and disruptive than treating lymphedema to prevent infections.

Effective lymphedema care reduces the risk of complications through:

• Complete Decongestive Therapy (CDT) including skin care, lymph drainage, compression, and exercise as explained starting on page 30.

• Modified activities of daily living, see "Risk Reduction" starting on page 247.

Several conditions may occur as complications of lymphedema including bacterial and fungal infections, orthopedic complications, fibrosis, and (less commonly) lymphangiosarcoma. Each of these is explained below.

Bacterial Infections

Lymphedema creates an ideal breeding ground for bacteria because the acid mantle that normally protects against bacteria entering the skin is disrupted, the affected area is flooded with stagnant protein-rich fluid where bacteria can multiply, and the lymphatic system mechanisms that normally fight infection are ineffective.

Bacteria live harmlessly on the surface of healthy skin. Infections of the skin or lymphatic vessels are rare in people without lymphedema with an incidence of 1 case per 100,000 people. Lymphedema significantly increases the risk of infection and this risk rises with swelling and tissue changes in each stage of lymphedema (see "Stages of Lymphedema" on page 20):[5]

• Stage I infection incidence is 1 per 100 patients, or 1,000 times greater than the normal population.

• Stage II infection incidence is 27 per 100 patients, or 27 times greater than Stage I.

• Stage III infection incidence is 72 per 100 patients, or about 3 times greater than Stage II.

Prompt medical treatment at the first sign of an infection (see "Recognizing Infections and Irritation" on page 49) is essential to minimize tissue damage and the risk of death from a systemic infection. Treatment may include hospitalization to administer intravenous antibiotics. Any skin or soft tissue infection could be MRSA (methicillin-resistant *Staphylococcus aureus*), a type of infection that is resistant to many broad-spectrum antibiotics and potentially fatal.

Note that many doctors use the terms cellulitis and erysipelas interchangeably.

Cellulitis

Cellulitis is an acute bacterial infection that can spread freely and uncontrollably through the tissues below the surface of the skin. Cellulitis is characterized by redness, warmth, swelling, and pain; additional symptoms can include fever, chills, and enlarged lymph nodes. Cellulitis of the legs is most common followed by the face, arm, breast and trunk or other affected tissues.

Acute Lymphangitis

Acute lymphangitis is a bacterial infection of the superficial lymphatic vessels characterized by painful, red streaks below the surface of the skin. These bacteria normally live harmlessly on the surface of the skin. However, if the bacteria get through the skin they cause a potentially serious and rapidly spreading infection.

Erysipelas

Erysipelas is a superficial bacterial infection of the skin with symptoms that include blisters, skin lesions with raised borders plus painful, swollen red skin under the lesions. Additional symptoms include fever, shaking, and chills. These painful infections can spread rapidly and occur most frequently on the lower legs.[6]

These bacteria invade rapidly through any break in the skin and spread through the lymphatic vessels. This infection further disrupts the flow of lymph by damaging the lymphatic vessels and by increasing the fibrosis within the infected tissues. Erysipelas is a serious infection that requires prompt medical treatment.

Fungal Infections

Tissues affected by lymphedema are at increased risk for fungal infections, especially if the patient is taking antibiotics that kill the bacteria that normally keep fungus in check. Although most fungal infections are not serious, they break down the skin and can contribute to serious bacterial infections.

Fungal infections that most commonly affect tissues with lower extremity lymphedema include athlete's foot (*tinea pedis),* jock itch (*tinea cruris*), and toenail fungus (*onychomycosis*). Fungal or yeast infections (*candida*) of the skin are especially common in skin folds of obese patients.

Orthopedic Complications

Lymphedema can cause problems in muscles, tendons, and joints. This includes muscle strain due to the added weight of the swelling, the associated loss of symmetry, and changes in balance. Tendons that are flooded with excess fluid lose their flexibility and ability to glide smoothly, resulting in irritation and inflammation. Joints in the shoulder or pelvis can become unstable (hypermobile) due to accumulated fluid.

Fibrosis

Fibrosis is the replacement of normal tissues by an accumulation of fine scar-like protein structures that further restrict lymph drainage. Fibrosis is evaluated by a therapist based on the firmness of the tissues and their flexibility. The amount of swelling is not an indicator of the risk for developing fibrosis or the degree of fibrosis. Fibrosis is not well understood, some patients progress to fibrosis quickly and others do not.

Without treatment, fibrosis will increase and cause further tissue degeneration. Effective lymphedema treatment will slow this degenerative process. If your patient has fibrotic tissue, his or her therapist should give you directions for treating these tissues. This can include specialized skin manipulation or specialized compression for hardened areas.

Lymphangiosarcoma

Lymphangiosarcoma, also known as angiosarcoma or *Stewart-Treves syndrome*, is a rare but deadly form of cancer that can develop in tissues affected by long-standing lymphedema. These are aggressive tumors with a high local recurrence rate and a tendency to spread quickly.

Lymphedema and Other Conditions

Patients with lymphedema frequently have other medical conditions. Some of these conditions can cause lymphedema or make it worse. Understanding these disorders and their interactions is important because it impacts the treatment and potential outcome of both conditions.

These conditions are discussed below: obesity, lipedema, congestive heart failure, chronic venous insufficiency, diabetes, and peripheral neuropathy. Readers can skip conditions that are not relevant to their situation.

Obesity and Morbid Obesity

Obesity is an excess of fat in proportion to lean body mass resulting in a weight that is considered to be unhealthy for a given height, age, and gender. Body mass index (BMI) is a measure of body fat calculated based on weight and height, see www.nhlbisupport.com/bmi/ for more information. For adults, obesity is defined as a BMI of 30 or more and morbid obesity is a BMI of 40 or more.

Although lymph is dense and swelling causes weight gain, not everyone with lymphedema becomes obese. Lymphedema may contribute to obesity through the formation of subcutaneous fat in affected areas, limits on mobility and exercise, and stress that can lead to overeating.

Not everyone with obesity develops lymphedema. Lymphedema can develop as a complication of obesity when weight gain is combined with a lack of exercise, loss of mobility, and unhealthy eating patterns. Obesity also increases the risk of venous disease which can lead to secondary lymphedema (see "Chronic Venous Insufficiency" on page 27).

Weight gain generally makes lymphedema worse, especially in the lower extremities.

Lipedema

Lipedema, also known as 'painful fat syndrome,' is a metabolic disorder that affects mostly women and is characterized by abnormal fatty deposits below the skin of the hips and legs with symmetrical swelling of both legs. These fatty tissues are very resistant to diet and exercise. Affected areas can be painful, touch-sensitive, and bruise easily. Initially, the fatty deposits stop in a cuff-like ring around the ankle and the feet are not involved. [7]

Lipedema develops around puberty, can be hereditary, and may be associated with hormonal disorders. Many persons with lipedema also have eating disorders such as anorexia or bulimia.

Lipedema can cause lymphedema when the size and density of the fat deposits interferes with lymph flow. When lymphedema develops, the feet begin to swell and the swelling extends upward toward the ankles. The combination of lipedema, obesity, and lymphedema is known as *lipo-lymphedema.* Compression can reduce the pain of lipedema and may reduce the risk of lipo-lymphedema.

Lymphedema does not cause lipedema.

Congestive Heart Failure

Congestive heart failure (CHF) is a condition where the pumping action of the heart is greatly reduced and this causes blood to back up into certain areas of the body. CHF occurs most often in the elderly and can lead to edema and lymphedema in the feet and lower legs.

Lymphedema does not cause congestive heart failure.

If a patient has CHF, the CHF must be treated before considering lymphedema treatment. Lymphedema treatment should progress cautiously, and under medical supervision, to prevent pulmonary or cardiac edema.

CHF treatment includes medications to control blood pressure and strengthen the heart beat. Diuretics are used to remove excess fluid from the cardiovascular system (see "Common Misunderstandings" on page 41 for information on diuretics and lymphedema). Patients may be advised to keep their legs elevated and to wear compression stockings to minimize swelling.

Chronic Venous Insufficiency

Chronic venous insufficiency (CVI) is a condition in which the veins of the legs do not efficiently return blood to the heart. This may be due to improper functioning of the valves in the veins, the partial blockage of one or more veins in the lower legs, or a combination of these conditions. CVI results in the pooling of fluid in the legs and feet, and causes symptoms that include dull aching pain and a feeling of heaviness or cramping. Swelling of the legs with low-protein fluid is also present. This swelling usually occurs in the second half of the day and is known as *dependent edema* or *orthostatic edema*. This swelling is often the result of standing for long periods of time; in the early stages of CVI, the swelling often goes down overnight.

CVI is the most common cause of lymphedema and the combination is sometimes called *phlebo-lymphedema, chronic venous-lymphatic insufficiency, phlebo-lymphostatic edema,* or *venous stasis.*

Lymphedema does not cause chronic venous insufficiency.

Diabetes

Diabetes is a chronic endocrine disorder in which the body does not produce or use insulin properly resulting in elevated blood sugar levels. Lymphedema does not cause diabetes and diabetes does not cause lymphedema; however both conditions can be present at the same time.

Elevated blood sugar levels make infections more likely and damage the cardiovascular system leading to reduced oxygen levels in the skin, the tissues under the skin, and the deeper connective tissues. This makes these tissues extremely fragile, prone to infection, and slow to heal. Diabetes can also cause nerve damage (see below). When lymphedema is also present, it further damages the tissues, increases the risk of infections, and impedes the normal healing process.

Peripheral Neuropathy

Peripheral neuropathy is damage to the nerves in the hands and arms or feet and legs. This damage can be caused by diseases such as alcoholism or diabetes; as a side-effect of chemotherapy, medication, or radiation therapy; as the result of surgery or an injury; or for unknown reasons (*idiopathic*). The initial symptoms of peripheral neuropathy are tingling, pins and needles, or numbness in the hands or feet. As the damage progresses the sensations are described as burning, throbbing, aching, and feelings "like frostbite" or "walking on a bed of coals."

Lymphedema can cause peripheral neuropathy when swelling causes pressure on nerves (nerve entrapment). Patients who have had chemotherapy or have diabetes can develop both conditions. Chronic swelling may intensify the symptoms of neuropathy. Peripheral neuropathy complicates lymphedema treatment because the nerve damage can cause numbness, touch sensitivity, or pain.

Notes

1   **Textbook of Lymphology for Physicians and Lymphedema Therapists** by M. Földi, E. Földi, and S. Kubik, eds. Urban & Fischer, 2003.

2   **Lymphedema: Diagnosis and Treatment** by B.B. Lee, et al. Springer, 2008.

3   International Society of Lymphology. The diagnosis and treatment of peripheral lymphedema. Consensus document of the International Society of Lymphology. *Lymphology* 2003; 36(2): 84-91.

4   **Lymphedema: Diagnosis and Treatment** by B.B. Lee, et al. Springer, 2008.

5   **Lymphedema Diagnosis and Therapy, Third Edition** by H. Weissleder, and C. Schuchhardt. Viavital Verlag, 2001, p.126.

6   **Erysipelas** www.nlm.nih.gov/medlineplus/ency/article/000618.htm Update date: 10/09/2006.

7   "Understanding Lipedema" by Gunter Klose and Roman Strossenreuther. *Lymph Link* January-March 2007.

Chapter 2

How is Lymphedema Treated?

Lymphedema treatment is conservative therapy designed to remove the stagnant protein-rich fluid, slow or stop the progression of lymphedema by improving lymphatic circulation, and minimize the risk of complications. Treatment should be provided and coordinated by a professional lymphedema therapist (as defined below) in combination with home care.

Patients may also need psychosocial support to help them address the emotional aspects of lymphedema and to increase or sustain motivation for care activities. Support can be provided by the patient's lymphedema therapist, other health care professionals, or a support group. We discuss the caregiver's role in the chapter on "Emotional Care and Support" (page 189). For more information on emotional issues and support see **Overcoming the Emotional Challenges of Lymphedema.**[1]

This chapter covers:

- Who treats lymphedema, what is a lymphedema therapist, and the roles of the therapist and caregiver.

- Complete Decongestive Therapy, which is the standard of care for lymphedema treatment, and the components of this treatment.

- Phases of treatment, the importance of daily care, types of care, and care goals.

- Other treatments and common misunderstandings about lymphedema treatment.

Who Treats Lymphedema?

A *certified lymphedema therapist* (CLT) is a licensed health professional (doctor, physical therapist, physical therapist assistant, registered nurse, occupational therapist, occupational therapy assistant, massage therapist, or chiropractor) with at least 135 hours of postgraduate training in the pathology and treatment of lymphedema. The Lymphology Association of North America (LANA) has established training standards and certifies therapists as CLT-LANA based on a combination of education, experience, and a certification exam. For more information on lymphedema therapist training, finding lymphedema treatment, and reimbursement issues, see **Living Well With Lymphedema**[2] and the websites and organizations listed in Appendix B (page 417).

Professional therapists provide hands-on patient care including manual lymph drainage. They also provide education to enable the patient and/or caregiver to carry out the daily care routine.

A *caregiver* assists a patient who is unable to manage the daily care routine on their own. The caregiver follows the instructions provided by the patient's therapist.

Complete Decongestive Therapy

The most widely accepted method of lymphedema treatment is known as *Complete Decongestive Therapy* (CDT). This treatment involves four components used in combination:[3]

* Skin and nail care to minimize the risk of infection.

* Lymphatic drainage by manipulating the skin to increase the flow of lymph away from the affected area.

* Compression techniques to reduce or limit swelling.

* Decongestive exercise to increase lymph flow and pump lymph away from the affected area.

Home care involves all four components plus risk reduction during activities of daily living. Professional treatment focuses on skin care, lymphatic drainage (using advanced techniques), and compression. Some treatment centers offer specialized exercise programs for patients and support groups.

Intensive treatment with a series of daily therapy sessions may be used to reduce swelling when a patient is first diagnosed with lymphedema and later, as needed. For more information see "Phases of Treatment" on page 36.

Skin Care

Proper skin and nail care is essential for maintaining the health of the skin and preventing wounds or breaks in the skin that might lead to an infection. This involves keeping the skin clean and moisturizing the skin with lotions to support the acid barrier, or acid mantle, on the surface of the skin. Skin care also involves monitoring the skin for changes or signs of infection and obtaining medical care for any suspected infections.

Skin care is important for several reasons:

- Swelling causes the skin to become poorly nourished, dry, and unhealthy by interfering with the flow of oxygen carrying red blood cells and nutrients into the skin, and oil production in the sebaceous glands under the skin.

- The body's ability to fight infection is slowed by stagnant fluid, inhibiting the immune response to bacteria, viruses, or fungi that enter the skin.

- Stagnant lymph fluid provides an ideal breeding ground where harmful microorganisms can multiply and spread.

Lymphedema disrupts the skin's defense mechanism known as the acid mantle. The acid mantle is a thin coating over the skin with a low pH created by skin oils and sweat (salt water). This skin coating is a natural antibiotic that slows the growth of harmful microorganisms, including bacteria, yeast, and fungus. Malnutrition of the skin disturbs the acid mantle and may result in overgrowth of microorganisms. Such overgrowth increases the opportunity for infectious materials to enter the body through breaks in the skin.[4] Using good skin care and controlling swelling keeps the skin healthier and reduces the risk of infection.

Lymphatic Drainage

Lymphatic drainage techniques are used to increase the flow, or drainage, of lymphatic fluid out of the affected area and back into the circulatory system.

There are three forms of lymphatic drainage using skin manipulation:

- *Manual Lymph Drainage* (MLD) is a more complicated technique performed by a trained lymphedema therapist. In addition to lymph drainage, MLD includes deeper tissue manipulations to soften fibrotic tissue.

- *Simple Lymph Drainage (SLD)* is based on the principles of MLD using simple hand movements that can be taught to a caregiver by the patient's therapist. The basics of this technique are explained starting on page 67.

- *Self-Massage,* or self-MLD, is a subset of simple lymph drainage that some patients are able to perform on themselves. The basics of self-massage are explained in **Living Well With Lymphedema**[5].

Lymph drainage is a specialized skill that should not be attempted by an untrained person. Estheticians are not trained or qualified to treat lymphedema, and lymphatic massage by an esthetician is not appropriate for a patient with lymphedema.

In some cases a mechanical device called a sequential compression pump can be used to facilitate lymph drainage in combination with these techniques. For more information see "Sequential Compression Pump" on page 240.

Principles of Lymphatic Drainage

All three lymph drainage techniques work by manipulating lymphatic vessels to promote the flow of lymph through the body. Light pressure and slow movements that mimic the natural movements of the lymphatic vessels are used along pathways that follow the normal flow of a healthy lymphatic system, or alternative pathways that avoid damaged areas.

Lymph drainage starts by clearing or draining the terminus. The terminus is the area at the base of the neck where the large lymphatic ducts empty into the subclavian veins. Draining the terminus creates space within the lymph vessels for the lymphatic fluid from other parts of the body.

Lymph drainage continues from the terminus down the trunk and out to the extremities, and then back to the terminus in the reverse sequence. If congestion develops during MLD, the therapist may clear the terminus and major lymph node clusters repeatedly.

Alternate Lymphatic Pathways

When the lymphatic system is working normally, lymph from each area of the body drains through the nearest lymph node cluster. When parts of the lymphatic system are not working normally, lymphatic drainage uses stroking techniques to reroute fluid from the swollen area towards working lymph nodes via alternate lymphatic pathways (anastomoses), if possible. These alternate pathways are shown in Figure 2-1 on page 34.

The alternate pathways include:

- Upper Front and Upper Back pathways towards the working axillary nodes.

- Right and Left Side pathways towards the working inguinal or axillary nodes.

- Lower Front and Lower Back pathways towards the working inguinal nodes.

Compression Techniques

Compression is an essential element of lymphedema treatment. Carefully controlled amounts of pressure and pressure differences (or gradients) are used to support and enhance lymphatic system function in the affected area. Although they look similar, most compression materials used for lymph-edema treatment are different from the bandages used to treat sprains or other orthopedic problems.

Compression techniques are used to:

- Facilitate the flow of lymph and drain lymph away from swollen tissues.

- Prevent or minimize additional swelling.

- Maintain the swelling reduction achieved through MLD treatment.

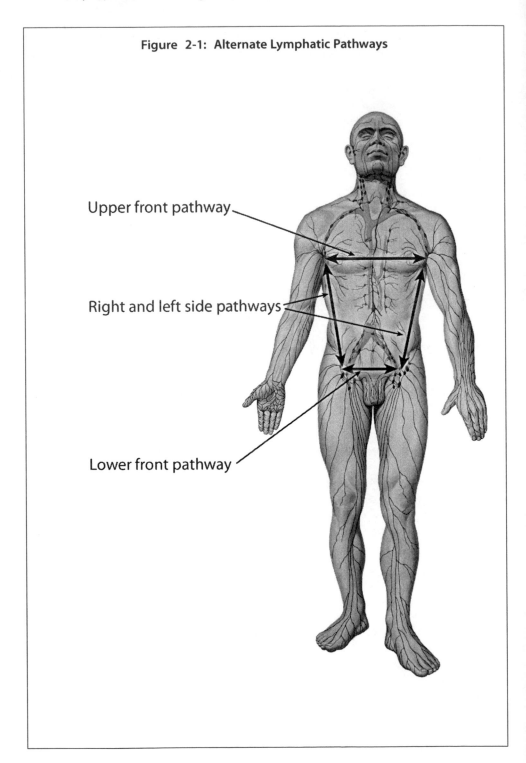

Figure 2-1: Alternate Lymphatic Pathways

Upper front pathway

Right and left side pathways

Lower front pathway

Different types of compression are used for specific purposes and it is important to understand the benefits of each method. The three types of compression are:

- *Bandaging,* or *wrapping,* is the most versatile form of compression because bandages conform to the shape of the limb and can be adjusted to meet the need for localized changes in pressure. Compression bandaging typically involves several layers and many patients need the assistance of a caregiver to place and remove wrappings or to learn self-bandaging, see page 95.

- *Compression garments* are specialized two-way stretch, knit, or woven garments including compression sleeves or stockings. This type of garment is worn during the day while the patient is up and about; compression garments are not typically worn while the patient is sleeping because they provide too much compression when the body is at rest. These garments can be difficult to put on (don) or remove (doff) and caregiver assistance may be required, see page 133.

- *Compression aids* are non-elastic devices that may be padded with foam or stitched into channels to aid in draining lymph. These aids are also called *night garments* because they are typically worn while the patient is sleeping; however, they can be worn both night and day. Depending on the type of compression aid, the help of the caregiver may be required to put on or remove these devices, see page 133.

Compression pumps are treatment devices to help with lymph drainage, not a compression method.

Bandaging is the most effective method for reducing swelling and may be used day and night during an intensive treatment series (see "Phases of Treatment" on page 36). Bandages are flexible and inexpensive but can be time-consuming and frustrating to apply.

Patients who are not undergoing intensive treatment will typically wear compression garments during the day and either bandages or a compression aid at night (if night compression is required). Night-time compression helps decrease any swelling which may have occurred during the day and also helps prevent further swelling as the patient sleeps.

Patients may use additional compression while exercising or traveling (see "Travel Tips" on page 255). Compression will help control swelling-related pain. Some patients use compression, or additional compression, as needed for pain control.

Decongestive Exercises

Exercise is an important part of lymphedema treatment because it encourages the flow of lymph out of the swollen area and maintain overall health, mobility, and quality of life. Compression is essential while exercising, except when exercising in shoulder-deep water. The caregiver may be required to guide the patient through the exercises and to help maintain the motivation to exercise.

Decongestive exercises activate the lymphatic system and help decrease swelling. Typically exercises start with the neck, trunk, and major joints (shoulders, elbows, hips, and knees), followed by the affected areas. As the muscles contract, they tighten around lymph vessels, which moves lymph out of the area. When the muscles relax, lymph vessels refill with more lymphatic fluid. This contract-relax cycle, known as a "muscle pump," is an important mechanism for moving lymph through the body.

Stretching- or flexibility-exercises stretch the skin, muscles, and other soft tissues, to minimize stiffness and scarring which may contribute to swelling by constricting lymph and blood flow. In addition, flexibility exercises stretch and relax lymph vessels of the skin further stimulating lymph flow.

Phases of Treatment

Lymphedema treatment can be described in terms of two phases, and therapists use several terms for each phase. These terms include:

- *Phase 1*, an *intensive phase, treatment phase,* an *intervention*, or *decongestive phase* is typically the first phase of treatment and is intended to reduce the swelling in, or decongest, the affected area.

- *Phase 2, maintenance phase*, the *optimization phase*, or *home management phase* focuses on maintaining the swelling reduction achieved during the treatment phase.

Typically, a patient will be diagnosed by a physician and referred to a qualified lymphedema therapist who begins treatment with an intensive series of treatments to reduce swelling. After the swelling is reduced, the patient enters the maintenance phase. If additional swelling reduction is required, the intensive treatment phase may be repeated, as needed.

Intensive Phase

During an intensive phase or an intensive treatment series, the patient has daily therapy sessions for two or more weeks where the therapist uses MLD and compression to reduce the swelling. Bandages are typically used during an intensive phase and the patient may be bandaged day and night.

Some hospitals offer in-patient treatment programs that may include more than one treatment per day. Some facilities can arrange for patients to stay nearby during an intensive.

During the patient's first intensive treatment series, the therapist will teach the patient the home care routine and care skills. Ideally the caregiver should attend at least some of these sessions to learn and practice care activities. During these sessions, the patient's home care routine can be worked out by the patient, therapist, and caregiver or care arranger and documented as described under "Weekly Care Plan" on page 333.

If the patient has a home care routine, the therapist may change the normal routine during an intensive treatment series and some care activities that are normally done at home may be done in the clinic or by the therapist.

Maintenance Phase

After the swelling has been reduced and the training is complete, the patient enters the *maintenance phase*, with a focus on maintaining the swelling reduction achieved during the treatment phase. During this phase, most patients choose to wear compression garments during the day, because they are less bulky and more cosmetic than bandages. At night patients who need compression may wear bandages, a compression aid, or a compression garment that provides less pressure. Compliance with garment wear during the maintenance phase is one of the most challenging aspects of lymphedema management.[6]

Throughout the maintenance phase, the patient and caregiver follow the weekly care plan worked out with the therapist (see "Weekly Care Plan" on page 333) to maintain, and improve upon, the progress achieved during the intensive phase. They should also monitor the condition of the affected area and contact the therapist or doctor if there is an increase in swelling or signs of an infection.

Follow-up therapist visits are typically scheduled every six months to monitor the patient's progress, though some patients may need more frequent monitoring. At times, patients may require additional therapist treatments or an intensive treatment series to reduce swelling or respond to other changes.

The Importance of Daily Care

Lymphedema therapy can be cumbersome, uncomfortable, time-consuming and expensive—even with insurance coverage. The need for care continues throughout the lifetime of the patient.

The vast majority of lymphedema treatment is daily care provided by the patient and caregiver. After an initial intervention or intensive treatment phase, therapist sessions become relatively infrequent. Typically, a patient has 1-3 therapist visits per year during the maintenance phase. Very few American patients have multiple intensive treatments.

Effective treatment requires close cooperation between the lymphedema therapist, the patient, and the caregiver. Some patients can manage lymphedema home care by themselves. Others need assistance, and this is where the role of the caregiver is so extremely important to the success of the treatment.

Not only is daily care essential to successful treatment, some insurance companies require a record of compliance with the daily care routine as a precondition for reimbursement for treatment.[7] Records based on the Weekly Care Plan should meet these requirements; see page 333.

Types of Care

Medicare and other insurance providers classify care as either:

- *Short-term care* following an illness, injury, or hospitalization and providing services to help the patient regain their ability to function and care for themselves.

- *Long-term care* to meet health or personal care needs over an extended period of time due to a chronic illness or disability.

- *Palliative* or *hospice care* provided for people with advanced illness who are only expected to live for six months or less.

The type of care depends upon the patient's overall condition—not just their lymphedema—and is not directly related to the phase of lymphedema treatment. A patient may receive different types of care at different times.

Understanding the patient's overall situation and type of care is important for:

- Care planning and estimating the expected duration of care services, see "Evaluating Care Needs" on page 331.

- Care resources and reimbursement options, as discussed in the chapter on "Finding and Paying for Care" (page 347).

- Care goals, as discussed below.

Care Goals

In general, the goal of lymphedema care is to minimize swelling and the risk of infection. The caregiver may have additional goals based on the type of care being provided (as defined above), the patient's age and physical condition, and the patient's cognitive abilities and willingness to cooperate. For example:

- Short-term care: help the patient learn to carry out the daily care routine independently, to the best of their abilities. In this situation, it is the need for assistance that is short term, not the need for daily lymphedema care.

- Long-term care: to encourage the patient to keep up the daily care routine.

- Palliative or hospice care: make the patient as comfortable as possible, given their situation. For more information see "Palliative Care" on page 237.

These additional goals will influence how a caregiver interacts with a patient as discussed in the chapter on "Roles, Goals, and Relationships" (page 395).

Other Lymphedema Treatments

Medications are not currently used for lymphedema treatment in North America.

Antibiotic and anti-fungal drugs are used to treat infections. Patients with a history of frequent infections may be prescribed preventative (prophylactic) low dose antibiotics on an on-going basis and/or standby antibiotics the patient can start taking at the first sign of an infection.

Surgical treatment of lymphedema is not common and is an area for further research. Surgery can be curative in cases of acute lymphedema caused by trauma, and may be required in rare cases to reduce the weight of the limb or the risk of secondary angiosarcoma.[8]

A variety of treatment devices are available but only a few have specific FDA approval for lymphedema and evidence of effectiveness based on randomized controlled trials with statistically significant results. The more promising devices include:

- Flexitouch System, a lymph preparation and drainage device from Tactile Systems Technology, see page 240.

- RianCorp (www.riancorp.com) low level laser therapy device has been FDA approved for therapist use in treating post-mastectomy lymph-edema. We do not cover this device because it is not approved for home care.

Common Misunderstandings

Common misunderstandings about lymphedema treatment include:

• *Taking diuretics or restricting fluid to reduce swelling.* Diuretics are not helpful for lymphedema patients unless fluid reduction is necessary to treat other medical conditions, such as congestive heart failure (see page 26). Adequate water intake and tissue fluid levels are essential for proper functioning of the lymphatic system, the skin, and the rest of the body (see "Water Intake" on page 268).

• *Eating less protein to make lymphatic fluid less protein-rich.* Adequate nutrition, including protein, is important for healing and fighting infections; see the chapter on "Diet and Nutrition" (page 265) for more information.

• *Applying tape to control swelling.* Although there are special elastic tapes that can be used to treat lymphedema (see "" on page 241), other types of tape can damage the skin, block the flow of lymph, and impede venous circulation.

• *Treating swelling with Rest, Ice, Compression, and Elevation (RICE).* Although this is standard treatment for acute swelling due to orthopedic injuries, ice and compression using long-stretch bandages can damage tissues with lymphedema; rest and elevation are safe and may be helpful.

• *Draining excess fluid with a needle.* A needle can be used to drain a pocket of fluid, such as a cyst or abscess. Lymphedema cannot be drawn out because the fluid is trapped in the tissues of the swollen area.

Notes

1   **Overcoming the Emotional Challenges of Lymphedema** by Elizabeth McMahon. Lymph Notes, 2005.

2   **Living Well With Lymphedema** by Ann Ehrlich, Alma Vinjé-Harrewijn, and Elizabeth McMahon. Lymph Notes, 2005.

3   "Guidelines for the Diagnosis Assessment and Management of Lymphoedema" by the Clinical Resource Efficiency Support Team (CREST). CREST Secretariat February 2008. Available from www.crestni.org.uk.

4   **Living Well With Lymphedema** by Ann Ehrlich, Alma Vinjé-Harrewijn, and Elizabeth McMahon. Lymph Notes, 2005, p. 120.

5   **Living Well With Lymphedema** by Ann Ehrlich, Alma Vinjé-Harrewijn, and Elizabeth McMahon. Lymph Notes, 2005.

6   "The Garments We Wear" by Paula Stewart. *Lymph Link* April-June 2007.

7   Aetna Clinical Policy Bulletin: Lymphedema Treatments at www.aetna.com/cpb/medical/data/1_99/0069.html accessed on June 16, 2008.

8   Position Statement of the National Lymphedema Network Topic: Treatment, NLN Medical Advisory Committee, 2006.

Lymphedema Care Skills

Lymphedema patients typically receive home care one or more times per day based on a schedule and activity descriptions developed in cooperation with the patient's therapist. See "Evaluating Care Needs" (page 331) for tips on determining and documenting the care routine. The frequency of care and the mix of care activities depend upon the affected area(s), the patient's condition, and available care resources. Head and neck edema may require care two to three times per day, genital or hand edema may require care four or more times per day.

The daily care routine typically includes:

- Skin care, see page 45.

- Simple lymph drainage, see page 67. Some patients use a sequential compression pump to help with lymph drainage, see page 240 for more information on pump usage.

- Compression bandaging (page 95), or helping the patient put on compression garments or aids (page 133), as recommended by the patient's therapist. A patient may use different compression during the day, at night, or during exercise. In some situations, the patient's therapist may recommend using Kinesio Tape instead; see page 242 for more information.

- Decongestive exercise, see page 143.

Skin condition is monitored daily as part of skin care. Measurements of limb size, temperature, and weight are typically scheduled once a week but may be done more frequently if necessary. See "Taking Measurements" (page 59) for instructions.

The normal care routine may change during an intensive treatment series (see "Phases of Treatment" on page 36). The therapist may handle some of the care activities that are normally done at home while the patient is receiving frequent professional treatments.

Caregivers also provide emotional care and support for their patients. For specific suggestions on how to do this, see the chapters on "Emotional Care and Support" (page 189) and "Communicating Effectively" (page 205).

Care activities can be modified based on patient needs. We provide suggestions for:

- Treating infants and children in the chapter on Infant and Child Care, see page 217.

- Working with elders, obese patients, wheelchair bound patients, or providing palliative care in the chapter on Special Situation, see page 229.

Depending on the situation, a caregiver may also be responsible for managing supplies, medications, and equipment (see the section that starts on page 269) or arranging and managing care (see page 329).

Chapter **3:**
Skin Care

Skin care to keep the affected area clean, moisturized, and protected is important for all individuals with lymphedema (see page 31) and is especially important for patients with severe swelling, fibrosis, or a history of infections. Skin care is performed one or more times per day in accordance with the Weekly Care Plan and instructions provided the Care Activity Forms.

Skin care includes:

- Removing any compression bandages (see page 126), compression garments (page 138) or compression aids (see page 140). Kinesio tape does not have to be removed for skin care (see page 241).

- Inspecting the skin for signs of infection or irritation, as described on page 47.

- Washing and drying the skin as described on page 55.

- Moisturizing the skin with lotion or cream as described on page 56.

- Applying topical medications, if required, as described on page 57.

Measurement of limb size can be done after skin inspection and before washing the skin, see "Taking Measurements" (page 59) for instructions.

Monitoring and record keeping can be informal if the patient's condition is stable and there is only one caregiver. More frequent monitoring is recommended if the patient's condition is fluctuating. More formal records will improve problem recognition and coordination in situations with multiple caregivers.

Routine monitoring should be done at least once a day as part of skin care and any change in condition noted on the Weekly Care Plan Form. The general guidelines are:

- Monitor swelling and skin condition every time you do skin care.

- Measure the circumference of the affected area and the patient's temperature and weight once a week, as indicated on the care plan (see page 59).

More frequent monitoring is recommended when:

- The patient doesn't feel well but there are no objective symptoms of an infection. Inspect the skin and check the patient's temperature every four hours or less while the patient is awake. Start standby antibiotics (if they have been prescribed for the patient) or seek treatment, at the first sign of redness, fever, or other symptoms of infection (see page 49).

- Swelling appears be increasing. Measure the affected area and the patient's weight daily, if possible. Contact the patient's therapist if there is a significant unexplained increase in limb circumference (more than 1 centimeter or ½ inch) or weight (more than one pound (0.45 kg) per day).

Caregivers should always have clean hands and use medical gloves when handling an area where there is a wound or open sore. Gloves may also be used when applying lotoins and should be used when applying topical medications.

Skin care for wounds—such as pressure ulcers or other injuries—is not covered in this book, and normal lymphedema care procedures are not used on wound areas. If the patient has a wound, ask the patient's physician or wound care specialist for care instructions. Care for areas that are known to have weeping lymphedema is discussed in on page 238.

First aid tips for minor injuries (see page 259) and protecting the skin to avoid injuries (page 247) are covered in the section on "Activities of Daily Living." Seek medical attention for more serious injuries.

Preparing for Skin Care

Before starting skin care the caregiver should:

- Assemble the supplies listed on the Care Activity Form. For example, soap, moisturizer, towels, cotton swabs, medical gloves, topical medications, etc.

- Wash their hands with soap and water.

- Put on medical gloves before handling any area with a known skin infection, open wound, or sore.

Inspecting the Skin

When an individual has a compromised lymphatic system, daily skin and nail inspection is recommended so the caregiver or patient can quickly respond to any injury, infection, or other issues. See page 49 for signs of infection and recommended actions. Foot care and inspection is especially important for patients with lower extremity lymphedema and diabetes or peripheral neuropathy.

If the patient has a minor scratch or skin irritation, clean the area well, apply an antibiotic ointment, add a note to the care record (see below), and continue as usual. First aid for lymphedema affected areas is covered on page 259.

Check the fingernails and toenails for signs of infection—such as redness or soreness—or ingrown nails. If the patient has lower extremity lymphedema, consider having a podiatrist or other foot care professional trim their toenails regularly, especially if the nails are thickened due to a fungal infection.

Note on the Week Care Plan form (see page 424):

- Changes in skin condition or color, especially any signs of infection.

- Any changes in swelling or size of each affected area.

Patients who are doing (or learning) self-inspection may need long handled mirrors or anti-fog mirrors that can be used in the shower to help them see the soles of the foot, between the toes, the back of the legs, the armpits and other areas.

By monitoring the affected areas, the caregiver can respond to any changes in the patient's swelling and minimize any increase. This enables the caregiver to be:

- *Proactive* in recognizing activities that trigger an increase in swelling and suggesting precautions to minimize swelling.

- *Reactive* by responding to increased swelling once it has occurred.

The caregiver can monitor the affected area for changes in these ways:

- **See for Size (Fullness):** look and see if each affected area is smaller or larger than it was previously.

- **Press for Pitting:** in areas with pitting edema (see page 18), gently press your finger or thumb into the swollen area and hold for several seconds. Upon release of the pressure, note any change in skin indentation; an increase in the depth of the indentation usually indicates more swelling.

- **Feel for Fibrosis:** in areas with fibrosis, feel the difference, if any, in skin texture between the involved and uninvolved limbs. Note any increase or decrease in firmness (the skin may feel harder or leathery) that indicates a change in fibrosis.

- **Look for Changes:** in skin texture, color, tissue fluid seeping through the skin in an area that has not had weeping before, new wounds, or warty growths (papillomas), especially in leg lymphedema.

Make a record of any change in size, pitting, fibrosis, or other changes on the Weekly Care Plan Form, along with the time and date.

Photographs of the involved limb(s) can be an excellent way to monitor changes in swelling or skin condition over the course of time, especially with young children or irregularly shaped swelling. A digital camera that records the time and date for each image is ideal for this purpose. The camera should be close enough to show the area of interest clearly; you may have to use the macro setting if the camera has one. If possible, use the same camera position and lighting, and include a ruler in the image to show the scale. Each time you take photographs, add a note to the Weekly Care Plan Form.

Contact the patient's medical care provider and lymphedema therapist if you notice:

- A new wound such as a pressure ulcer or other break in the skin.

- Weeping lymphedema in an area that has not had weeping before.

- Signs of a skin infection (see below).

- Significant changes in swelling (size), skin color, or texture.

Recognizing Infections and Irritation

The goal of minimizing skin infections and preventing illnesses through good skin care may seem self-explanatory; however, there are greater implications for the lymphedema patient. Complications associated with multiple infections include an increase in swelling and fibrosis, increased scar tissue, and potential damage to the remaining healthy lymphatics. Repeated infections may affect the person's ability to work and their overall quality of life.[1]

Check the patient's skin completely—including the soles of the feet, sides of the fingers and toes, and the spaces between the fingers and toes—for signs of bacterial or fungal infection or skin irritation. As a caregiver, your responsibility is to recognize a change that needs attention and help the patient take corrective action. You are not expected to distinguish between the different types of infections.

Color versions of the images for this section are available on the book website and show the changes in the skin more clearly than the printed images.

Bacterial Infections

Skin or lymph vessel infections are relatively common in people with lymphedema (see page 22). Typically an infected area turns bright or "angry" red, quickly feels hot, swollen, itchy, and is painful when touched. See Figure 3-1 on page 50 .

Within hours, the infection may worsen with the redness spreading over a large area. Cellulitis and lymphangitis can spread to the rest of the body and become a systemic infection characterized by aching joints, flu-like symptoms, fever, and chills. Severe headache or vomiting can accompany a systemic infection or may occur up to 24 hours before any redness develops.[2] Serious systemic infections often require hospitalization and severe cases can be fatal.

Mycobacterium marinum is a slow growing bacterium. This type of infection typically appears as a slowly developing raised bump (nodule) at the site where the bacteria entered the body. This nodule can enlarge and become an ulcer-like sore. As the disease progresses, nearby lymph nodes swell and multiple sores may form along the lymphatic vessels that drain the site.

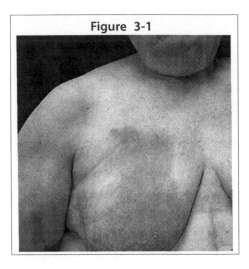

Figure 3-1

If a patient has a history of infections, their doctor may prescribe:

- Standby antibiotics to keep on hand so the patient can start taking them at the first sign of an infection.

- Low dose antibiotics, also known as prophylactic antibiotics, on an ongoing basis to prevent infection. Low dose antibiotics may be discontinued if the patient starts taking standby antibiotics or other antibiotic therapy, check the doctor's instructions.

As a caregiver, it is important for you to know:

- What medications have been prescribed for the patient and how the medication should be taken (how much, how often, when, etc.).

- If the patient is known to have any medication allergies.

This information should be provided and maintained in the Patient Notebook (see page 372).

When a bacterial infection is suspected:

- **Stop simple lymph drainage and compression** since this may spread the infection further. Do not resume these treatments until advised to do so by the patient's physician or lymphedema therapist.

- **Seek medical attention immediately** by contacting the patient's primary care physician or an emergency department physician. Systemic infections spread quickly—do not wait to see if the patient gets better.

- **Start antibiotics as directed**, if standby antibiotics have been prescribed for the patient. Also request replacement antibiotics.

- **Update the Weekly Care Plan Form** with:

  - Information on the signs of infection and the size of the infected
    area. Make a note if any pictures were taken of the infected area.

  - Medications given, including dose and time, if the patient was
    given standby antibiotics or other medications.

  - Changes in the medication routine, if any, according to the
    instructions provided by the patient's doctor. For example,
    antibiotic therapy to treat an infection may continue for a specified
    number of days and low-dose preventative antibiotics may be
    discontinued during this period.

  - Changes in the care routine, if any. For example, discontinue SLD
    of the infected area or changes in bandaging or compression.

Fungal Infections

Athlete's foot, jock itch, and nail fungus are frequently observed in patients
with lymphedema. Athlete's foot causes dry cracked skin of the toes and
soles of the feet, allowing bacteria to enter the body and increasing the risk
of cellulitis.[3]

Symptoms of athlete's foot include red, dry, flaking or scaly skin, itching and
pain, cracking skin between the toes, blisters or pustules (small raised areas
containing pus), and weeping sores. Treatment of athlete's foot typically
involves over the counter antifungal ointments such as Lamisil, Lotrimin,
Micatin, or Whitfield's ointment.[4] If these are not effective, a prescription-
strength anti-fungal ointment may be required.

Jock itch causes a discolored rash on the groin, buttocks, and inner thigh
areas, accompanied by itching. Anti-fungal cream or spray, good hygiene,
and loose-fitting cotton underwear are used to treat this condition.

Nail fungus symptoms include nails that are thickened, brittle, distorted,
and have a foul odor. Nail fungal infections can persist indefinitely if not
treated and can spread to the skin. Fungus can be difficult to cure without
prescription-strength medication.

Discuss all infections with the patient's primary care physician, podiatrist, or dermatologist for the best form of treatment.

Yeast Infections

Yeast or fungal infections of the skin often occur in warm, moist environments such as breast folds, armpits, large abdominal skin folds, and hip bends. Yeast infections look like diaper rash and can be identified by redness and a characteristic pattern where each larger red bump (lesion) is surrounded by numerous smaller red bumps (satellite lesions).[5] Contact the patient's health care provider for treatment if you think the patient has developed a yeast infection.

Recurring yeast infections can be prevented by keeping the skin clean and dry. Powder, such as non-talc baby powder or corn starch, can be used to help absorb moisture.

Skin Irritation

Areas that have been bandaged, or covered by compression garments or aids, may show signs of skin irritation when compression is removed. This subsection explains common signs of irritation, related causes, and steps to avoid future irritation. Any skin irritation should be noted on the Weekly Care Plan form.

Swelling reduction causes skin changes, including a darker appearance and changes in texture, that can be difficult to distinguish from irritation. Textured padding material, such as Komprex II, can leave a harmless impressions on the skin surface that look like blisters. Check with the patient's therapist if you not sure if a change in the patient's skin is irritation.

Redness between Fingers or Toes

Small red areas in the finger or toe web spaces, or at the underside of the toes, may occur when a patient in bandages has frail skin or is generally quite active. If the skin is irritated, decrease the stretch tension of the bandages as the fingers or toes are being wrapped.

Streaks of Redness

Streaks of redness going around the limb and following the edges of bandages (shown in Figure 3-2) can be caused by over pulling the bandage as

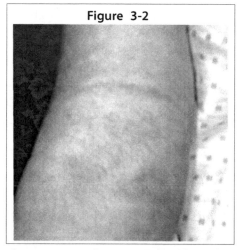

Figure 3-2

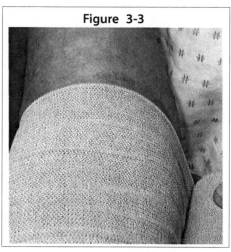

Figure 3-3

the patient is being wrapped, as demonstrated in Figure 3-3. To avoid this, keep the bandage roll close to the patient's body and decrease the stretch during application. Additional protective padding may be required.

Vertical streaks of redness along a limb may indicate a bacterial skin infection (lymphangitis) that requires immediate medical attention. See page 49.

Small Red Dots

Small red dots or freckles (*petechiae*), as shown in Figure 3-4, are caused by breakage of the small blood capillaries in the skin. There are several possible causes of these red dots, if a patient develops them in an area that is not treated with compression, or over a large area of skin, they could indicate a

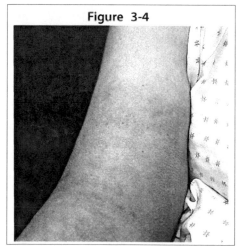

Figure 3-4

serious medical problem, contact the patient's health care provider.

In areas that are bandaged, or covered by a compression garment, these red dots can be caused by high pressure relative to the degree of swelling and padding used. The patient shown in this photo also had horizontal streaks of redness at the elbow, a sign of too much tension and insufficient padding at this sensitive skin area. Less bandage pressure and more cotton or foam padding should alleviate this problem. Excessive bandage tension and insufficient padding are frequent causes of bandage tightness, skin irritation, and overall discomfort.

Rash

A rash is a change in skin color and texture that may be accompanied by itching. If the patient develops a widespread rash, or a rash that starts in a location that is not being treated for lymphedema, contact the patient's health care provider for advice.

A rash that is related to bandaging, or other lymphedema treatment, typically starts in the area being treated. The rash will initially appear light red and spread out over the limb, the patient may report that the area of the rash feels itchy or warmer than surrounding areas. See Figure 3-5.

Both bandage pressure and increased skin temperature under the bandages may produce a reaction in the skin that results in a rash.[6] Rashes may also result from reactions to skin lotion, padding, or bandaging materials. First aid for treating rashes is described on page 260.

When a patient is sensitive to padding or bandaging materials, a rash and redness may appear within three to four days after a patient starts wearing bandages day and night, or less commonly, wearing bandages 8-10 hours per day. After several days, the area may become darker red and blisters may develop. If a rash like this develops, ask the patient's therapist about replacing synthetic cotton-like padding with 100% cotton or foam rolls such as Rosidal Soft.

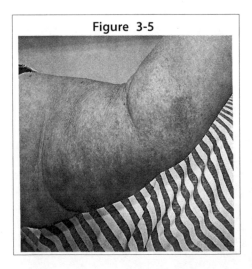

Figure 3-5

Washing the Skin

Regular washing is important to remove dead skin cells, dirt, and micro-organisms from the skin's surface. Use a clean washcloth and towel each day. Clean linens are important to prevent the spread of skin infections, especially when the patient has open sores. Soiled towels and washcloths should be sanitized between uses by bleaching them during the wash cycle. Careful attention to these details will help prevent the spread of infection. Disposable washcloths and towels may be an easier alternative to use, and are available at most drug and retail stores.

When cleaning, keep the following suggestions in mind:

- **Use moisturizing or antibacterial soap**. See page 286.

- **Use warm or lukewarm water.** Avoid hot water as this dries the skin and may cause an increase in swelling.

- **Consider rinsing the skin with a mild vinegar water solution** made by adding 1 teaspoon of white vinegar to 1 cup of water. Vinegar lowers the pH of the skin and helps to maintain the acid mantle.

- **Gently wash and dry all skin areas.** When washing and drying the skin, pay close attention to hard to reach areas such as between the toes, deep skin folds, and tight (contracted) joints of hands, armpits, knees, or hips. Pat dry particularly sensitive or fragile skin areas. Soft washcloths and towels are best for this since they will not scratch the skin. Hard rubbing or scrubbing should be avoided. Nylon scrubbers, loofa pads, and similar skin exfoliators are not recommended; however, patients with relatively healthy skin may use them lightly, taking care not to scratch the skin.

- **Stroke in the direction of the desired lymph flow while washing and drying affected areas.** Stroke towards the heart (in general) to reduce the swelling by following the stroke directions used for SLD (see page 67); avoid motions that move fluid toward swollen areas of the arm, leg, face, trunk or genitals. For example: when cleaning the leg, stroke from the foot towards the knee or hip (see Figure 3-6 ; when cleaning the arm, stroke from the hand towards the shoulder (see Figure 3-7).

Moisturizing the Skin

Moisturizing lotions and creams are used to prevent the skin from getting overly dry and cracked. For most patients, moisturizer should be applied twice a day; adjust this schedule as needed:

- Exposed areas with dry skin may require more frequent applications.

- Do not moisturize broken skin or skin that is infected, irritated, or weeping. Skin irritation in areas where moisturizer has been applied may indicate an allergic reaction to the moisturizer.

- Lotions may keep Kinesio tape from sticking. Either skip moisturizing areas where tape will be applied or allow the moisturizer to dry thoroughly before taping.

Rub the lotion or cream in gently, stroking towards the heart or working lymph nodes to promote lymph flow out of the affected area. See page 285 for information on selecting a lotion or cream.

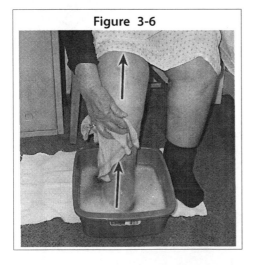

Figure 3-6

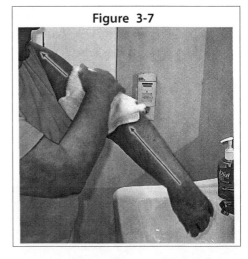

Figure 3-7

Applying Topical Medications

Depending on the patient's needs, the caregiver may be responsible for applying medications to the skin to prevent, or treat, existing conditions. For example, applying cream, powder or spray medication for athlete's foot or jock itch, or drying powder. Consult the Weekly Care Plan and Care Activity description for details. To minimize risk of infection, wear medical gloves while applying cream or handling infected limbs. A cotton swab may be used to apply cream between the patient's toes.

Cleaning Up

After completing skin care the caregiver should:

*   Clean up the area, dispose of disposable supplies and put used wash-cloths and towels in the laundry.

*   Wash their hands with soap and water.

*   Update the Weekly Care Plan Form to show that skin care was completed.

*   If there are any supplies that have been used up, make a note on the Item Needed Form (see page 283).

Frequently Asked Questions

Why do blisters on the patient's leg look white?

When a blister has a white color, it may be infected. If you smell any type of foul odor, contact the patient's health care provider right away for an appointment.

If there is no foul odor or any other signs of infection, the white color of a water blister may be related to a condition known as chylous reflux. *Chylous reflux* occurs when the lymphatic system in the patient's trunk is not effectively transporting fluid.

Lymph in the trunk contains fats that have been absorbed through the digestive system. This lymph has a milky white appearance and can back up into the genitals or legs with severe lymphedema. When this happens, any lymphatic blisters will have a watery white appearance. The patient's lymphedema therapist should be made aware of the problem and will suggest treatment to properly drain the trunk. Most likely this will emphasize deep breathing as part of the home care routine.

How can I tell an infection from inflammation?

Skin infections caused by bacteria are distinguished by a sudden color change from normal flesh color to a bright red color (similar to severe sunburn) within hours or days. Skin that is inflamed will also be red but the change occurs gradually over several weeks to months. Additionally, inflamed skin due to chronic edema will gradually become less red with consistent compression. Bacterial infections will not resolve without antibiotics. If there is any concern, let the physician evaluate the patient's condition to determine the best course of treatment.

Notes

1   "A Guide to Lymphedema" by K. D. Gordon and P. S. Mortimer. *Expert Rev Dermatol*. 2007;2(6):741-752.

2   "A Guide to Lymphedema" by K. D. Gordon and P. S. Mortimer. *Expert Rev Dermatol*. 2007;2(6):741-752.

3   **Lymphedema Management The Comprehensive Guide for Practitioners** by J. E. Zuther. Thieme 2005, p. 247.

4   "A Guide to Lymphedema" by K. D. Gordon and P. S. Mortimer. *Expert Rev Dermatol*. 2007;2(6):741-752.

5   "A Primer of Skin Diseases Associated With Obesity" by Noah S. Scheinfeld; Daniel H. Parish; Lawrence Charles Parish, *Expert Rev Dermatol*. 2007;2(4):409-415. Available at www.medscape.com/viewarticle/564201 accessed on June 20, 2008.

6   www.netdoctor.co.uk/diseases/facts/nettlerash.htm.

Chapter **4:**

Taking Measurements

The condition of the affected area, and the patient's overall health, should be monitored daily as part of skin care. Routine measurements should be taken according to the Weekly Care Plan, typically once a week. More frequent measurements may be needed if changes in the patient's condition are suspected.

Measurements include:

- Size, or circumference, of the affected area to monitor swelling. Instructions for arm and leg measurements are provided below. If the patient has lymphedema in other areas, ask the patient's therapist if these areas should be measured and how to take and record the measurements.

- Temperature, which can be a symptom of infection.

- Body weight, if practical, to check for fluid retention or other weight related health issues.

Limb size measurements are tracked on arm or leg measurement forms that are kept in the Patient Notebook. Temperature and weight are recorded on the Weekly Care Plan form.

General instructions are provided below. There may be a Care Activity form with specific measurement procedures and instructions.

Arm and Leg Measurements

When record keeping starts, take baseline measurements with the help of the patient's therapist and record them on the appropriate Arm Measurement Form (page 428) or Leg Measurement Form (page 429).

Measuring the patient's arms or legs regularly helps the caregiver recognize changes in lymphedema-related swelling. Current measurements can be compared to baseline measurements to monitor the effectiveness of lymphedema care.

The baseline used for comparing measurements varies with the affected area(s):

- Patients with lymphedema in one arm or one leg (unilateral lymphedema) use the uninvolved limb as the baseline and monitor the difference between limbs.

- Patients with lymphedema in both arms or both legs (bilateral lymphedema) use the same limb as the baseline and monitor changes in the size of each limb.

The ideal goal is for the involved limb(s) to be close to their "normal" or pre-swollen size. Normal is a relative term, and is sometimes difficult to accurately determine. The next best goal is for the involved limb to be as close to the size of the uninvolved limb as possible. This is one of the goals used by lymphedema therapists.

Once arm or leg swelling has been reduced through intensive treatment, the aim of home care is to maintain the swelling reduction. The baseline measurements are the size of the limb on the day of maximum reduction or "best day."

The therapist can advise the patient and caregiver of the Goal and Best Day measurements. If the arm or leg edema continues to decrease in size, the Best Day measurements may be adjusted accordingly. Optimally, the Best Day measurements will be equal to the Goal measurements of the uninvolved side or the near-normal size of the same limb prior to any swelling.

For accurate comparison, measure the same locations each time. The choice of location is individual and may be taken at standard locations (as explained below) or at unique spots, such as freckles, birthmarks, or scars.

Take measurements at the same time of day, if possible, and have the patient in the same position. Find a place where the elbow or knee can be relaxed during measurement such as resting on a table (for arm measurement), bed, or massage table.

You will need the following equipment and forms:

- A cloth tape measure or a specialized tape measure sold by lymphedema supply companies. Ask the patient's therapist if they use centimeters or inches and use the same units if possible (the conversion factor is 2.54 cm per inch).

- A washable marker, ballpoint pen, or eyebrow pencil for marking positions.

- A calculator for comparing past and present measurement values.

- Copies of the Arm Measurement Form (page 428) or Leg Measurement Form (page 429) for each affected limb.

The information in the top part of each measurement form stays the same. You can save time by making a master copy of the form for each affected limb (as explained below) and copying the master to make additional forms as needed. Current measurement forms, master copies, and spare measurement forms should be kept in the Patient Notebook (page 372).

To make a master arm or leg measurement form:

1. Fill in the patient's name, affected limb, and measurement units.

2. For limbs with unilateral lymphedema, measure the uninvolved arm or leg at the locations noted below and write these measurements in the first row labeled Goal. If both limbs are involved, leave this row blank since the Best Day measurements substitute for the Goal measurements.

3. Next, take measurements of the involved arm or leg at the locations noted below. If this is the first time measuring the involved limb(s) after the patient has undergone treatment, place this set of measurements in the Best Day row (unless the therapist has provided a specific set of measurements).

Record measurements on a copy of the arm or leg measurement form as follows:

1. Record the date and time in the Date column of the Measurement row.

2. Record measurements in the appropriate columns of the same row.

3. Calculate the *Difference* in measurements of the involved arm or leg by subtracting the Best Day measurements from the current day's Measurements. A positive (+) *Difference* indicates an increase in swelling and a negative (-) *Difference* indicates a decrease in swelling.

4. Use the Notes area to record by date any change in activities, diet, or weather that may contribute to an increase or decrease in swelling.

Contact the patient's doctor or therapist if there is any increase in swelling of more than 1 centimeter (or ½ inch) that cannot be reduced within a few days by elevating the arm or leg, extra compression, SLD, and exercise.

When all measurement rows on the page are filled, make a new copy from the master form and add the new sheet to the Patient Notebook in front of the old sheet. If the master form does not include the Goal and Best Day measurements, copy these to the new form.

Arm Measurement

The arm measurements are recorded on the Arm Measurement Form (page 428). Measure the arm at the:

- **Hand:** wrap the tape measure around the middle of the hand and read the measurement where the tape measure begins to overlap (that is, at the zero point of the tape measure). See Figure 4-1.

- **Wrist:** wrap the tape measure around the wrist at the crease and read the measurement where the tape measure begins to overlap.

- **Mid-Forearm:** wrap the tape measure around the mid-forearm and read the measurement where the tape measure begins to overlap. To be more accurate, the caregiver may draw a line at the mid-forearm 15 centimeters (or 6 inches) above the wrist to ensure the same spot is measured each time. Place the tape measure over the line.

- **Upper Arm:** wrap the tape measure around the middle of the upper arm and read the measurement where the tape measure begins to overlap. To be more accurate, the caregiver may draw a line on the upper arm 30 centimeters (or 12 inches) above the wrist to ensure the same spot is measured each time. See Figure 4-2 below.

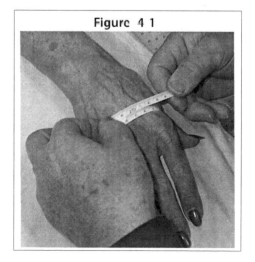

Figure 4-1

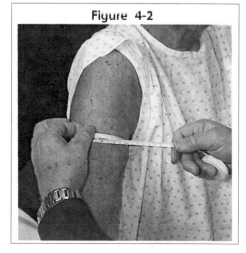

Figure 4-2

Leg Measurement

Leg measurements are recorded on the Leg Measurement Form (page 429). Measure the leg at the:

- **Arch of the foot:** wrap the tape measure around the middle of the foot and read the measurement where the tape measure begins to overlap (that is, at the zero point of the tape measure).

1. **Ankle:** wrap the tape measure around the smallest part of the ankle and read the measurement where the tape measure begins to overlap. To be more accurate, the caregiver may draw a line at the ankle 10 centimeters (or 4 inches) above the heel to ensure the same spot is measured each time. Place the tape measure over the line.

- **Mid-Calf:** wrap the tape measure around the largest part of the calf and read the measurement where the tape measure begins to overlap. To be more accurate, the caregiver may draw a line at the calf 30 centimeters (or 12 inches) above the heel and measure at the line.

- **Mid-Thigh:** wrap the tape measure around the middle of the thigh and read the measurement where the tape measure begins to overlap. To be more accurate, the caregiver may draw a line at the thigh 60 centimeters (or 24 inches) above the heel and measure at the line.

If the patient's swelling is irregularly shaped you may need to adjust measurement locations or add more measurement points. Note any changes in procedure on the Care Activity form and customize the measurement form so that future measurements can be made consistently.

Body Temperature

A thermometer can be used to measure temperature in the mouth (oral), rectum, or under the armpit to see if the patient has a fever. Always use the same measurement location for reliable results. Glass and mercury thermometers are not recommended for children.

Adults or cooperative children can have their temperature taken with a thermometer under the tongue as follows:

- Wait at least 15 minutes after the patient has any hot or cold food or drink.

- Prepare the thermometer:

    - Digital thermometer: cover the thermometer with a disposable cover and turn the thermometer on. Follow the instructions provided with the thermometer.

    - Mercury or other analog thermometer: clean the thermometer with soapy water or rubbing alcohol and rinse. Shake the mercury down, if necessary.

- Place the tip of the thermometer as far back under the tongue as possible and have the patient close their mouth gently.

- The thermometer should remain in place for about one minute. Some digital thermometers will beep when they are ready.

- Check the temperature reading and record it in the patient record.

Contact the patient's doctor if the oral temperature is more than 100°F (37.8°C) or 2°F (1.1°C) above the patient's baseline temperature. Note that elderly patients may have a smaller temperature increase due to an infection and children show larger temperature variations.

Weight

Ideally you should be able to weigh the patient at the same time of day and with similar clothing (or lack of clothing) every time. It may not be practical for a caregiver to weigh a morbidly obese patient or a patient with limited mobility.

It is important to maintain a record of your patient's weight and to track weight changes over time. Record the weight at the bottom of the Weekly Care Plan Form.

As long as things are going smoothly, weighing once a week should be enough. If weight changes by more than one pound per week up or down, or if there are signs of a problem, weight should be checked daily and the weight change should be brought to the attention of the doctor and the therapist. Gaining more than one pound (0.45 kg) per day could be a sign of congestive heart failure or kidney problems.

If the patient is gaining weight, it may be due to one of these causes:

- **Increased swelling.** Weight gain due to increased swelling is usually matched by increased measurements of the affected limb or changes in the trunk. This may be an indication that treatment is not as effective as it could be, contact the patient's lymphedema therapist.

- **Fluid retention.** Rapid weight gain may indicate a fluid imbalance or other medical problem, contact the patient's doctor.

- **Overeating.** If the patient is gaining weight that is not associated with increased swelling or fluid retention, this may be due to overeating or a lack of exercise. You may want to ask the patient's physician about appropriate weight goals for the patient; if weight management is an issue the doctor may refer the patient to a dietitian or a weight control program.

Chapter 5

Simple Lymph Drainage

Simple Lymph Drainage (SLD) is a gentle skin manipulation technique used by the caregiver to increase the flow of lymph toward functioning lymph node clusters. For an overview of SLD, patient self-massage, and manual lymph drainage by a therapist see page 32.

SLD should only be provided by individuals trained by the patient's therapist. Areas affected by lymphedema *should never be* massaged by an individual without appropriate training.

SLD is typically provided 1-3 times per day as specified in the Weekly Care Plan (see page 333) and Care Activity description developed in cooperation with the patient's therapist. The activity description should specify which SLD sequence to use and any special instructions.

The therapist will check with the patient's doctor to be sure that SLD is appropriate and personalize the SLD routine for the patient's current condition and medications.

Routine SLD should be suspended or modified if there is a change in the patient's condition; for example, an untreated infection, an acute kidney or heart condition, or a recent blood clot. Check with the patient's doctor or therapist if you have any question about the safety of continuing SLD or when to restart SLD.

If the patient uses a pain patch (Duragesic or Fentanyl Transdermal System), check with the patient's doctor before doing SLD or applying compression near the patch, or using anti-fungal medications.

SLD begins with stationary circles over the functioning lymph node clusters (see page 72) followed by specific sequences of strokes and circles to guide lymph towards the functioning lymph nodes (see page 78).

The SLD routine provided by the therapist should be tailored to the needs of the patient, taking into account areas where lymph flow is blocked and directing fluid towards working lymphatic pathways. We have provided SLD sequences for common conditions that can be adapted by the patient's therapist (starting on page 78). If your patient is an infant or a child, see also page 220.

Tailoring the SLD for a patient requires detailed knowledge of lymphatic anatomy, an understanding of the patient's condition, expert judgment based upon years of experience, plus some trial and error. Documenting the SLD sequence in the care plan and following the instructions will maximize the effectiveness of this treatment.

This chapter explains SLD in terms of:

- Preparing for SLD.

- Basic SLD techniques: stationary circles, strokes, and deep breathing, starting on page 69.

- Techniques for making circles over working lymph node clusters in a specific way, starting on page 72.

- SLD sequences for specific swelling conditions, starting on page 78.

- Frequently asked questions about SLD, see page 91.

Preparing for SLD

Select a location for SLD that is quiet, private, and at a comfortable temperature. The area of the body that is being manipulated should be uncovered. You may want to cover other areas with a sheet or blanket to keep the patient warm and comfortable.

The patient may be seated or lying on a massage table or bed that is accessible from the sides. The patient position should be high enough for the caregiver to work comfortably without having to reach or bend down too far. See the chapter on "Body Mechanics" (page 383) for suggestions on safe and comfortable working positions.

Typically, SLD is performed after skin care and before applying compression. Any moisturizing lotions or creams should be fully absorbed so the skin is not slippery. Massage oils or lotions are not used for SLD.

Basic SLD Techniques

SLD uses combinations of stationary circles, strokes, and deep breathing as explained below. Treatment begins with stationary circles over the major lymph node clusters that are working properly followed by a sequence of strokes and circles, and deep breathing, to guide lymph towards the working lymph nodes. While providing SLD, be careful not to aggravate the lymphatic system by using too much hand pressure.

Stationary Circles

When making stationary circles, or simply circles, the caregiver keeps the hand in one spot, while gently moving the patient's skin in a circular motion. Each circle has two equally important parts:

- *Working phase* is the first half of the circle where the caregiver's hand moves and stretches the patient's skin. This movement causes the muscles surrounding the lymph vessels in the skin to contract and moves lymph fluid in the direction of the hand motion.

- *Resting phase* is the second half of the circle where the caregiver releases their hand pressure, allowing the patient's skin to return to the start position. This allows the lymph vessels to relax and refill with more fluid.

To develop the proper rhythm for this technique, it may help if you talk through the timing as "work-rest, work-rest, work-rest" or "pump-refill, pump-refill, pump-refill," either aloud or to yourself. This will help you maintain a speed of one circle per second.

When performing circles, the caregiver should keep these five points in mind:

1. *Location*: Place the hands so they completely cover the area to be stimulated. The hand should rest flat on the patient's skin and be relaxed, not stiff. Avoid cupping the hand while making a circle; this raises the palm so that only the fingertips touch the skin.

2. *Pressure*: Make a circle using just enough pressure to gently stretch the patient's skin.

   - *Pressure should not be so light* that the hand simply slides over the skin.

   - *Pressure should not be so hard* that the patient's skin turns red. Redness indicates increased blood flow which can increase swelling.

3. *Direction*: Circles are usually directed "towards the heart" or towards intact lymph node clusters during the working phase.

4. *Speed*: Circles should be slow with one complete work-rest cycle per second.

5. *Order*: The sequence of the circles is initially from the center of the body moving out along the arms or legs. This empties the lymphatic vessels nearest the terminus first, making room for fluid from the affected area.

Strokes

Strokes are very gentle brush-like motions with the caregiver's finger tips or the palm of the hand softly touching the patient's skin to stimulate lymph vessels within the skin. All strokes should be very light, like stroking a cat or a child's head, taking care not to scratch the patient's skin.

You may see goose bumps or narrow white streaks on the patient's skin indicating that the area has been stimulated. Also, the patient may report a chill or tingling sensation in the swollen area. These are not causes for concern.

Deep Breathing

The third element of SLD is deep breathing, or abdominal breathing, which enhances the pumping action of the thoracic duct. The thoracic duct is the largest lymphatic vessel in the body and drains both legs, the left arm, and the left side of the body. See Appendix A (page 399) for more information.

As the patient breathes in and out, the diaphragm relaxes and contracts around the thoracic duct and this helps to pump lymph fluid. Deep breathing has the added benefit of relaxing the body.

Patient position: The patient can be in any position; however, lying on their back with the knees bent and feet on the bed is best. The caregiver or patient places a hand on the patient's stomach just above the belly button and should feel the stomach rise on the inhale.

Working phase:

- Ask the patient to breathe in deeply and slowly to a count of 5.

- Tell the patient to relax the stomach to allow it to rise up with the full inward breath.

Resting phase:

- Ask the patient to breathe out slowly to a 5-10 count and note that the patient's stomach lowers as air leaves the body.

- As the patient breathes out, ask the patient to purse their lips (as if to whistle) to provide some resistance as they exhale. Each breath should be slow and steady.

- Do not apply pressure to the patient's stomach as the patient blows out unless specifically advised by the patient's therapist; this can be problematic for some patients.

Repeat: 5 times.

Circling Lymph Node Clusters

Stationary circles (see page 69) are used to promote the flow of lymph through clusters of lymph nodes. Therapists refer to this as clearing or draining the nodes.

Specific lymph drainage techniques for these lymph node clusters are explained below:

- *Terminus* or *supraclavicular nodes* located above the collarbone.

- *Cervical nodes* located at either side of the neck.

- *Occipital nodes* located at the back of the head.

- *Auricular nodes* around the ears.

- *Axillary nodes* in the armpits.

- *Antecubital nodes* in the folds of the elbows.

- *Inguinal nodes* in the groin located below the crease where the legs join the trunk.

- *Popliteal nodes* located at the backs of the knees.

These clusters are summarized in Figure 1-1 on page 14 and shown in more detail in Appendix A (page 399).

Terminus/Above the Collarbone

Supraclavicular lymph nodes at the base of the neck drain fluid from the head, neck, and collar area of the shoulders. From this area lymph flows to the terminus or end point where it re-enters the bloodstream. See Figure 5-1 on this page and Figure 5-2 on page 73.

Patient position: Lying on their back or sitting in a chair.

Starting position: Place the flat of the hand just above the collarbone

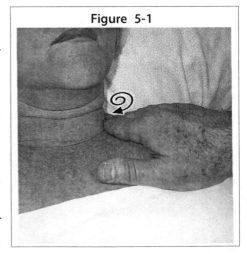

Figure 5-1

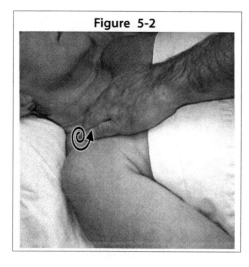

Figure 5-2

in the small hollow of the neck and shoulder.

Working phase: Move the hand in a circle from the patient's shoulder forward and in toward the front of the body. Gently pull the skin while moving the hand.

Resting phase: Relax the hand to release the pressure allowing the patient's skin to return to the start position.

Repeat: 5-7 times.[1]

Cervical/Side of the Neck

Cervical lymph nodes located at each side of the neck drain fluid from the head and neck. See Figure 5-3 .

Patient position: Lying on their back or sitting in a chair.

Starting position: Place the flat of the hand on each side of the patient's neck.

Working phase: Move the hand in a circle from the patient's head down and forward toward the front of the body. Gently pull the skin while moving the hand.

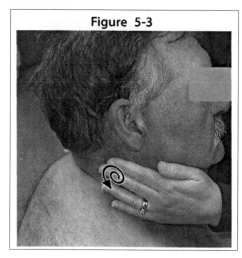

Figure 5-3

Resting phase: Relax the hand to release all pressure and allow the patient's skin to return to the start position.

Repeat: 5-7 times.

Occipital/Back of the Head

Occipital lymph nodes located at the back of the head near the base of the skull drain fluid from the top and back of the head. See Figure 5-4.

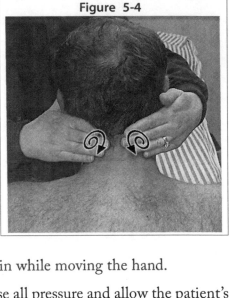

Figure 5-4

Patient position: Lying on their back or sitting in a chair.

Starting position: Place the flat of the hand behind the patient's neck at the base of the skull.

Working phase: Move the hand in a circle from the patient's head down toward the shoulder. Gently pull the skin while moving the hand.

Resting phase: Relax the hand to release all pressure and allow the patient's skin to return to the start position.

Repeat: 5-7 times.

Auricular/Around the Ears

Auricular lymph nodes in front of and behind the ears drain fluid from the head and face. See Figure 5-5.

Patient position: Lying on back or sitting in a chair.

Starting position: Place the flat of the hand in front of or behind the ear, or both, splitting the fingers so that the ear is in between.

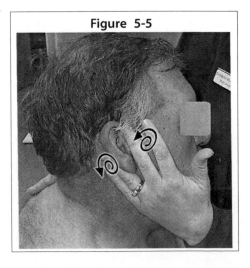

Figure 5-5

Working phase: Move the hand in a circle from the ear to the back of the patient's head, then down towards the neck. Gently pull the skin while moving the hand.

Resting phase: Relax the hand to release all pressure and allow the patient's skin to return to the start position.

Repeat: 5-7 times.

Axillary/Armpits

Axillary lymph nodes, which are located in the armpits, drain fluid from the chest, upper back, and arms. See Figure 5-6 and Figure 5-7.

Patient position: Lying on their back or sitting in a chair.

Starting position: Place the flat of the hand on the chest wall at the armpit, as if warming a cold hand.

Working phase: Circle the hand up into the armpit and forward toward the front of the patient's body. Gently pull the skin while moving the hand up.

Resting phase: Relax the hand to release all pressure and allow the patient's skin to return to the start position.

Repeat: 5-7 times.

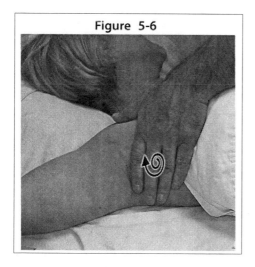

Figure 5-6

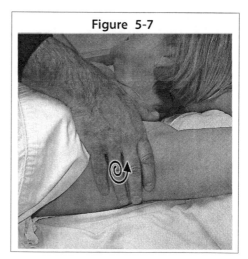

Figure 5-7

Antecubital/Elbow

Antecubital lymph nodes, which are located at the front (palm) side of the arm in the elbow bend, drain fluid from the lower arms and hands. See Figure 5-8 and Figure 5-9.

Patient position: Lying on their back or sitting in a chair.

Starting position: Place a flat hand over the crease at the bend of the patient's elbow.

Working phase: Circle the hand toward the upper arm, gently pulling the patient's skin while moving the hand up and slightly in.

Resting phase: Relax the hand to release all pressure and allow the patient's skin to return to the start position.

Repeat: 5-7 times.

Inguinal/Upper Thigh

Inguinal lymph nodes, which are located at the front of the upper thighs near the groin, drain fluid from the stomach, lower back, and legs, including the feet. See Figure 5-10 on this page and Figure 5-11 on page 77 .

Patient position: Lying on their back.

Starting position: Place the flat of one or both hands on the patient's upper leg near the bend of the front hip with the fingers parallel to the hip bend.

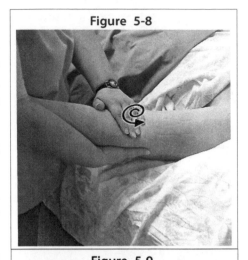

Figure 5-8

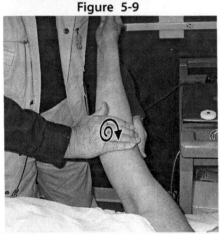

Figure 5-9

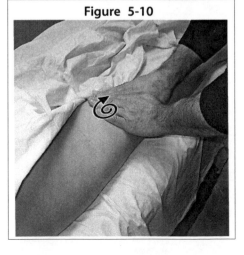

Figure 5-10

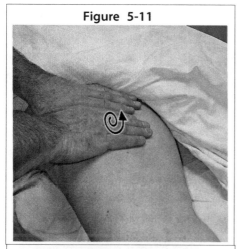

Figure 5-11

Working phase: Circle the hand up from the lower thigh toward the patient's stomach and heart. Gently pull the skin while moving the hand up.

Resting phase: Relax the hand to release all pressure and allow the patient's skin to return to the start position.

Repeat: 5-7 times.

Popliteal/Back of the Knee

Popliteal lymph nodes, which are located at the back of the knee, drain fluid from the calves and feet. See Figure 5-12 and Figure 5-13.

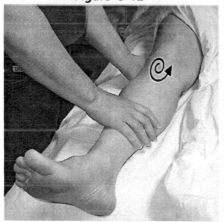

Figure 5-12

Patient position: Lying on their back with knees slightly bent.

Starting position: Place the flat of one, or both, hands behind the knee at the knee crease.

Working phase: Circle the hand up from the foot toward the upper thigh. Gently pull the skin while moving the hand up.

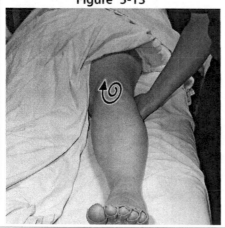

Figure 5-13

Resting phase: Relax the hand to release all pressure and allow the patient's skin to return to the start position.

Repeat: 5-7 times.

Specific SLD Sequences

Sequences provide combinations of the basic SLD techniques and the lymph node cluster circling methods described above that are specific to each affected area. One or more of these SLD sequences may be used to address the patient's affected area(s). For example, a person with right arm lymphedema post-mastectomy should be treated with the SLD sequences for the right upper body and breast and for the right arm.

Variations in SLD technique are common and the patient's therapist may provide a different SLD sequence that is more effective. Always defer to the therapist's professional expertise when performing home treatment with your patient.

Specific sequences for each patient should be listed in the Weekly Care Plan and associated Care Activity Forms created in cooperation with the patient's therapist.

Sequences are provided below for lymphedema in the:

- Head and Neck, page 79.

- Right or Left Upper Body and Breast, pages 79 and 82.

- Right, Left or Both Arms, pages 81, 84, and 85.

- Lower Body, Stomach, Genitals, and Buttocks, page 86.

- Right, Left, or Both Legs, pages 87, 88, and 90.

For each of the sequences given below:

- **Begin working with the patient resting on their back**. If this is not possible, use the position that is most comfortable for the patient and modify the treatment accordingly.

- **Complete the entire treatment** sequence by performing the circles, deep breathing, and strokes approximately 5-7 times each area.

- **If time permits,** repeat the sequence once or twice during a session; each sequence usually only takes 5-10 minutes. Optionally include the advanced SLD variation provided the end of each sequence; advanced SLD sequences may take up to 60 minutes to complete.

- Record the treatment on the Weekly Care Plan Form.

Head and Neck

This complete sequence is for patients whose lymph nodes have been removed or irradiated on one side. Check with the patient's therapist if both sides are affected or if fluid must be transferred through damaged areas. You may be able to transfer fluid to the occipital nodes and then the axillary nodes by performing only steps 2, 3, 6, 8, and 9.

1. **Circles** at the terminus above the collarbone. **Note:** Skip the side where the patient's lymph nodes have been removed or irradiated.

2. **Circles** at the left and right axillary nodes/armpits.

3. **Deep breathing.**

4. **Circles** at the cervical nodes/sides of the neck.
   Note: Skip the side where the patient's lymph nodes have been removed or irradiated.

5. **Circles** at the auricular nodes in front of and behind the ears.
   Note: Skip the side where the patient's lymph nodes have been removed or irradiated.

6. **Circles** at the occipital nodes/back of the head.

7. **Strokes** along the non-swollen side of the face to the ear and jaw on the same side and then from the side of the ear and jaw down the neck on the non-swollen side.

8. **Strokes** across the chest, upper back and shoulder to the armpit on the side with the swelling. See Figure 5-14 on page 80 .

9. **Strokes** along the swollen side of the face, around the ear and jaw to the back of the head, and then down the neck to the armpit on the same side. See Figure 5-15 on page 80.

10. **Intraoral** (inside the mouth) lymph drainage may be performed by the patient as suggested by the patient's therapist.

Advanced SLD: Perform circles along the stroke routes. The direction of the working phase of the circles should be the same as the stroke direction.

Figure 5-14

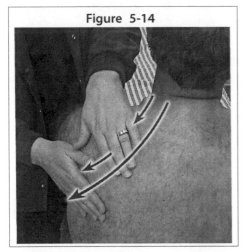

Figure 5-15

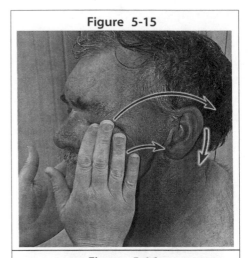

Right Upper Body and Breast

1. **Circles** at the terminus above the collarbone.

2. **Circles** at the left axillary nodes/ armpit.

3. **Deep breathing.**

4. **Circles** at the right inguinal nodes/upper thigh.

5. **Strokes** along the right outer shoulder to the neck. See Figure 5-16.

6. **Strokes** from the right armpit across the chest and/or upper breast (above the surgical scar) to the left armpit (the upper front pathway).

7. **Strokes** from the back of the right armpit down the side of the body in a slight diagonal to the front of the right hip (the right side pathway). See Figure 5-17.

Figure 5-16

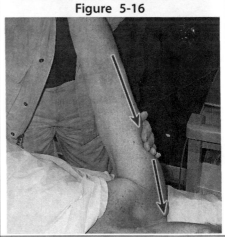

Figure 5-17

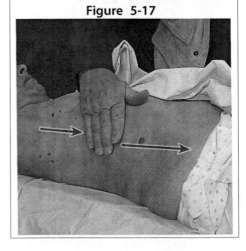

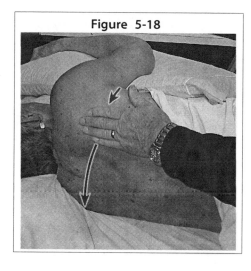

Figure 5-18

8. **Strokes** from the lower breast (below the surgical scar) and front lower ribs/chest to the side pathway.

9. **Change Patient Position:** Have the patient roll onto their non-swollen left side for the following strokes.

10. **Strokes** from the right armpit across the upper back to the left armpit (the upper back pathway). See Figure 5-18.

11. **Strokes** from the back lower ribs out to the side and towards the side pathway Alternative: strokes from the back lower ribs to the left armpit. Choose only one stroke path, not both.

If the patient also has right arm swelling, have the patient roll back onto their back and perform steps #8 and 10 of the right arm treatment sequence below.

Advanced SLD: Perform circles along the stroke routes. The direction of the working phase of the circles should be the same as the stroke direction.

Right Arm

1. **Circles** at the terminus above the collarbone.

2. **Circles** at the left axillary nodes/armpit.

3. **Deep breathing.**

4. **Circles** at the right inguinal nodes/upper thigh.

5. **Circles** at the right antecubital nodes/elbow bend.

6. **Strokes** along the right outer shoulder to the neck.

7. **Strokes** from the right armpit across the chest to the left armpit (the upper front pathway).

8. **Strokes** from the palm-side of the wrist along the front of the right arm to the front side of the armpit as shown in Figure 5-19. *Avoid stroking into the armpit since this is the affected area.* Alternative: combine strokes by doing step 8 before step 7.

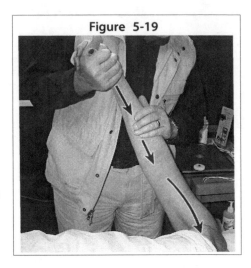

Figure 5-19

9. **Strokes** from the back of the right armpit down the side of the body in a slight diagonal to the front of the right hip (the right side pathway).

10. **Strokes** from the back side of the hand along the back of the right arm to the back of the armpit. Figure 5-26 on page 86 shows the left arm version of this stroke. *Avoid stroking into the armpit.* Alternative: combine strokes by doing step 10 before step 9.

11. **Change patient position:** Have the patient roll onto their non-swollen left side for the following stroke. Patient returns to lying on their back after the stroke is completed.

12. **Strokes** from the right armpit across the upper back to the left armpit (the upper back pathway). See Figure 5-18 on page 81.

Advanced SLD: Strokes are advanced by first stroking the upper arm, then the lower arm, then the hand. Circles can be performed along the stroke routes. The direction of the working phase of the circles should be the same as the stroke direction.

Left Upper Body and Breast

1. **Circles** at the terminus above the collarbone.

2. **Circles** at the right axillary nodes/armpit.

3. **Deep breathing.**

4. **Circles** at the left inguinal nodes/upper thigh.

5. **Strokes** along the left outer shoulder to the neck.

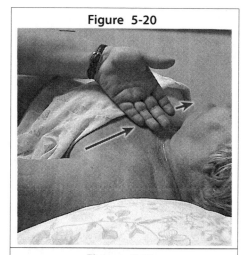

Figure 5-20

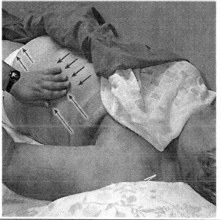

Figure 5-21

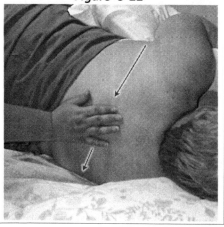

Figure 5-22

6. **Strokes** from the left armpit across the chest and/or upper breast (above the surgical scar) to the right armpit (along the upper front pathway). See Figure 5-20.

7. **Strokes** from the back of the left armpit down the side of the body in a slight diagonal to the front of the left hip (along the left side pathway). See Figure 5-21.

8. **Strokes** from the lower breast (below the surgical scar) and lower ribs/chest to the side pathway.

9. **Change Patient Position:** Have the patient roll onto their non-swollen right side or stomach for the following strokes.

10. **Strokes** from the left armpit across the upper back to the right armpit (along the upper back pathway). See Figure 5-22. Optionally, stroke with the patient sitting up; see Figure 5-23 on page 84.

11. **Strokes** from the back lower ribs out to the side and toward the side pathway. Alternative: strokes from the back lower ribs to the right armpit. Choose only one stroke path; do not do both.

If the patient also has left arm swelling, have the patient return to their back and perform steps #8 and 10 of the left arm treatment sequence below.

Advanced SLD: Perform circles along the stroke routes. The direction of the working phase of the circles should be the same as the stroke direction.

Left Arm

1. **Circles** at the terminus above the collarbone.

2. **Circles** at the right axillary nodes/armpit.

3. **Deep breathing.**

4. **Circles** at the left inguinal nodes/ upper thigh.

5. **Circles** at the left antecubital nodes/elbow bend.

6. **Stroking** along the left outer shoulder to the neck. See Figure 5-24.

7. **Stroking** from the left armpit across the chest to the right armpit (along the upper front pathway).

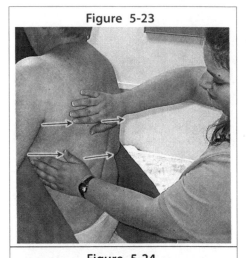
Figure 5-23

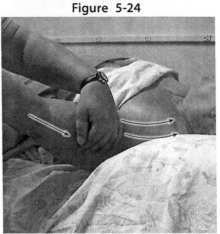
Figure 5-24

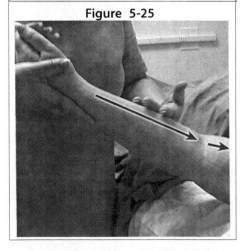
Figure 5-25

8. **Stroking** from the palm-side of the wrist along the front of the left arm to the front side of the armpit as shown in Figure 5-25 on page 84. *Avoid stroking into the armpit since this is the affected area.* Alternative: combine strokes by doing step 8 before step 7.

9. **Stroking** from the back of the left armpit down the side of the body in a slight diagonal to the front of the left hip (along the left side pathway).

10. **Stroking** from the back side of the hand along the back of the left arm to the back of the armpit as shown in Figure 5-26 on page 86. *Avoid stroking into the armpit.* Alternative: combine strokes by doing step 10 before step 9.

11. **Change** patient position. Have the patient roll onto their non-swollen right side for the following stroke. Patient returns to back lying position after the stroke is completed.

12. **Stroking** from the left armpit across the upper back to the right armpit (along the upper back pathway).

Advanced SLD: Advance by first stroking the upper arm, then the lower arm, then the hand. Circles can be performed along the stroke routes. The direction of the working phase of the circles should be the same as the stroke direction.

Both Arms

1. **Circles** at the terminus above the collarbone.

2. **Deep breathing.**

3. **Circles** at the left and right inguinal nodes/upper thighs.

4. **Circles** at the left and right antecubital nodes/elbow bends.

5. **Stroking** along the outer shoulders to the neck.

6. **Stroking** from the palm-side of the wrists along the front of the arms to the front side of the armpits and continuing to the terminus. See Figure 5-19 on page 82. *Avoid stroking into the armpits since these are affected areas.*

7. **Stroking** from the back side of the hands along the back of the arms to the back of the armpits. See Figure 5-26. *Avoid stroking into the armpits.*

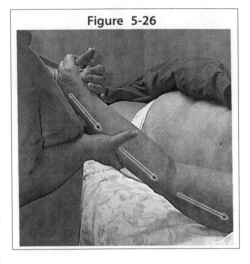

Figure 5-26

8. **Stroking** from the back of the armpits down the left and right sides of the body in a slight diagonal to the front of the hips (the right and left side pathways).

Advanced SLD: Advance by first stroking the upper arms, then the lower arms, then the hands. Circles may be performed along the stroke routes. The direction of the working phase of the circles should be the same as the stroke direction.

Lower Body, Stomach, Genitals, and Buttocks

Note: Medical gloves are recommended for SLD on the genital area.

1. **Circles** at the terminus above the collarbone.

2. **Circles** at the right and left axillary nodes/armpits.

3. **Deep breathing.**

4. **Circles** at the left and right inguinal nodes/upper thighs. Note: skip these circles if the patient's lymph nodes have been removed or irradiated in the inguinal or pelvic areas.

5. **Stroking** from the front of the right and left hips up the sides of the body in a slight diagonal to the armpits on the same side (the right and left side pathways).

6. **Stroking** from the swollen areas on the right or left lower body, stomach, genitals, and buttocks towards the side pathway on the same side. Have the patient roll onto their side or stomach to treat the buttock area.

Advanced SLD: Perform circles along the stroke routes. The direction of the working phase of the circles should be the same as the stroke direction.

Right Leg

1. **Circles** at the terminus above the collarbone.

2. **Circles** at the right axillary nodes/armpit. Optional circles at the left axillary nodes/armpit.

3. **Deep breathing.**

4. **Circles** at the left inguinal nodes/upper thigh. If the patient has primary lymphedema, only circle one time.

5. **Circles** at the popliteal nodes at the back of the right knee.

6. **Stroking** from the front of the right hip up the side of the body in a slight diagonal to the right armpit (the right side pathway).

7. **Stroking** from the front of the right hip along the front of the lower stomach to the front of the left hip (the lower front pathway). Note: this step may be skipped if the patient has primary lymphedema or secondary lymphedema from radiation or lymph node removal in the pelvic area.

8. **Change patient position:** Have the patient roll onto their non-swollen side or stomach for the following stroke. Patient returns to back lying position after the stroke is completed.

9. **Stroking** along the back of the right hip and buttock to the left buttock and hip (the lower back pathway). Note: this step may be skipped if the patient has primary lymphedema, secondary lymphedema from radiation or lymph node removal in the pelvic area, or if it is too difficult for the patient to change positions.

10. **Stroking** from the foot to the outer hip along the front and side of the right leg, then into the side pathway. *Stroke around but not through the inguinal lymph nodes at the front hip since this is the affected area.*

11. **Stroking** from the foot to the buttock along the back of the right leg and around to the front of the abdomen, then into the side pathway. Have the patient bend their knee to allow the caregiver to stroke the back side of the leg and buttock.

Advanced SLD: Advance by stroking first the thigh, then the knee, the lower leg, and the foot and toes. Perform circles along the stroke routes.

The direction of the working phase of the circles should be the same as the stroke direction.

Left Leg

1. **Circles** at the terminus above the collarbone.

2. **Circles** at the left axillary nodes/armpit. Optional circles at the right axillary nodes/armpit.

3. **Deep breathing.**

4. **Circles** at the right inguinal nodes/upper thigh. If the patient has primary lymphedema, only circle one time.

5. **Circles** at the popliteal nodes at the back of the left knee.

6. **Stroking** from the front of the left hip up the side of the body in a slight diagonal to the left armpit (the left side pathway). Figure 5-27 shows this with the patient on their stomach.

7. **Stroking** from the front of the left hip along the front of the lower stomach to the front of the right hip (the lower front pathway). Note: this step may be skipped if the patient has primary lymphedema or secondary lymphedema from radiation or lymph node removal in the pelvic area.

8. **Change patient position:** Have the patient roll onto their non-swollen side or stomach for the following stroke. Patient returns to their back after the stroke is completed.

9. **Stroking** along the back of the left hip and buttock to the right buttock and hip (lower back pathway). Note: this step may be skipped if the patient has primary lymphedema, secondary lymphedema from radiation or lymph node removal in the pelvic area, or if it is too difficult for the patient to change positions.

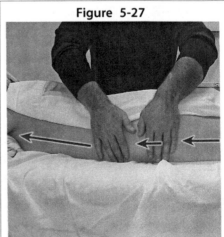

Figure 5-27

Figure 5-28

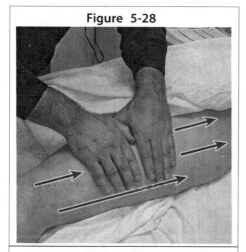

10. Stroking from the foot to the outer hip along the front and side of the left leg, then into the side pathway. See Figure 5-28. *Stroke around and not through the inguinal lymph nodes at the front hip, since this is the affected area.*

11. Stroking from the foot to the buttock along the back of the left leg and around to the front of the abdomen into the side pathway. Have the patient bend their knee to allow the caregiver to stroke the back side of the leg. Figure 5-29 shows this with the patient on their stomach.

Figure 5-29

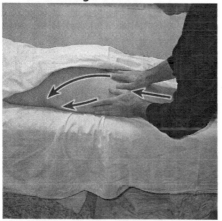

Advanced SLD: Advance by first stroking the thigh, then the knee, the lower leg, and the ankle, foot, and toes. See Figure 5-30. Circles can be performed along the stroke routes. The direction of the working phase of the circles should be the same as the stroke direction.

Figure 5-30

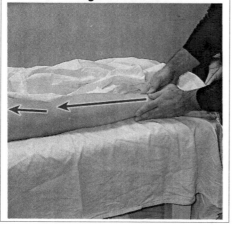

Both Legs

1. **Circles** at the terminus above the collarbone.

2. **Circles** at the right and left axillary nodes/armpits.

3. **Deep breathing.**

4. **Circles** at the left and right inguinal nodes/upper thighs. Note: this step may be skipped if the patient has primary lymphedema or the patient's lymph nodes have been removed or irradiated in the inguinal or pelvic areas.

5. **Circles** at the right and left popliteal nodes/knee bends.

6. **Stroking** from the front of the right hip up the right side of the body in a slight diagonal to the right armpit (the right side pathway).

7. **Stroking** from the front of the left hip up the left side of the body in a slight diagonal to the left armpit (the left side pathway).

8. **Stroking** from the foot to the outer hips along the front and side of the each leg, then into the side pathways. *Stroke around and not through the inguinal lymph nodes at the front hips, since these are the affected areas.*

9. **Stroking** from the foot to the buttock along the back of the each leg and around to the front of the abdomen into the same side pathways. Have the patient bend their knees to allow the caregiver to stroke the back sides of the legs.

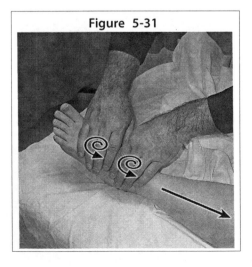

Figure 5-31

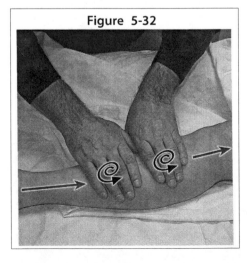

Figure 5-32

Advanced SLD: Advance by first stroking the thighs, then the knees, the lower legs, and the ankles, feet and toes. See Figure 5-31 and Figure 5-32 on page 90. Perform circles along the stroke routes. The direction of the working phase of the circles should be the same as the stroke direction.

Frequently Asked Questions

Should I circle the lymph nodes in the swollen area?

There is some debate among lymphedema specialists about manipulating lymph nodes in an area where swelling is related to lymph node removal or radiation. Some therapists do not circle remaining lymph nodes because these nodes are already overwhelmed and unable to drain lymph fluid effectively. Alternatively, some therapists believe that circling remaining lymph nodes will help process fluid out of the swollen area. Ask the lymphedema therapist which is best for your patient.

How can I tell if I'm circling with the right pressure?

Take your finger and gently press into the patient's skin at the forearm with very light pressure until the patient's skin under your finger begins to change color. As soon as the finger is removed, the skin returns to its normal color as the blood flows back into the area. This very gentle pressure is enough to affect the blood capillaries. Use the same light pressure to perform circles.

How can I tell if I'm stroking with the right pressure?

Strokes are lighter than circles. The caregiver's hand should move easily over the patient's skin very little pressure, almost like a feather.

What if there is a scar in a stroke pathway?

When there is a scar in the stroke pathway, stroke around the scar and not through it, since lymph vessels within the scar tissue have been disrupted and the transfer of fluid across a scar is usually ineffective.

How can I overcome the embarrassment of doing SLD?

SLD can be uncomfortable when the caregiver or the patient is not used to such personal contact. To overcome this discomfort or embarrassment, remember that you are doing SLD (and other treatment activities) to help the patient with their swelling.

Be confident in your skills. If this is the first time working with a patient, practice on yourself, or someone who you are comfortable touching, to become familiar with the motions.

Tell the patient what you are going to do before you perform each step of the sequence. For example, you may say "now I will circle the lymph nodes at your upper thigh." This helps both you, and the patient, be more comfortable and know what to expect.

If the patient is able to help, let them do the SLD (or self massage) in sensitive areas.

How can I do SLD on an obese or large-breasted patient?

When you have trouble reaching lymph node clusters because the patient has extra skin folds or a large breast, ask the patient to help lift the stomach or breast out of the way or directly move the flesh yourself, so that you can reach the lymph node location. Stroking an area with increased skin folds is somewhat difficult, try not to worry if the strokes seem imperfect; some stimulation is better than none. The patient's therapist may also be able to provide more individualized instruction.

How can I explain the proper breathing technique?

Ask the patient to place one hand on their abdomen and the other hand on their chest. Have them practice breathing "normally" and pay close attention to any rise and fall of the stomach and lower ribs (sometimes the movement may be very slight). Once the patient is able to feel even the smallest movement in the stomach and lower ribs with a normal breath, ask the patient to take a fuller breath by raising the stomach more.

If the patient converts back to upper chest breathing, start over. Keep practicing this until the patient is able to take full (deep) breaths easily. Don't despair if this takes a week or two, the benefit of properly taking deep breaths is well worth the effort.

What if the patient gets dizzy during deep breathing?

It is not unusual for a person to get dizzy when first learning to breathe deeply. If this happens, have the patient take a few normal breaths until the dizziness goes away, then finish the number of recommended deep breaths.

If the patient continues to get dizzy, make sure the patient is not breathing too quickly and hyperventilating; if they are, ask the patient to breathe more slowly. Usually dizziness occurs only the first few times a person takes larger than normal breaths. If dizziness persists, contact the patient's therapist or physician.

Can SLD be overdone?

Yes, this may occur if the caregiver presses too hard while performing the circles or repeats the circles in one area for an extended period of time. If you notice the patient's skin becoming red, lighten your hand pressure. Excessive pressure or repetition can dilate blood capillaries, causing more fluid to transfer from the blood to the tissues. Excessive stimulation can also cause the smooth muscles encircling the lymph vessels to spasm, which decreases the lymph vessels' ability to absorb and transport fluid.[2]

Notes

1   **Lymphedema Management The Comprehensive Guide for Practitioners** by J. E. Zuther. Thieme Medical Publishers, Inc. 2005. pp. 104, 135.

2   **Lymphedema Management, The Comprehensive Guide for Practitioners** by J. E. Zuther. Thieme Medical Publishers, Inc., 2005. p 134.

Chapter 6

Compression Bandaging

Compression is an important part of lymphedema treatment as explained on page 33. Bandaging, or wrapping, is used to reduce swelling, especially during the early phases of treatment and during an intensive treatment series (see page 36). Once the swelling is controlled, bandages may be replaced by compression garments and aids (see page 133).

Properly applied bandages create a gentle pressure gradient with more pressure at the foot or hand, and less pressure closer to the body. Pressure on the skin and underlying tissues helps excess fluid enter the lymph vessels and blood vessels so the fluid can be transported out of the swollen area. Compression (bandages, garments, or aids) also minimizes fluid accumulation in affected areas and improves the ability of the muscle and joint pumps to move fluid out of the limb during exercise and other activities.

Compression is not recommended for all patients with swelling issues. The patient's physician determines the need for compression, and when to resume compression after a hiatus. The lymphedema therapist decides what form of compression—bandages, compression garments, compression aids, or a combination— is appropriate for the patient during the day, at night, and while exercising. The therapist may modify the use of compression as the patient's condition changes.

Typically, the therapist bandages the patient during the first intensive treatment series (see page 37). After the intensive, the therapist will recommend a home care routine and train the patient or caregiver in applying bandages. Typically patients use compression garments during the day and bandages at night.

The home care routine outlined in the Weekly Care Plan (see page 333) should cover compression usage, including when to apply or remove compression bandages. There should be a Care Activity Form describing how to bandage each affected area. This form should include a list of bandaging materials and supplies, and instructions that refer to this book or alternate procedures provided by the patient's therapist.

The normal bandaging routine (or other compression usage) may need to be adjusted or suspended if the patient has an untreated infection, blood clot, wound, or other skin changes, see Skin Care (page 49) for more information. Any other changes in the bandaging schedule should be discussed with the therapist before implementation.

Bandages can be worn day and night if the patient does not have a properly fitted compression garment, or has more swelling than usual. Bandages should be removed at least once a day for skin care and then reapplied, unless directed otherwise by the patient's therapist.

Caregiver responsibilities may include:

- Applying bandages (or helping the patient apply bandages), checking and adjusting bandages, and giving the patient certain instructions based on the procedure outline below (starting on page 97) and the Care Activity forms.

- Removing bandages as specified in the Weekly Care Plan, see page 126.

- Washing, inspecting, and rolling bandages as described in "Bandage Care" on page 292.

- Managing bandages (see page 287) and related supplies (page 281).

Bandages come in multiple types and sizes and are used with several kinds of padding. Caregivers who are not familiar with the materials used for compression bandaging should read the description starting on page 294 before they start applying bandages.

You may also want to read about:

- Common bandaging problems and solutions, page 126 .

- Frequently asked questions, page 129.

- Bandaging infants and children (page 222).

> ### *The Cardinal Rules of Bandaging*
>
> - Pressure should be firmest at the hand or foot and softest near the body.
> - Less pressure is better than more pressure to minimize bandage complications.
> - A well-applied wrap should be comfortable and "feel good" on the swollen limb.

- Working with obese (page 235) or wheelchair-bound patients (page 236).

Untrained individuals should not apply compression bandages because incorrectly applied wraps can harm the patient.

The Steps of Bandaging

Every therapist develops his or her own bandaging style over time and each therapist in a clinic may bandage differently and yet be equally effective. The steps of bandaging described below are guidelines and are not meant to replace the instruction of a skilled therapist. Ideally, the caregiver will attend several treatment sessions to learn compression bandaging and other aspects of treatment.

The steps of bandaging include:

1. Organize supplies and prepare tape.

2. Inspect the skin before bandaging (if not done as part of skin care).

3. Apply bandages, as explained below for different affected areas. See "Specific Bandaging Procedures" on page 99.

4. Check the bandages for firmness and make adjustments, if necessary; see "Post-Wrap Check" on page 121.

5. Tell the patient what to watch out for, see "Post-Bandaging Instructions" on page 125.

6. Updating records, see "Update Records" on page 126.

Organize Supplies and Prepare Tape

The Care Activity Form that describes applying bandages should show:

- Supplies and equipment needed, such as bandage scissors, medical gloves, lotion, and masking or cloth tape.

- Bandaging materials required and the sequence in which they are applied. Bandaging materials may include tubular bandage or stockinette, finger or toe bandages, cotton and/or foam rolls, foam pads, bandages, and shoe(s).

- The number of tape pieces required and the type of tape. Masking tape can be used for most bandages; cloth tape is recommended for the trunk and lower extremities (see page 286).

To simplify the bandaging process, collect all the bandaging materials and arrange them in the order they will be used. See Figure 6-1.

To prepare tape, tear four-inch strips of tape, fold one end over for easy removal, and place the strips within easy reach. This is an easy task for the patient, helps incorporate them into the process, and saves time. If you are unsure how much tape you need, start with 10 pieces.

When securing a bandage, do not let tape touch the cotton or foam padding since tape may damage these materials. Also, tape should never stick directly to the patient's skin since the adhesive can irritate or tear fragile skin (if you do get tape on the skin see page 131).

Pre-Bandaging Skin Inspection

If skin care has not been done recently, inspect the skin before bandaging and deal with any changes such as scratches or skin irritation (see page 45).

When there are signs of infection or a sudden increase in swelling, defer compression bandaging and seek advice from the patient's health care provider immediately. A sudden in-

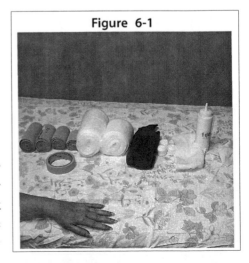

Figure 6-1

crease in swelling may indicate an infection or other serious problem such as a blood clot, tumor, or acute congestive heart failure. Once any serious medical condition has been ruled out or controlled, the patient's physician will advise when it is safe to resume using compression. When bandaging is resumed following an interruption, the therapist may need to modify the bandaging procedure, especially if the patient's swelling has increased.

Specific Bandaging Procedures

This section discusses specific procedures for bandaging different affected areas. You should bandage each affected area using the procedure provided here and the specific instructions in the Weekly Care Plan and Care Activity Forms. After bandaging each area do the checks described on page 120.

Bandaging procedures for these affected areas are discussed below:

- Arm Swelling, page 99.

- Trunk Swelling, page 108.

- Leg Swelling, page 109.

If the patient is an infant or child, see also page 222. If the patient uses a wheelchair or crutches, see also page 236.

Note: we do not cover bandaging for head and neck or genital lymphedema because these procedures are customized for each patient and incorrect application can cause serious complications. Bandaging for these conditions should be based on specific instructions from the patient's therapist.

Tips from the Clinic

- For ease of application, position the bandage so the end is under the roll and next to the patient's limb (the roll should be 'barrel up'). If the end of the bandage is at the top of the roll (barrel down), the bandage must be lifted away from the limb as it is applied, potentially increasing bandage tension.

- Alternate the direction of each bandage as it is applied. The change in the bandage fiber direction is thought to increase overall bandage strength.

- Fold the end of the tape under, as you finish applying it to the bandage. This tab makes it easier to remove the tape.

Arm Swelling

Bandages: The number of bandages and the amount of padding will vary depending on the severity of the patient's swelling and their body size. The caregiver should use the number of bandages suggested by the patient's lymphedema specialist. The instructions below use these bandages for one arm:

- Stockinette and padding.

- Finger bandages: three or four rolls of 2.5 or 5.0 cm wide gauze bandages. Figures show 2.5 cm Elastomull.

- Cotton or foam rolls: one each 10 cm and 15 cm wide.

- Short-stretch bandages: one each 6 cm, 8 cm, 10 cm, and 12 cm wide by 5 meters in length.

Estimated Time: 20-30 minutes.

Patient position: Sitting comfortably in a firm chair with the swollen arm resting on a table.

Caregiver position: Sitting on a firm chair in front of the patient.

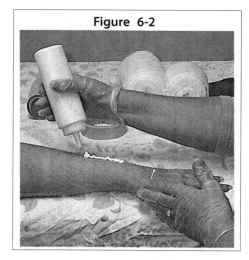

Figure 6-2

Apply Moisturizing Lotion

Before bandaging, gently massage a generous amount of lotion over the patient's arm to keep the skin from drying out while the arm is wrapped. Remember to stroke from the hand toward the shoulder. The caregiver may choose to wear medical gloves while applying lotion. See Figure 6-2. The lotion does not have to fully soak in before continuing with the bandaging.

Place Stockinette on Arm

Stockinette that is 1.5 to 2 times the length of the patient's arm is sufficient to cover the swollen area and provide three to four inches of stockinette to extend over the completed bandage. Reuse an existing piece that is clean or cut a new piece and cut a 1/2 inch (1 cm) hole for the thumb, approximately one inch (2.5 cm) from one end of the stockinette. Place the stockinette smoothly on the arm, allowing the thumb to come through the hole as shown in Figure 6-3.

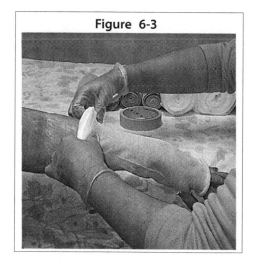

Figure 6-3

Apply Finger Bandages

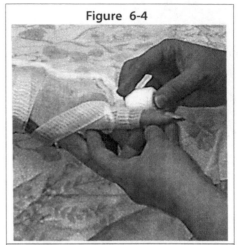

Figure 6-4

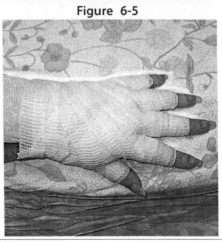

Figure 6-5

1. First, wrap the finger bandage very lightly (no pull) around the wrist, and secure the bandage by wrapping over the loose end.

2. Continue rolling out the finger bandage, bringing it across the knuckle of one finger, then wrap around the same finger starting at the web and moving in a spiral toward the nail bed. Overlap 50-75% of the bandage width with each circle of the wrap. The caregiver may use their index fingers as pulleys to weave the bandage between the patient's fingers as shown in Figure 6-4.

3. The tension of the bandage should be minimal (that is, very little pull on the bandage).

4. Once at the nail bed, change the direction of the spiral and bandage back toward the finger web.

5. A fully covered finger should be bandage colored without flesh showing through. If necessary, add a second layer of bandages to obtain good finger coverage.

6. After completing the first finger, cross over the knuckle and around the wrist before wrapping the next finger.

7. Repeat steps 2-6 above until all fingers have been wrapped, see Figure 6-5. If the bandage roll runs out, start a new bandage by wrapping one end of the new bandage around the wrist first, then cover the end of the old bandage to secure it in place (tape is not usually needed). Continue wrapping each finger as described above until all fingers are fully wrapped.

If the knuckles do not seem adequately covered, wrap another layer of bandage around the base of each finger. Remember to wrap around the wrist before transitioning between the fingers, otherwise the patient will have "webbed" fingers.

Ask the patient to open and close the fingers (making a fist) several times to loosen the finger bandages slightly before continuing to bandage. This will give the patient an opportunity to determine if the finger bandages are too tight. As the patient is flexing their hand check that:

- Fingertip color is normal. Bluish fingertips are a sign that bandages are too tight.

- All areas are sufficiently covered. If flesh shows through the finger wraps, add another layer or two of finger bandages as necessary.

If finger bandages are difficult to apply, ask the patient's therapist about replacing them with a therapeutic glove (Isotoner is one example, see www.totes-isotoner.com) or a light compression glove. Continue with bandaging as described below.

Apply Cotton or Foam and Padding

See Figure 6-6. Loosely wrap the cotton or foam roll in a spiral pattern around the patient's arm beginning at the knuckles and continuing up to the armpit. Avoid covering the thumb so it can be moved and used.

Cover the limb with at least two layers by overlapping the layers by 50% with each circle around the limb. Use as many rolls of cotton or foam as needed. Cotton is not very flexible so open gaps are expected. Do not pull on the cotton or it will become very long and narrow, making it harder to use.

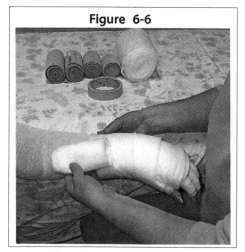

Figure 6-6

If needed, place extra cotton or foam padding over bony or sensitive skin areas as the cotton is applied. Padding will protect the skin and minimize irritation. Bony areas of the arm include the knuckles, the wrist bone, and back of the elbow; sensitive skin areas include the palm side of the wrist and the elbow.

If you notice a swelling bulge at the base of the thumb after removing hand bandages, there probably was not enough compression on this area. Cover the area with low density foam padding (over or under the cotton) to help keep the bandages in place, provide more pressure, and minimize any swelling bulge.

Bandage the Hand

1. Hold the narrowest short-stretch bandage (usually a 6 cm bandage) close to the wrist and begin rolling the bandage around the wrist moving in a spiral toward the base of the thumb. Overlap the bandage by 50% with each spiral.

2. Once the base of the thumb is covered, the next spiral of the wrap will pass by the thumb to cover the thumb web space. Do not cover the thumb. Fold the edge of the bandage next to the patient's thumb; this will narrow the bandage to help prevent it from covering any part of the fingers. See Figure 6-7.

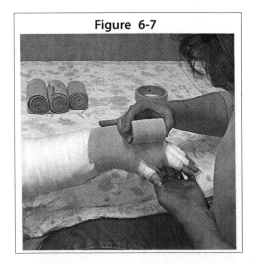

Figure 6-7

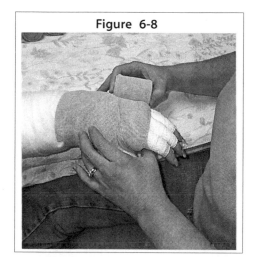

Figure 6-8

3. Have the patient spread their fingers apart and continue rolling out the bandage across the back of the hand, covering all of the knuckles. Avoid angling the bandage at the knuckles because areas that are uncovered or not adequately covered may have increased swelling. See Figure 6-8.

4. Next, spiral around the palm of the hand and back toward the thumb base.

5. Alternate spiral wraps between the thumb base and the thumb web space three to four times according to how much hand swelling there is (less swelling needs fewer layers of bandage, more swelling requires more layers).

6. After the fourth wrap over the knuckles, spiral toward the thumb base and continue to the wrist until the bandage has been completely rolled out.

Check the number of layers at the knuckles, there should be four. See Figure 6-9.

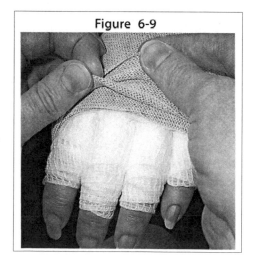

Figure 6-9

Bandage to the Forearm

1. With the second bandage (usually 8 cm wide), start at the wrist and wrap down to the knuckles adding one more layer (for a total of 5 layers at the knuckles). See steps 1-3 above for detail. The final fold at the web space may be made by pinching the middle part of the bandage as shown in Figure 6-10.

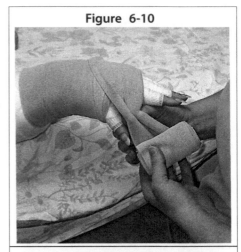
Figure 6-10

2. Reverse directions (see step 4 above for detail) and continue with a spiral wrap past the wrist and up the forearm toward the elbow. Stop below the elbow bend unless there is enough bandage remaining to wrap past the elbow. In Figure 6-11 the caregiver's thumb is at the elbow bend.

3. Once the bandage is completely unrolled, secure the end with tape.

Figure 6-11

Bandage the Forearm to the Upper Arm

Have the patient bend their arm approximately 90 degrees (a right angle) while bandages are applied to the elbow; this helps make the wrapped arm flexible enough for daily activities. Beginning at the lower forearm, take the third bandage (usually 10 cm wide) and spiral wrap from the lower forearm over the bent elbow to the upper arm. See Figure 6-12.

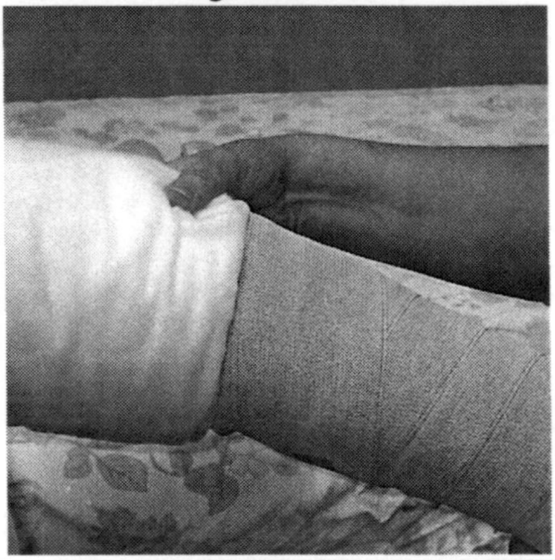

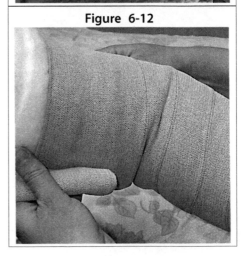
Figure 6-12

Figure 6-13

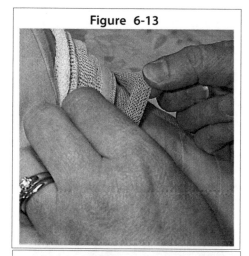

Bandage the Elbow to the Upper Arm

With the last bandage (usually 12 cm), wrap from the lower elbow to the armpit.

Wrap in a small upwards angle at the outer shoulder, alternating between the upper outer arm and mid arm using a figure eight pattern until the upper arm has three layers covering it. Count the number of layers as shown in Figure 6-13.

Fold any remaining bandage in front of the arm (try not to end the bandage in a spot that the patient cannot easily reach to remove the wrap if necessary) and secure the final bandage in place with several pieces of tape. See Figure 6-14 and Figure 6-15.

Fold over any remaining stockinette.

Figure 6-14

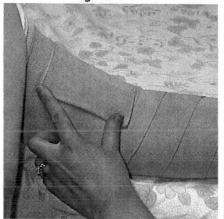

Figure 6-15

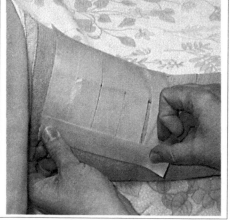

Trunk Swelling

Bandages:

- Stockinette or a T-shirt and foam padding may be used, see below.

- Medium-stretch bandages: 2-4 rolls of 12 cm Lenkelast are used in the instructions below. Wider (15-20 cm) Lenkelast may be needed for large affected areas.

Note: Bandages listed above are 5 meters in length. Bandages in 12 cm width come in two lengths; one 10 meter bandage can replace two 5 meter bandages.

Estimated Time: 5-10 minutes.

Patient position: Standing.

Caregiver position: Standing.

Apply Moisturizing Lotion

Before bandaging, the patient or caregiver should gently massage a generous amount of lotion over the area to keep the patient's skin from drying out while the trunk is wrapped. The caregiver may choose to use medical gloves to apply the lotion.

Place Underwear or Stockinette

Have the patient cover the affected area with a soft bra (for upper body swelling), a cotton T-shirt, or a length of stockinette. Stockinette is a stretchy tube; the patient may pull the stockinette over their head or step into it. Stockinette should be loose and may not fit large patients.

Other underwear may be put on before or after bandaging according to the patient's preference.

Apply Foam Padding

Apply padding to the swollen areas of the trunk according to the therapist's instructions. Depending on the patient's needs, the therapist may make a custom pad or use a manufactured pad. Manufactured pads that are specialized for the trunk include JoViPak breast, chest wall, or genital pads, Peninsula Medical OptiFlow packs, and Solaris Swell Spots.

Bandage the Trunk

Taking a bandage roll, begin at the lower part of the trunk area and bandage in a spiral toward the upper part of the trunk, covering the swollen area.

For upper trunk and chest edema, begin at the waist and finish at the upper trunk near the armpits, wrapping over the breast or chest wall.

For lower trunk edema, begin at the hips or lower abdomen and wrap to the waist.

Repeat this process with the remaining bandages. Secure the bandages in place with tape.

Leg Swelling

Some patients with leg swelling are bandaged from the toes to the thigh and some are only bandaged up to the knee. For a patient who is only bandaged to the knee, use only the materials for the foot and up to the knee and skip from "Bandaging the Lower Leg to the Knee" to "Put on a Shoe" as explained below.

Bandages: The quantity of bandages and padding vary depending on the severity of the patient's swelling and their body size. The caregiver should use the number of bandages suggested by the patient's lymphedema therapist.

These instructions use the following bandages for one leg:

- Stockinette and padding.

- Toe bandages: one or two rolls of 2.5 cm (1 inch) wide gauze bandage. A 5 cm wide bandage can replace two rolls of 2.5 cm wide gauze if the bandage is folded in half lengthwise and re-rolled.

- Cotton or Foam Rolls:

  - Up to the knee: one roll of 10 cm and one roll of 15 cm.

  - From the knee to the thigh: two more rolls of 15 cm.

- Short-stretch bandages:

  - Up to the knee: one each 6, 8, and 10 cm, and two 12 cm bandages. For men with large feet, use two 8 cm bandages instead of one each 6 and 8 cm; for a long leg use two each 8, 10, and 12 cm bandages.

- – From the knee to the thigh: two 10 cm and two 12 cm bandages.

• A post-operative shoe or oversized tennis shoe.

Note: Bandages listed above are 5 meters in length. Bandages in 10 and 12 cm width come in two lengths; one 10 meter bandage can replace two 5 meter bandages.

<u>Estimated Time:</u> 30-60 minutes.

<u>Patient position:</u> Sitting comfortably in a hardback chair. Alternative position: lying down close to the edge of the bed. Use a blanket roll or wedge under the patient's knee and mid-calf to elevate the foot for bandaging.

<u>Caregiver position:</u> Sitting on a low stool in front of the seated patient or standing at the foot of the bed.

Apply Moisturizing Lotion

Gently massage a generous amount of lotion over the area to be bandaged. Remember to stroke from the foot toward the heart. The caregiver may choose to wear medical gloves while applying lotion as shown in Figure 6-2 on page 101. The lotion does not have to fully soak in before continuing with the bandaging.

Place Stockinette on Leg

A piece of stockinette that is 1.5 to 2 times the length of the patient's leg (or the area to be bandaged) is sufficient to cover the swollen area and to provide 3-4 inches (8-10 cm) of stockinette to extend beyond the bandage. Reuse an existing piece that is clean or cut a new piece of stockinette. Place the tubular stockinette smoothly over the patient's foot and leg as shown in Figure 6-16.

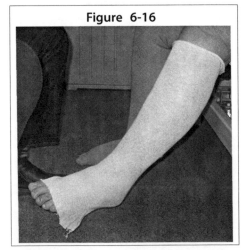

Figure 6-16

Figure 6-17

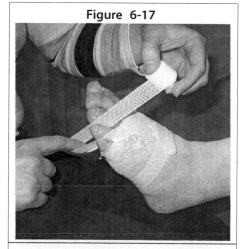

Figure 6-18

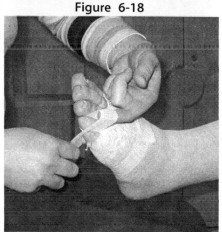

Apply Toe Bandages

1. Wrap the toe bandage very lightly (no pull) around the arch of the foot; secure the end by covering it with the bandage.

2. Continue rolling out the bandage bringing it across one toe, then wrapping around the same toe starting at the web and moving in a spiral toward the nail bed. The caregiver may use their index fingers like pulleys to weave the bandage between the patient's toes. See Figure 6-17 and Figure 6-18.

3. The tension of the bandage should be minimal, with very little pull on the bandage. Be very careful with bandage tension under and between the toes to avoid irritating tender skin.

4. When you reach the nail bed, change the direction of the spiral and continue bandaging back toward the web space. End the bandage at the top of the foot.

5. A fully covered toe should be the color of the bandage without any flesh showing through. Add a second layer of bandages if required to completely cover the toe or if there is severe swelling.

6. After completing the first toe, cross over the previous bandage at the top of the foot and wrap around the foot arch before continuing with the next toe. Note: all toes should be wrapped in the same direction.

7. Repeat steps 2-5 above until the first four toes have been wrapped (the little toe is optional). See Figure 6-19 on page 112.

If the top of the foot near the web spaces does not seem adequately covered, wrap another layer of bandage around the base of each toe. Remember to wrap around the foot arch before transitioning between the toes, otherwise the patient will have "webbed" feet.

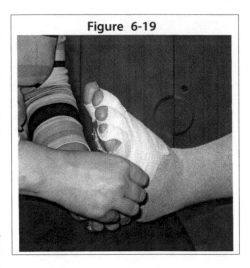

Figure 6-19

Apply Cotton or Foam and Padding

See Figure 6-20 and Figure 6-21. Loosely wrap the cotton or foam roll in a spiral pattern evenly around the patient's limb beginning at the ball of the foot and continuing up to the knee or upper thigh. Cover the limb with at least two layers by overlapping the cotton by 50% with each circle around the limb. Use as many rolls of cotton or foam as needed. Cotton is not very flexible and may gap away from the body. These gaps may be folded over to lie smoothly against the skin as the bandages are applied. Do not pull the cotton or it will become very long and narrow, which will make it harder to use.

Place any extra padding for bony or sensitive skin areas under or between the layers of cotton as you apply it. Padding will protect the skin and minimize irritation. Bony areas of the leg are the sides of the toes near the forefoot,

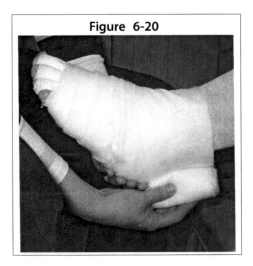

Figure 6-20

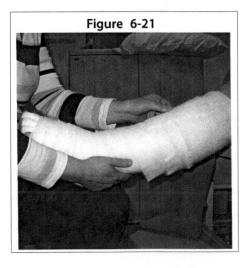

Figure 6-21

Figure 6-22

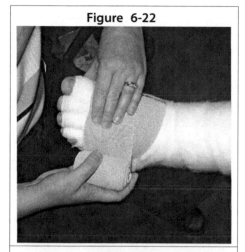

Figure 6-23

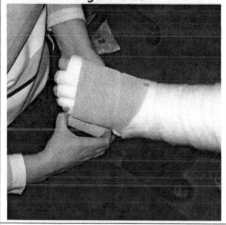

Figure 6-24

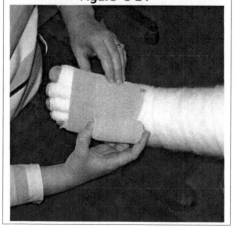

sides of the ankle, and the kneecap; sensitive skin areas are at the front of the ankle, behind the knee, and at deep skin folds.

Bandage the Foot

1. Hold the smallest short-stretch bandage (usually a 6 or 8 cm bandage) close to the arch of the foot and begin rolling the bandage around the arch moving in a spiral toward the ball of the foot. Cover 50% of the bandage with each spiral. See Figure 6-22.

2. As you bandage across the top of the foot near the toes, the bandage should be straight from the first to the fifth toe; do not angle the bandage near the toes since this may leave an area with inadequate bandage layers that could swell.

3. Next, spiral around the ball of the foot and back toward the arch.

4. Alternate spiral wraps between the ball and the arch of the foot 3-4 times depending on the amount of forefoot swelling (less swelling requires fewer layers of bandage, more swelling requires more layers). See Figure 6-23 and Figure 6-24.

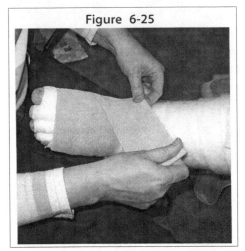
Figure 6-25

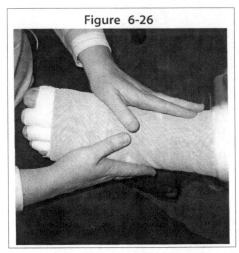
Figure 6-26

5. After the fourth wrap at the ball of the foot, spiral toward the arch and continue to the ankle until the bandage has been completely rolled out. This first bandage may transition from the arch of the foot to the ankle without covering the heel. See Figure 6-25 and Figure 6-26.

6. Count the number of layers at the forefoot; there should be 4. See Figure 6-27.

7. Tape can be placed starting at the fifth toe and extending along the side of the foot to secure the bandage in place. See Figure 6-28.

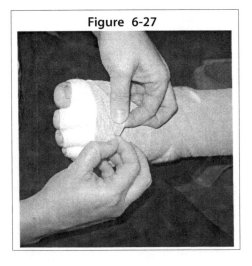
Figure 6-27

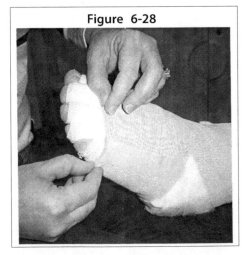
Figure 6-28

Figure 6-29

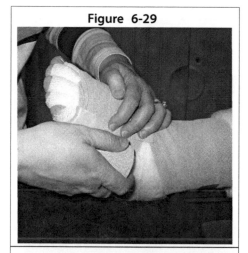

Figure 6-30

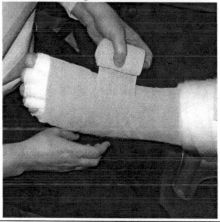

Figure 6-31

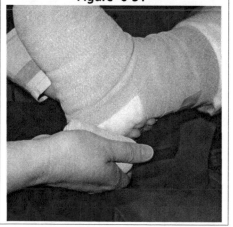

Bandage the Heel and Ankle

1. With the next smallest bandage (usually 8 cm), start at the arch of the foot and spiral wrap one time around the forefoot the same way the first bandage was applied. See Figure 6-29.

2. Spiral toward the heel of the foot and cover the bottom of the heel. See Figure 6-30.

Note: Have the patient bend their ankle and point their toes toward their nose while the foot and ankle are being wrapped, this helps prevent too much pressure at the front of the ankle.

3. Continue spiraling to cover the point of the heel. See Figure 6-31. At the front of the ankle, the bandage layers will be close together (~75% overlap) and at the heel the layers will be wider apart (~40-50% overlap), like the spokes on a wheel. Keep the pressure very light at the front of the ankle by not pulling on the bandage, since this area will have more pressure.

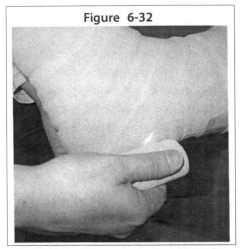

Figure 6-32

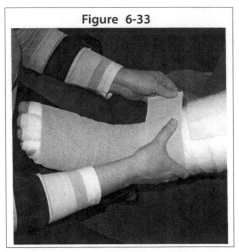

Figure 6-33

4. Wrap in a spiral, covering the back of the heel and ankle. See Figure 6-32.

5. Finish the bandage spiraling up the leg, covering 50% of the last spiral of the wrap. See Figure 6-33.

6. With the next bandage (either another 8 cm or a 10 cm), start wrapping at the ankle and spiral down toward the heel. See Figure 6-34.

7. Cover the heel in the reverse order: cover the back of the heel, then the point of the heel, followed by the bottom of the heel. See Figure 6-35 on this page and Figure 6-36 on page 117.

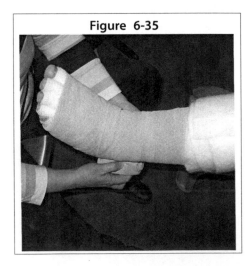

Figure 6-34

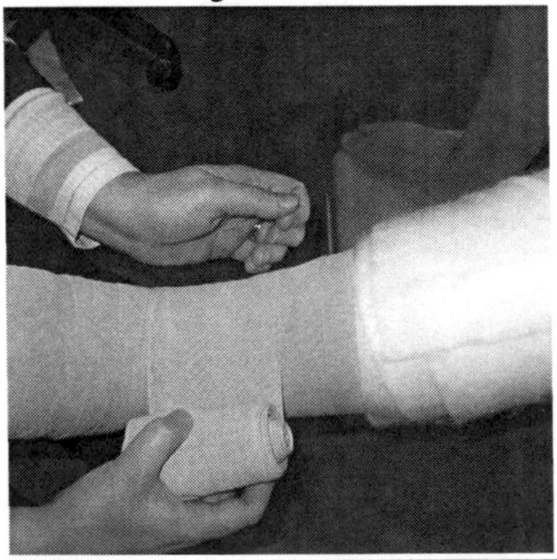

Figure 6-35

Figure 6-36	**Figure 6-37**
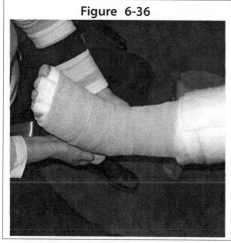	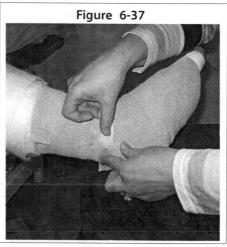

8. Finally, change directions and spiral to the point of the heel, followed by the back of the heel and proceed up the leg until the bandage has been fully applied. Secure with tape. See Figure 6-37.

Change Patient Position

If the patient is sitting, have them remain sitting until the lower leg is completely wrapped. If the patient is lying down, reposition the blanket roll or wedge under the foot to elevate the leg, or remove the roll or wedge and

Wrapping a Figure-Eight Pattern

Figure 6-38

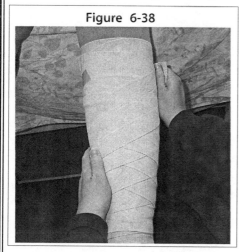

A figure-eight or herringbone pattern can be used at the knee or elsewhere to make bandaging more comfortable for the patient.

A figure-eight pattern is created by angling the bandage up and around the leg, and then angling the bandage down and around the leg, weaving the bandaging instead spiraling it.

Figure 6-39

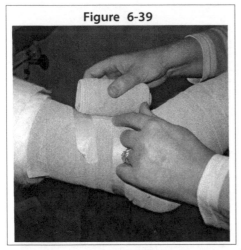

Figure 6-40

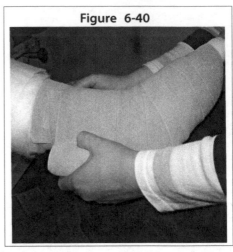

have the patient bend their knee and place their foot on the bed, so the rest of the leg may be wrapped.

Bandage the Ankle to the Knee

1. With the next bandage (10 or 12 cm), begin at the ankle and cover the end of the previous bandage. See Figure 6-39 and Figure 6-40.

2. Wrap in a simple spiral covering 50% of the previous spiral until the bandage is completely rolled out close to the upper calf. The bandages should stay below the knee bend. See Figure 6-41 and Figure 6-42.

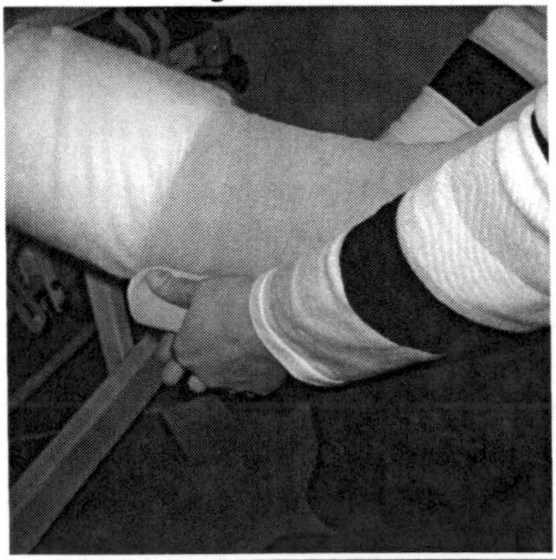

Figure 6-41

Figure 6-42

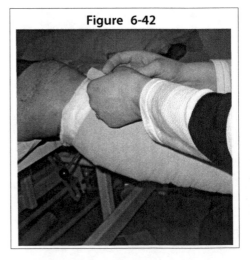

Figure 6-43	Figure 6-44
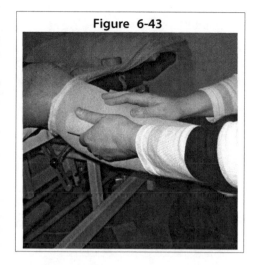	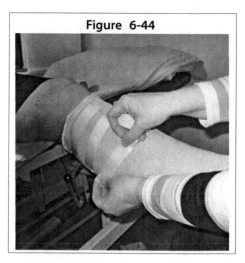

Bandage the Lower Leg to the Knee

1. Squeeze the bandage to determine where the bandage transitions from firm to relatively soft (usually around the upper ankle or mid-calf) and begin the next 12 cm bandage at this spot. See Figure 6-43.

2. Spiral wrap the bandage up to the knee, making sure the bandage stays below the bent knee. If necessary, wrap loosely below the knee in a figure-eight pattern (see "Wrapping a Figure-Eight Pattern") until the bandage is completely rolled out.

If only the lower leg is being bandaged, secure the final bandage with several pieces of tape. Fold any remaining stockinette down over the top of the bandage as shown in Figure 6-44 and continue with "Put on a Shoe" on page 120.

Change Position

If the patient is sitting, have them stand with the knee bent to complete the bandaging. If the patient is lying down, they should remain in the same position with the knee bent and their foot on the bed.

Bandage the Knee

With the next bandage (usually 10 or 12 cm), start the spiral at the lower part of the knee and wrap up to the upper knee, covering 50% of the last spiral with each circle around the leg.

Repeat with the next two bandages.

Optional: bandages may be more comfortable if a figure-eight pattern is used at the knee, see "Wrapping a Figure-Eight Pattern" on page 117.

Note: it is important to have the patient's knee bent approximately 90 degrees during bandage application so the patient may bend the knee and sit down without difficulty after the leg is wrapped.

Bandage the Thigh to the Groin

Wrap the final one or two bandages (usually 10 or 12 cm) in a spiral from the lower thigh to the upper thigh near the groin.

If there is extra bandage after the thigh is wrapped, roll out the remaining bandage lightly in a figure-eight pattern, alternating between the mid and upper thigh so the bandage does not become too firm.

Secure the final bandage with extra tape.

Fold the stockinette over the final wrap.

Put on a Shoe

Have the patient put on a post-operative shoe with Velcro straps or an oversized tennis shoe (about 2 sizes larger and wider than normal shoe size) when the bandages are worn outside of the house to prevent bandages from becoming soiled or damaged. Post-op shoes, such as Darco "Softie," may be found at most drugstores and medical supply companies, or online at www.Darcointernational.com.

After Bandaging

After bandaging: do a post-wrap check and adjust bandage tension (if necessary), give the patient post-bandaging instructions, and update care records as explained below.

Post-Wrap Check

Since it is easy to apply too much pressure, the caregiver should always check the wrapped limb by squeezing the completed wrap in several places to assess the general firmness (from soft or light to very firm) and to make sure there is a gradual decrease in pressure from the hand/foot to the upper arm/leg. See "Adjusting Bandage Tension" on page 122 for details.

Other ways to monitor pressure include:

- **Asking the patient directly how the bandages feel immediately after completing the bandage application and again 30-60 minutes later.** Direct feedback from the patient is often the best way of monitoring the bandage pressure.

- Checking the color of the patient's finger or toe tips and nail beds.

  - A flesh-tone color indicates good circulation.

  - Darker skin discoloration indicates that venous circulation has slowed down. Have the patient move their arm or leg for several minutes and see if the color of the finger/toe tips improves. Usually the discoloration disappears after a few minutes. If the color persists after 10-15 minutes, or the arm or leg becomes painful, remove one or more bandages and reapply them with less pressure.

  - Lighter skin color indicates arterial circulation has been cut off. **If you suspect that arterial circulation has been impaired, remove the bandages immediately** since this can have very severe adverse effects. Bandages should be reapplied at a lighter pressure.

- **Checking capillary refill.** Press the patient's finger or toe tips and note if the color changes to a lighter (white) color with pressure, then back to normal color within one or two seconds after the pressure is removed. On a dark-skinned person, press the nail bed. Pressure will naturally stop circulation in the blood capillaries briefly, changing the patient's skin color; when the pressure is removed, capillaries refill with blood and the color returns to normal. Quick capillary refill indicates that the fingers or toes have normal arterial blood circulation. If the return to normal color is delayed by more than a few seconds, it indicates that arterial capillary flow has been delayed. When this happens, the bandages should be removed and reapplied with less tension.

Adjusting Bandage Tension

The degree of bandage tension needed to maintain or decrease limb swelling will vary from patient to patient, depending upon the severity of the swelling, the patient's ability to tolerate bandages, and the general health of the patient's skin. The tension will range from very light to very firm. Usually mild swelling requires only light pressure and severe swelling requires firm to very firm pressure. Normal healthy skin will be able to tolerate more pressure than the thin, fragile skin of elderly patients.

Bandage pressure must be estimated by both patient and caregiver, since the tension cannot be accurately measured. After the patient has been bandaged, the caregiver should squeeze the wrapped area in several places to check for firmness, as shown in Figure 6-45, Figure 6-46, Figure 6-47, and Figure 6-48.

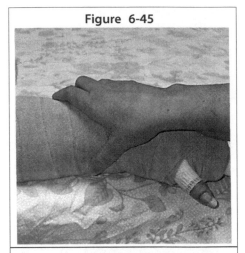

Figure 6-45

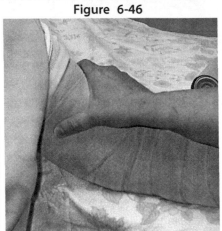

Figure 6-46

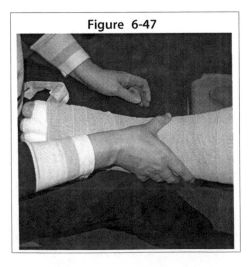

Figure 6-47

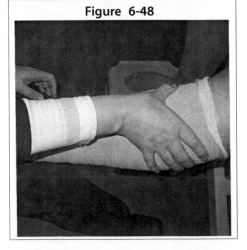

Figure 6-48

The firmness of the bandages should be graduated with lighter pressure closer to the trunk. This means that bandage pressure or firmness should be higher at the hand or wrist than at the armpit and higher at the foot and ankle than at the groin. If too firm, not firm enough, or unevenly firm, the caregiver should remove one or more of the bandages and readjust the pressure.

Bandages that are applied too tightly can impair circulation by:

- **Creating a tourniquet.** When bandages are too tight in one area they act as a light tourniquet that stops lymph flow, and possibly blood flow. If lymph flow is blocked, the patient will have puffiness or bulging in the area below the tight bandage. If blood circulation is restricted, the patient may not tolerate the wrap and will usually ask to have some or all of the bandages removed.

- **Damaging lymph and blood vessels.** Applying bandages too firmly can break delicate lymph and blood capillaries in the wrapped area. This may result in increased swelling due to leakage from the broken capillaries and ineffective absorption and transportation of tissue fluid. Furthermore, as broken capillaries are repaired, scar tissue develops around the lymph and blood vessels, reducing the vessels' ability to function properly.[1]

There are several ways to adjust the bandage tension to assure the patient's comfort while the wrap remains effective. The techniques described below may be combined, as needed.

If possible, have the therapist demonstrate these tension adjusting techniques. The caregiver (and the patient if they will be self bandaging) are encouraged to practice these techniques and get feedback from the therapist.

Add or Remove a Bandage

Adding more layers is the best way to apply extra pressure while keeping the bandages comfortable for the patient and minimizing skin irritation. By removing a bandage, the bandage pressure will decrease making a "lighter" or less firm wrap.

Increase or Decrease the Overlap

Covering approximately 50% of the bandage as it is rolled out (see Figure 6-49 will give a light to moderately firm wrap. Covering less than 50% will decrease the amount of pressure (see Figure 6-50). Overlapping the bandage by more than 50% will increase the amount of pressure (see Figure 6-51).

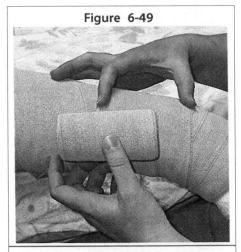

Figure 6-49

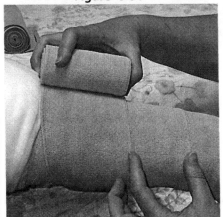

Figure 6-50

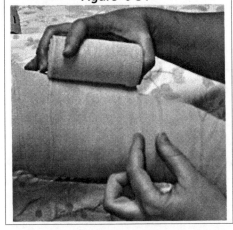

Figure 6-51

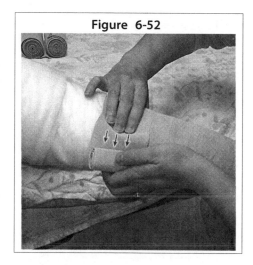

Figure 6-52

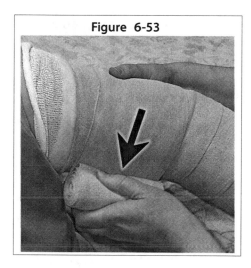

Figure 6-53

Stretch or Don't Stretch the Bandage

Stretching a bandage increases the bandage tension; applying the bandage more loosely will decrease the bandage tension. Stretching the bandage is done in one of two ways:

- **Iron the bandage.** When applying a bandage over padding, the best way to stretch the bandage is to "iron" or smooth it toward the bandage roll with your hand as shown in Figure 6-52.

- **Short firm pulls of the bandage.** When wrapping one bandage over another, stretch the outer bandage by a series of short firm pulls on the bandage roll at the sides of the limb. See Figure 6-53. Be careful not to pull a bandage too tightly over sensitive areas such as the front of the ankle or elbow and the back of the knee. Sometimes, the inside of the armpit or the back of the thigh can also be sensitive to excessive pressure.

Post-Bandaging Instructions

Remind the patient that newly applied bandages should never cause numbness, tingling, burning, or any other unusual sensation; nor should the patient feel as if the bandages are "cutting off" their circulation. If the patient complains of an unusual discomfort, have the patient move their arm or leg to loosen up the bandages. If the discomfort persists for more than 10-15 minutes (less if the discomfort is great), remove one or more bandages until the problem resolves. The bandages should then be reapplied at a lighter pressure. See "Adjusting Bandage Tension" on page 122. With experience, the caregiver should be able to apply the bandages more quickly and effectively with little or no problems for the patient.

Update Records

Update records after bandaging as follows:

- Mark the Weekly Care Plan Form to show that bandaging was completed. Add notes about any condition changes or other issues.

- Update the Item Needed Form if any supplies were used up or bandages need to be replaced. See page 287 for more information.

Removing Bandages

Bandages can be removed by peeling off and discarding the tape used to hold the bandages and then unwrapping each bandage. Also remove any padding or stockinette. Do not cut bandages off, even if you know that they are not going to be reused.

Bandages that are going to be washed do not have to be rolled before washing.

Common Bandaging Problems

Even a highly skilled therapist will make adjustments in their bandaging techniques when he or she first begins working with a new patient. The therapist will inspect the skin after removing the bandages and look for any signs of a problem. Minor problems are not unusual. Recognition and proper response to any problems is the most important key to continued success with compression bandages. Common bandage problems and possible solutions are listed below.

Slipping Bandages

A frequent problem for patients is slippage of the bandages after application. Even well-applied wraps normally slip down an inch or two as the patient moves around. The more active a person is, the more the bandages may slip. If the bandages slide down more than two inches over the course of the night (or day), consider the following options:

- Check to make sure that there are at least three layers of bandages at the upper part of the wrap to prevent the bandages from becoming too loose and sliding down. Add one or more layers if necessary. When applying extra layers, make sure the pressure is not too tight and consider adding more padding to avoid skin irritation.

- Apply a cut-off section of extra large (Queen-size) nylon stocking over the person's arm or leg wraps. See Figure 6-54. This helps to hold the bandages in place and the slickness of the nylon will allow clothing to slide smoothly over the bandages, avoiding unnecessary pulling on the bandages as clothing is removed and replaced.

- Consider using Spandage, which is open-webbed tubular retainer netting that can be cut into strips the length of the arm or leg and placed over the top of the bandage. Spandage was specifically designed to hold bandages in place and can be re-used multiple times before requiring replacement. Spandage is available in various widths and may be found on-line or at local medical supply shops. See www.spandage.com for more details.

Bulging Areas

The skin is usually wrinkled after bandages are removed. If the patient or caregiver notices an area where the skin is bulging out (more swelling), this suggests the bandages may have been applied unevenly. The next time the bandages are applied, the caregiver should make sure the pressure is more evenly applied and gradually decreases from the far end of the limb to the part closest to the body.

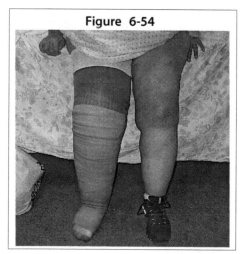

Figure 6-54

Occasionally, bulges are due to slippage of the bandages as they are worn. If this is a problem, see "Slipping Bandages" on page 126 for possible solutions. The bulge may also occur above the level of the wrap at the upper arm, knee, or upper thigh. If this occurs, try bandaging a little higher on the patient's limb to respond to this swelling area.

Skin Irritation

Bandages may cause several types of skin irritation including streaks of redness, tiny red dots, or a rash that are observed when bandages are removed. Bandages that are too tight or do not have sufficient padding are more likely to cause irritation. Signs of common irritation and ways to avoid them are described on page 52 . First aid for treating rashes is described on page 260.

Patient Reactions

Patient's reactions to bandages vary. Some find that they are comfortable or give relief from lymphedema related pain. Other patients find bandages difficult to wear and may comment that bandages are hot, itchy, tight, heavy, or cumbersome. Bandages also restrict the patient's ability to do daily activities including writing, typing, eating, washing their hair, going to the bathroom, walking, wearing shoes, doing chores, and driving. In general, it is not easy to wear bandages.

The caregiver may need to gently remind the patient of the reasons for wearing bandages including controlling the patient's swelling, decreasing swelling-related skin tightness and discomfort, and reducing the risk of skin infections and sores.

Frequently Asked Questions

Can the patient wear compression at night only?

Some patients can but, unfortunately many patients need compression day and night. Swelling is caused by the body's inability to remove excess tissue fluid. Fluid builds up more quickly during the day when the patient is active, than at night when the patient is resting. Compression during the day helps minimize fluid build up and enhance fluid removal.

Is it OK to only wrap part of an arm or leg?

Continue to wrap according to the therapist's instructions and check with the patient's therapist about any swelling changes in an unwrapped area. Some patients will only have part of a limb wrapped for specific reasons.

When only part of a limb is wrapped, swelling can occur in the unwrapped area. For example, if the arm is wrapped but not the hand, the hand usually swells due to constriction of lymph flow out of the hand. In patients with full leg edema, bandaging only the foot and lower leg may result in more swelling at the knee or thigh.

What if the patient has trouble keeping bandages on?

Some patients have trouble keeping bandages on because of discomfort or limb pain and complain that the bandages are "too tight." The most common cause is bandage pressure that is greater than the patient's swelling. Start by reviewing the instructions for adjusting bandage tension, see "Adjusting Bandage Tension" on page 122.

If the bandage tension is reduced and the patient still reports that the bandages are too tight, examine the overall application of the bandages. A common mistake is to extend the bandage roll away from the arm or leg and pull the bandage around the area being wrapped. Pulling overstretches the bandage and the bandage becomes very restrictive and tourniquet-like.

Keep the bandage roll close to the body to prevent overstretching as shown in Figure 6-55 and Figure 6-56.

If the bandage tension remains too tight, try using fewer bandages. Finally, consider scheduling a follow-up appointment with the patient's therapist to review the bandaging process and solve any persistent problems.

On rare occasion, the inability to tolerate compression (bandages, garment, or aid) is a sign of active cancer. If this is suspected, contact the patient's physician as soon as possible for an appointment.

How does the patient bathe with bandages?

If the bandages are only used overnight, the patient may bathe or shower after removing the bandages in the morning or in the evening before bandages are applied. If the bandages are on for longer than a day, the patient may take a sponge bath or use a garbage bag over the bandaged arm or leg while showering. Some patients put plastic wrap (Saran Wrap) around the upper part of the garbage bag to seal out water. The patient must be very careful not to slip while showering with a garbage bag on their foot. For safety, it may be best to take a sponge bath or remove the bandages prior to showering.

Figure 6-55

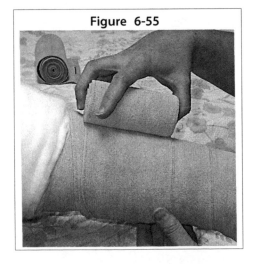

Figure 6-56

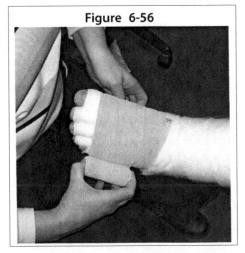

How can I tell a rash from an allergic reaction or infection?

A rash, an allergic reaction, and a skin infection look similar and are often difficult to distinguish. Redness and skin irritation caused by an allergic reaction to lotion or bandaging material will initially appear only in areas that were in contact with the allergen. See also page 49 for signs of infection. If you are unsure of the cause of the patient's skin redness, seek medical attention.

How can I monitor if someone else does bandaging?

If bandages have been applied by the patient or another caregiver, you can do a post-wrap check (see page 121) to see if the bandages were applied correctly and with even, graduated pressure. It may also be beneficial to inspect the patient's skin just after bandages are removed (see page 47). This may require scheduling a visit with the patient at the time when bandages are being changed.

How can I remove tape without damaging the skin?

Tape used to secure bandages should never touch the patient's skin because the skin of the affected area can be very fragile. If you do get tape on the skin, remove it carefully by pressing the patient's skin away from the tape as the tape is gently lifted. If necessary, use olive oil or medical adhesive remover (available from medical supply stores) to make the tape easier to remove. Thoroughly cleanse the skin after using adhesive remover.

Notes

1   "Pediatric Lymphology: Diagnosis and Treatment" by Ethel Földi and Güenter Klose. *Lymph Link*, Vol. 18, No 2, April-June 2006 pages 1-3.

Chapter 7

Compression Garments and Aids

Compression to help control swelling is an essential part of lymphedema treatment (see page 30). Three different forms of compression are used:

- Bandaging or wrapping with short stretch bandages, see page 95.

- Compression Garments made of stretchy fabrics are typically worn during the day and include sleeves, gloves, vests, knee-high, thigh-high, and waist-high stockings, etc. For more information see page 308.

- Compression Aids constructed of foam, fabric, and elastic can be used at night or during the day and may include features designed to soften fibrotic tissues. For more information see page 313.

Compression is prescribed by the patient's physician. The patient's therapist recommends the appropriate forms of compression and wearing schedule for each patient taking into account the severity of the swelling, the patient's medical condition and allergies, physical abilities, body shape, and other factors. A patient may use a different form or amount of compression during the day, while exercising, and at night. Compression garments and aids are sometimes used in combinations.

Compression garments and aids are available over-the-counter (OTC) in standard sizes or they can be custom made to fit a specific patient. The therapist may measure the patient for compression garments or aids or refer the patient to a certified fitter. A fitter is a person with special training in measuring and fitting compression garments or aids. Fitters are certified by manufacturers for their products. See page 307 for more information.

Garments and aids wear out and must be replaced periodically. They may also be replaced if the patient's condition changes and the garment or aid no longer fits properly or provides the appropriate amount of pressure. See "Managing Compression Garments and Aids (page 299) for more information.

Compression garments are typically worn from the early morning to the end of the evening. Compression levels may be changed during exercise, travel (see page 255), or other activities (see page 254). Patients with moderate to severe lymphedema may wear compression at night to prevent or reduce swelling; typically this will be bandages, a compression aid, or a lower-pressure compression garment.

The Weekly Care Plan (see page 333) worked out with the patient's therapist should reflect the wearing schedule and include activities for putting on or removing compression garments or aids. Occasional schedule variations are not problematic but check with the patient's therapist before making any major changes in the use of compression since time without compression can lead to increased swelling.

The Weekly Care Plan and Care Activity Forms should define the caregiver's responsibilities and provide specific instructions. Caregiver responsibilities may include:

- Helping the patient put on (called 'donning') and take off (called 'doffing') compression garments (see page 134) or compression aids (see page 140) based on the schedule established with the patient's therapist and the instructions provided on the Care Activity Form or in this chapter.

- Washing and inspecting garments (see page 305) or aids (see page 307).

- Managing compression garments or aids (see page 299 and purchasing associated clothing.

See also frequently asked questions on page 140.

Putting on a Compression Garment

This section includes guidelines for helping a patient put on:

- Arm sleeve and glove for arm lymphedema, see below.

- Compression top for breast or trunk lymphedema, see page 136.

- Toe caps and leg stockings for leg lymphedema, see page 136.

In addition to these guidelines, you should also check any instructions that came with the garment. Many vendors provide instructional videos on their web sites. Record the best procedure for each patient on the Care Activity Form, including any helpful tricks or things to avoid.

Compression garments for head-and-neck lymphedema or genital lymph-edema should be put or removed on according to the instructions provided by the patient's therapist.

Prepare for putting on compression garments based on the instructions in the Care Activity Form. Typically this will include:

- Collecting the compression garment(s); smoothing out each garment, making sure it is right side out, and checking for damage before applying.

- Collecting any donning aids (see page 312) or other equipment needed.

Applying an Arm Sleeve and Glove

Donning aids: rubber gloves for the caregiver and, optionally, for the patient.

Donning Time: 3-5 minutes.

There are several ways to put on an arm sleeve, also check the instructions provided with the garment. This method is one of the easiest:

1. Put on rubber gloves. It may be helpful to have the patient put a rubber glove on their non-swollen hand.

2. Place the compression garment over the patient's hand.

3. Have the patient stand (or sit) in front of you and gently push their closed hand (fist) against your chest or stomach. This helps to stabilize their arm.

4. Slowly inch the arm sleeve up the arm, being careful not to pinch the patient. The patient may help as they are able.

5. At the upper arm, have the patient place their arm on your shoulder; or you may gently hold and pull at their lower forearm (near the wrist but not over it), as you pull the sleeve into the armpit. Be sure the patient is looking away from you in case your hand slips, otherwise you may find yourself accidentally punching the patient in the jaw!

6. Remove your gloves for better finger dexterity and smooth out the sleeve at the armpit.

7. Inspect the arm sleeve, check to see that it covers the entire arm evenly and smooth out any folds or bunched-up areas.

8. Ask the patient to put on their own compression glove if they are able; if some assistance is needed, gradually inch the glove onto the hand. Work slowly to make sure each finger is in the proper finger sleeve as the glove is applied.

It may help to turn half of the sleeve inside out before donning.

Donning a Compression Top

If the patient finds it difficult to get a support top over their head, it may be easier for them to step into the top and pull it up and on. Start with the patient seated and ask the patient to place their feet inside the garment. Then have the patient stand up and assist the patient in pulling the garment up into position.

Donning Toe Caps and Leg Stockings

Donning aids: rubber gloves, foot slip, and non-slip rubber pad (see page 312). May also need a stool to support the patient's foot and a stool or chair for the caregiver.

Donning Time: less than 5 minutes.

There are many ways to put on stockings, also check the instructions provided with the garment. This method is one of the easiest:

1. Find a good spot for you and the patient to sit; for example, at the edge of the bed with your chair in front of the patient, or with the patient on a firm-back chair and you on a similar chair or lower stool in front of the patient. Have the patient place one foot or both feet on a stool so that you can reach their foot comfortably.

2. Sit in front of the patient and gradually slide the toe caps or foot glove onto the foot. Work slowly to make sure each toe is in the proper sleeve.

3. Place a foot slip over the patient's foot.

4. Put on rubber gloves. It may be helpful to have the patient put rubber gloves on as well.

5. Begin by "inching" the stocking onto the foot and leg, avoiding excessive bunching. Bunching makes the garment more difficult to put on and may hurt the patient.

6. Continue to gradually inch the stocking onto the leg, working the garment up as it begins to bunch in an area. Ask the patient to "pull up" the stocking as he or she is able.

7. The patient may also rub the heel of the foot forwards on a rubber pad placed on the floor to help get the stocking onto the foot.

8. Pull the stocking all the way up to the bend of the knee (but not into the bend) for a knee high, or up to the upper thigh or groin for a thigh high compression garment.

9. Smooth out any wrinkles or places where the garment appears to be bunched up. Wrinkles will cause too much pressure and restrict lymph flow, leading to an increase in swelling. Smoothing the upper part of the garment may be easier without gloves.

10. Remove the foot slip from the foot by pulling on it. Wiggling the foot slip from side to side as it is pulled may make removal easier.

11. Apply outer socks if desired.

What if you cannot get the sleeve or stocking on?

There are many reasons why an arm sleeve or leg stocking may be difficult to put on. Contact the patient's therapist if the solutions below do not solve the problem. See also "How can I tell if a garment doesn't fit?" on page 140.

• The garment bunched up as it was put on making it difficult to open up sufficiently to fit over the arm or onto the foot, over the heel, or up the leg. Solution: Avoid the bunch! Review steps 5 and 6 above to help with this. Alternatively, turn the hose inside out down to the heel.

• The arm or leg is sticky because the patient was not fully dried after washing or because lotion has just been applied. Solution: Wait 5-10 minutes and try again. Consider using non-talc baby powder or silicone fitting lotion to make the stocking slide more easily.

- The caregiver or the patient does not have sufficient strength to pull the garment up. Try a different position (such as standing) to gain leverage. Also, make sure the patient's limb is stable, since it is much more difficult to put the garment on if the limb is moving. The patient's arm can be stabilized by pushing against a wall or the caregiver's shoulder and the patient's leg can be stabilized by having the patient scoot forward in the chair, lean forward to put weight on their leg, or stand up.

- The stocking may be the wrong size or because of increased swelling, the stocking is now too small.

A stocking with the correct size and pressure that cannot be put on by the patient and caregiver may not be the right stocking after all. Sometimes, compromises are needed. Ask the therapist to assist you with this; it is better to have a lighter stocking *on* than a firmer stocking sitting in a drawer. If a lighter stocking is needed, the therapist may suggest a second garment to be placed over the first to ensure that the limb has adequate pressure to control swelling.

Removing a Compression Garment

Prepare for removing garments by collecting any doffing aids that are required (see page 312) and reviewing the instructions below.

Doffing an Arm Sleeve and Glove

Doffing aids: rubber gloves for the caregiver and, optionally, for the patient.

Removing a sleeve and glove is usually easier than donning one:

1. Put rubber gloves on both hands; the patient should put a rubber glove on the non-swollen hand if they are able to assist.

2. Remove the compression glove from the patient's hand first, by either inching it off the fingers, hand, and wrist, or by turning the glove inside-out as it is peeled off.

3. Remove the arm sleeve by either inching it down the arm or by peeling it off, turning the sleeve inside-out.

Doffing a Compression Top

Reverse the procedure used to put on a compression top to remove it.

If the patient was able to step into the top and pull it up in order to put it on, reverse the process by sliding the top down and having them step out of it. Start with the patient standing next to a chair and have the patient sit down once the top is far enough down.

Doffing a Leg Stocking and Toe Caps

Doffing aids: rubber gloves, rubber mat.

To take a stocking off the leg, simply reverse the order of putting it on. Use rubber gloves and inch the garment off. Remember to avoid bunching, which makes it nearly impossible to remove the stocking, especially at the heel.

Leg stockings may also be peeled off by turning the garment inside out as it is removed; however, this method tends to cause bunching of the garment at the lower leg. The caregiver should experiment with the two techniques to determine which is easiest. If necessary, contact the patient's therapist to assist with any complications in garment removal.

Remove toe caps or foot glove after removing the stocking.

Compression Aids

Although bandages are considered to be the best way to reduce swelling and maintain swelling reduction during sleep, compression aids are easier to use and do help reduce swelling and soften fibrotic tissues. Compression aids are a useful alternative for patients who cannot undergo intensive treatment with compression bandaging for various reasons such as distance from a treatment facility, health issues, or advanced age.

Compression aids are designed to provide consistent gradient pressure along the limb. Inside the device, padding and channeling are used to direct fluid flow.

For more information on compression aids, see page 313 or contact the manufacturers listed on page 418. Figure 7-1 shows a Reid Sleeve Classic Arm Sleeve.

Putting on or Removing a Compression Aid

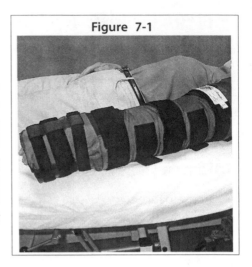

Figure 7-1

The procedure for putting on or removing a compression aid varies depending on the make and style of the compression aid. The caregiver should apply and remove the aid according to the manufacturer's instruction. The patient's therapist or the fitter should be able to demonstrate the correct technique.

Frequently Asked Questions

How can I tell if a garment doesn't fit?

Garments do not fit properly (or were put on incorrectly) if they are significantly uncomfortable to the patient, impair circulation or sensation in the limb, cause deep indentations in the skin, or do not control the patient's swelling as expected. First, check to make sure that the garment has been put on correctly and that there are no wrinkled areas. If the problem remains after adjusting the garment for comfort, contact the patient's therapist.

Garments usually do not fit properly if the garment size was incorrect initially, the garment is worn out or misshapen, or if the patient's limb size has changed.

How long does the patient have to use compression?

Some patients have a short term (acute) episode of swelling and may only need to wear compression garments or aids briefly. Other patients have more serious, chronic swelling which necessitates lifelong use of compression. The caregiver should follow the instructions of the physician and therapist for optimal management of the patient's swelling.

What if a garment is too tight at the wrist or the knee?

After washing, stretch the tight part of the garment over a plastic bottle as it dries. Usually within 3-4 days, the garment should be stretched out enough to be more comfortable. Contact the garment supplier or the patient's therapist if the garment remains too tight.

What if garments get uncomfortable by mid-afternoon?

Pulling up garments to adjust them will help rejuvenate their elasticity, resulting in more comfortable wear for the remainder of the day. Another option is for the patient to change their garments in the late afternoon; similar to a change in clothing, sometimes it just feels better. If the patient is continually pulling up their garments, this may be an indication that the garments need to be replaced.

Will a run in the garment affect the compression?

A run in the garment may affect the amount of compression the garment provides. When possible, avoid runs by taking your time putting the garment on and by wearing rubber gloves. If a serious run occurs, the garment will need to be replaced.

Is a garment required if the limb is not swelling?

The caregiver should follow the direction of the patient's therapist. If the patient has not shown any signs of swelling—but has increased risk of swelling due to cancer treatment—compression garment use may be recommended for air travel and strenuous activities such as weight lifting, prolonged standing, or running.[1]

Why can't compression garments be worn at night?

Because activity, gravity, and muscle pump activity affect swelling, daytime compression is generally firmer than night-time compression. In addition, elastic garments may constrict lymph flow if they wrinkle or shift during sleep. The patient's therapist will advise if compression is needed at night and provide specific recommendations for compression bandages, garments, or aids. In some cases, lower-pressure compression garments may be recommended for night use.

What about finger swelling with a compression aid?

If the patient's fingers are not covered by the compression aid and finger swelling has been observed in the morning, the caregiver may either wrap the fingers overnight (see page 102) or have the patient wear a light compression glove, such as an Isotoner Therapeutic Glove (www.totes-isotoner.com), under the compression aid.

Notes

1   Lymphedema Risk Reduction Practices, National Lymphedema Network, 2008.

Chapter 8

Decongestive Exercises

Exercise is an integral part of lymphedema treatment (see page 30)[1] and beneficial for all individuals.[2] People with lymphedema who are more physically fit find it easier to participate in rewarding activities of daily living with family and friends, at work and at home, and while traveling.

Decongestive exercises are designed to encourage the flow of lymph and complement the more passive lymph drainage techniques (MLD, SLD, and self massage). Both techniques are valuable and the daily care routine may be varied based on the patient's other activities and energy level. For example, have the patient exercise more on days when they are mostly sitting or traveling (sedentary). On days when the patient has been shopping, gardening, participating in sports or community exercise programs, SLD and rest with limb elevation may be more appropriate.

These exercises should not cause unusual pain; if pain occurs, stop that exercise and continue with the next one.

Consult the patient's therapist or physician before starting any new exercise program.

Exercise routines use combinations of the specific exercises described below. Specific exercises include:

- Basic exercises for all affected areas, page 148.

- Head and neck exercises, page 163.

- Upper body and arm exercises, page 165.

- Post mastectomy stretching exercises for the chest and shoulder, page 171.

- Lower body and leg exercises, page 173.

- Advanced exercises including Casley-Smith exercises, page 177.

Planning Exercise

The patient's therapist should design an exercise plan based on the patient's needs and condition. This may include one or more of the exercise routines for different affected areas provided below starting on page 146. The advanced exercise routines incorporate SLD for added benefit using the SLD circle and stroke techniques explained earlier (starting on page 69).[3]

Most patients should exercise one or more times a day, in accordance with the Weekly Care Plan (see page 333) and Care Activity descriptions worked out in cooperation with the patient's therapist..

Patients should wear compression bandages or garments while exercising and may need additional compression to control any extra swelling which may occur. The Care Activity form for exercise should describe the entire process (see page 145) including:

- Putting on additional compression before exercise (if needed) with specific bandages or garments.

- Specific exercise routines and any equipment required.

- Removing additional compression after the patient has cooled down.

A worksheet is provided for each exercise routine listing the exercise and the page number for the instructions. These worksheets can be marked up to show the recommended position and number of repetitions for each patient. Space is provided for adding other exercises recommended by the patient's therapist. Letter sized versions of these forms can be downloaded from the book Web site (www.Lymphedema-Caregiver.com).

Make a master copy of the worksheet for each exercise routine recommended for the patient. Fill in the patient's name, circle the recommended position, and mark any other changes. Copies of the worksheet can then be used to track the patient's exercises during a week by checking off the day columns on the right. Keep these worksheets in the Patient Notebook.

As a minimum, most patients should do the basic exercise routine for their affected area(s) to encourage lymph flow through the nodes at the neck, armpits, trunk, and hips.

With practice, the patient should be able to complete a basic exercise routine in about 10 minutes and the advanced exercise routine in 30 minutes. If the patient needs more time to perform the exercises, consider scaling down the routine to 4-5 exercises by choosing one exercise per body area. For example, the caregiver may have the patient perform one neck exercise, one shoulder exercise, deep breathing, one hip exercise, and one specific exercise for the patient's affected area (such as arm press-ups, ankle pumps, or face exercises for head and neck swelling). This will stimulate the lymphatics at the neck, shoulders, trunk (with breathing), and hips prior to stimulating the arm, leg, or face.

On occasion, the patient may have limited time to exercise, but still desire to stimulate the lymphatics in some way. When this occurs, pick one or two exercises for the patient to do that would best meet their needs, or do one repetition of several exercises ("one minute exercise" routine). Most importantly, encourage the patient to move throughout the day to keep the lymph flowing.

Exercise Process

The exercise process includes preparation, guiding the patient through the exercises, and post exercise cool down as described below.

Preparing for Exercise

Typically, exercise will follow compression in the care plan. To get ready for exercise:

- Choose a convenient and comfortable location. If the patient does exercises on their back, you will need a firm bed or an exercise table with space around the sides for access, the height should be comfortable for both patient and caregiver.

- Gather any equipment that is required. A straight-backed chair is the only equipment for the basic exercises; some of the advanced exercises use a broomstick or weights.

- Have water available and encourage the patient to drink frequently.

- If required, help the patient put on additional bandages or compression garments.

Guiding Exercises

The caregiver's role includes guiding the patient through the exercises and helping the patient develop and maintain the motivation to exercise, see the chapter on "Emotional Care and Support" (page 189) for suggestions.

As you guide the patient through the exercises, help them:

- Stay relaxed because muscle tension inhibits lymph flow.

- Perform each exercise slowly and steadily to a one-second count per repetition unless otherwise suggested. Rushing diminishes the desired effect of increased lymph flow and can cause tissue damage.

After Exercise

Offer the patient water. Store any equipment used. Whenever possible, the patient should rest with the affected limb elevated for 5-10 minutes after exercising.

After the patient has cooled down, remove any extra bandages or compression added for exercise.

Record the completed exercises in the daily column of the sheet for the exercise routine and mark the relevant activities as completed on the Weekly Care Plan Form.

Exercise Routines

Example exercise routine worksheets are provided for:

- Head and neck swelling, see page 149.

- Post-mastectomy stretches for the chest and shoulder, see page 150. To maximize post-surgery improvement: perform these stretches two to three times per day until full range of motion is achieved; once a full range of motion has been achieved, continue stretches once a day for at least a year to minimize the risk of backsliding.

- Basic upper body and arm swelling, see page 152:

  - Equipment (optional): two 1-3 pound (0.5-1.5 kg) hand weights as directed by the patient's therapist for exercises marked with an asterisk.

  - Steps 13-23 may be performed by the patient according to the degree of swelling in the particular area. For example, omit finger exercises if the patient does not have finger swelling.

- Advanced upper body and arm swelling, see page 154:

  - Equipment: Broomstick

  - This routine combines exercise with SLD circles over the unaffected lymph node clusters and strokes along alternate pathways leading to the unaffected lymph node clusters (page 33). Patients should wear compression while exercising, as specified by the therapist. If the compression garments or bandages interfere with the SLD, skip that step and continue with the next exercise.

- Basic lower body and leg swelling, see page 151.

- Advanced lower body and leg swelling, see page 156:

  - This routine combines exercise with SLD circles over the unaffected lymph node clusters and strokes along alternate pathways leading to the unaffected lymph node clusters (page 33). Patients should wear compression while exercising, as specified by the therapist. If the compression garments or bandages interfere with the SLD, skip that step and continue with the next exercise.

  - *Note: Many of the advanced leg exercises are difficult and may be stressful to the lower back. These exercises should only be done when recommended by a certified lymphedema therapist and if the patient is well-conditioned.*

Most basic exercises can be done with the patient sitting, standing, or lying on their back; select the position that works best for the patient. The advanced routines require the patient to change positions one or two times. If more than one position is listed, select the position that will be easiest for the patient.

Basic Decongestive Exercises

Basic exercises are used in most exercise routines.

Head Turns

See Figure 8-1.

<u>Purpose:</u> To increase lymph flow through the neck and shoulders.

<u>Start Position:</u> Sitting facing forward, with good posture and relaxed shoulders. <u>Alternative Positions:</u> Standing or lying on back.

<u>Exercise:</u> The patient turns their head to the right and holds 1-2 seconds, then turns to the left and holds 1-2 seconds. Return to the start position.

Neck Side Bends

See Figure 8-2 and Figure 8-3

<u>Purpose:</u> To increase lymph flow through the neck and shoulders.

<u>Start Position:</u> Sitting facing forward, with good posture and relaxed shoulders. <u>Alternative Position:</u> Standing.

<u>Exercise:</u> The patient tilts their head to the right and holds 1-2 seconds, then tilts to the left and holds 1-2 seconds. Return to the start position.

Continued on page 158.

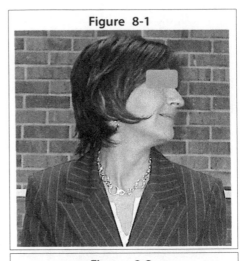

Figure 8-1

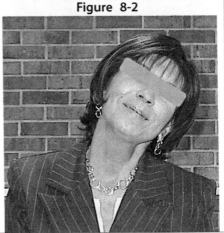

Figure 8-2

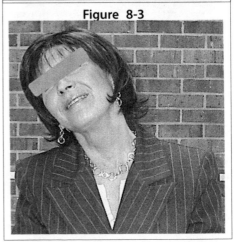

Figure 8-3

Exercise Routine for Head and Neck Swelling

Patient: _____   Week of: _____

Exercise	Pg	Position	Reps	M	T	W	T	F	S	S
1) Head Turns	148	Sit/Stand/Lie	5							
2) Neck Side Bends	148	Sit/Stand/Lie	5							
3) Forward Head Rolls	158	Sit/Stand	5							
4) Shoulder Shrugs and Presses	158	Sit/Stand/Lie	5							
5) Shoulder Points and Squeezes	159	Sit/Stand/Lie	5, squeeze 5 sec							
6) Bent Elbow Shoulder Squeezes	159	Sit/Stand/Lie	5, squeeze 5 sec							
7) Shoulder Rolls	160	Sit/Stand	5 each way							
8) Forward or Side Arm Raises	161	Sit/Stand/Lie	Optional, 5 each							
9) Deep Breathing	162	Sit/Stand/Lie	5							
10) Neck Back Bends	163	Sit/Stand	5, hold 10 sec							
11) Chin Tucks	164	Sit/Stand/Lie	5							
12) Jaw Open and Clench	164	Sit/Stand/Lie	5							
13) Lateral Jaw Relaxer	164	Sit/Stand/Lie	5							
14) Mouth Exercises	165	Sit/Stand/Lie	5							
15) Face Exercises	165	Sit/Stand/Lie	5							

Post-Mastectomy Stretch Exercise Routine

Patient:				Week of:							
Exercise	**Pg**	**Position**	**Reps**	**M**	**T**	**W**	**T**	**F**	**S**	**S**	
1) Forward Wall Walking	171	Stand	3, hold 30 sec								
2) Sideways Wall Walking	172	Stand	3, hold 30 sec								
3) Corner Wall Stretch	172	Stand	3, hold 30 sec								

Basic Exercise Routine for Lower Body and Leg Swelling

Patient: _____   Week of: _____

Exercise	Pg	Position	Reps	M	T	W	T	F	S	S
1) Head Turns	148	Sit/Stand/Lie	5							
2) Neck Side Bends	148	Sit/Stand	5							
3) Shoulder Shrugs and Presses	158	Sit/Stand/Lie	5							
4) Shoulder Points and Squeezes	159	Sit/Stand/Lie	5, squeeze 5 sec							
5) Shoulder Rolls	160	Sit/Stand/Lie	5 each way							
6) Forward Arm Raises	161	Sit/Stand/Lie	5							
7) Body Side Bends	162	Sit/Stand	5							
8) Deep Breathing	162	Sit/Stand/Lie	5							
9) Seat Squeezes	173	Stand/Lie	5, hold 3 sec							
10) Marching in Place	173	Stand/Sit	5							
11) Heel Slides/Knee to Chest	174	Lying on Back	5							
12) Bent Knee Hip Rotation	163	Sit/Stand/Lie	5							
13) Knee Extensions	174	Sit/Stand/Lie	5 each leg							
14) Ankle Pumps	175	Sit/Stand/Lie	5 each foot							
15) Ankle Circles	175	Sit/Stand/Lie	5 each foot							
16) Ankle Waves	175	Sit/Stand/Lie	5 each foot							
17) Toe Curls and Wiggles	176	Sit/Stand/Lie	5 each foot							

Basic Exercise Routine for Upper Body and Arm Swelling (1 of 2)

Patient:

Week of:

Exercise	Pg	Position	Reps	M	T	W	T	F	S	S
1) Head Turns	148	Sit/Stand/Lie	5							
2) Neck Side Bends	148	Sit/Stand	5							
3) Forward Head Rolls	158	Sit/Stand	5							
4) Shoulder Shrugs and Presses	158	Sit/Stand/Lie	5							
5) Shoulder Squeezes and Points	159	Sit/Stand/Lie	5, squeeze 5 sec							
6) Bent Elbow Shoulder Squeezes	159	Sit/Stand/Lie	5, squeeze 5 sec							
7) Shoulder Rolls	160	Sit/Stand/Lie	5 each way							
8) Forward Arm Raises*	161	Sit/Stand/Lie	5							
9) Side Arm Raises*	161	Sit/Stand/Lie	5							
10) Deep Breathing	162	Sit/Stand/Lie	5 , slowly							
11) Bent Knee Hip Rotation	163	Sit/Stand/Lie	5							
12) Body Side Bends	162	Sit/Stand	5, hold 3-5 sec							
13) Elevated Arm Circles	166	Sit/Stand/Lie	5 each way							
14) Arm Press-ups*	166	Sit/Stand/Lie	5							
15) Elevated Arm Twists	167	Sit/Stand/Lie	5 each way							

* optional 1-3 pound hand weights as directed by the patient's therapist

Basic Exercise Routine for Upper Body and Arm Swelling (2 of 2)

Patient:				Week of:						
Exercise	Pg	Position	Reps	M	T	W	T	F	S	S
16) Elbow Bends*	167	Sit/Stand/Lie	5							
17) Wrist Bends* (Palm up and down)	168	Sit/Stand/Lie	5 each way							
18) Wrist Circles	168	Sit/Stand/Lie	5 each way							
19) Hand Waves	169	Sit/Stand/Lie	5							
20) Hand Grips and Opens	169	Sit/Stand/Lie	5							
21) Finger Curls (Claw)	170	Sit/Stand/Lie	5							
22) Hand Puppet	170	Sit/Stand/Lie	5							
23) Finger Spread and Squeezes	171	Sit/Stand/Lie	5							

* optional 1-3 pound hand weights as directed by the patient's therapist

Advanced Exercise Routine for Upper Body and Arm Swelling (1 of 2)

Patient: _____   Week of: _____

Exercise	Pg	Position	Reps	M	T	W	T	F	S	S
1) Relaxation	177	Lying on Back	one minute							
2) Bouncing Knee To Chest	180	Lying on Back	16 gently							
3) SLD circles Terminus/Collarbone	72	Lying on Back	5							
4) Deep Breathing w/ Partial Sit-ups	177	Lying on Back	5							
5) Head Turns	148	Sit	5							
6) Forward Head Rolls	158	Sit	5							
7) Shoulder Shrugs and Presses	158	Sit	5							
8) Shoulder Points and Squeezes	159	Sit	5, squeeze 5 sec							
9) Shoulder Rolls	160	Sit	5 each way							
10) SLD circles unaffected Axillary/ Armpit	75	Sit	5							
11) Elevated Arm Circles	166	Sit	5 each way							
12) Deep Breathing w/ Body Curls	177	Sit	5							
13) SLD circles Inguinal/Upper Thigh (affected side)	76	Sit	5							
14) Bent Knee Hip Rotation	163	Sit	5							
15) Body Side Bends	162	Sit	5							

Advanced Exercise Routine for Upper Body and Arm Swelling (2 of 2)

Patient: _____   Week of: _____

Exercise	Pg	Position	Reps	M	T	W	T	F	S	S
16) SLD strokes upper body pathway toward unaffected axillary nodes		Sit	5 or up to 30 sec							
17) Pressing Hands Together	178	Sit	5, hold 3 sec							
18) Broomstick Arm Raises	178	Sit	5							
19) Elbow Bends	167	Sit	5							
20) Hand Grips & Opens (make a fist)	169	Sit	5							
21) Arm Twists (Rotating the arm)	167	Sit	5 each way							
22) Bent Elbow Shoulder Squeezes	159	Sit	5, hold 5 sec							
23) SLD strokes front upper pathway to unaffected axillary nodes, and side pathway to inguinal nodes		Sit	5 or up to 30 sec							
24) Bracing Against Wall with Hands	179	Stand	5, hold 3 sec							
25) Playing the Piano	179	Stand	5 taps/finger							
26) Deep Breathing w/Partial Sit-ups	177	Lying on Back	5							
27) Relax w/arm elevated on pillows	177	Lying	Up to 30 min							

Advanced Exercise Routine for Lower Body and Leg Swelling (1 of 2)

Patient: _____ Week of: _____

Exercise	Pg	Position	Reps	M	T	W	T	F	S	S
1) Relaxation	177	Lying on Back	1 min (optional)							
2) Deep Breathing w/Partial Sit-ups	177	Lying on Back	5 (optional)							
3) SLD circles Terminus/Collarbone	72	Sit	5							
4) Head Turns	148	Sit	5							
5) Forward Head Rolls	158	Sit	5							
6) Shoulder Shrugs and Presses	158	Sit	5							
7) Shoulder Points and Squeezes	159	Sit	5, squeeze 5 sec							
8) Shoulder Rolls	160	Sit	5 each way							
9) SLD circles Axillary/Armpits	75	Sit	5							
10) Bouncing Knee To Chest	180	Lying on Back	16, gently							
11) Deep Breathing w/Partial Sit-ups	177	Lying on Back	5							
12) SLD circles unaffected Inguinal/Upper Thigh	76	Lying on Back	5							
13) SLD strokes side pathway(s) to Axillary/Armpits		Lying on Back	5 or up to 30 sec							
14) Bouncing Both Knees to Chest	180	Lying on Back	10, gently							
15) Seat Squeezes	173	Lying on Back	5, hold 3 sec							
16) Bent Knee Seat Squeezes	181	Lying on Back	5							
17) Lower Back Contractions	181	Lying on Back	5							

Advanced Exercise Routine for Lower Body and Leg Swelling (2 of 2)

Patient:

Week of:

Exercise	Pg	Position	Reps	M	T	W	T	F	S	S
18) Bouncing Bent Knee Sideways	182	Lying on Back	16, gently							
19) SLD stroke side pathways to Axillary/Armpits and lower front and back pathways to unaffected Inguinal/Upper Thigh		Lying on non-swollen side	5 or up to 30 sec							
20) Leg Twists	182	Lying on Back	5							
21) Bouncing Knee	183	Lying on Back	16, gently							
22) Elevated Leg Stretches	184	Lying on Back	5							
23) SLD circles unaffected upper thigh and knee bend; stroke involved leg(s) from foot to hip	76,77	Lying on Back	5 or up to 30 sec							
24) Ankle Pumps w/Legs Elevated	175	Lying on Back	5							
25) Ankle Circles w/Legs Elevated	176	Lying on Back	5 each way							
26) Elevated Knee Bends Sideways	185	Lying on Back	5							
27) Elevated Legs Walking, Bicycles, and Scissors	186	Lying on Back	5 each, as able							
28) Bent Knee Side to Side	186	Lying on Back	5							
29) Bouncing Both Knees to Chest	180	Lying on Back	10, gently							
30) Deep Breathing w/ Partial Sit-ups	177	Lying on Back	5							
31) Relaxation with legs elevated	177	Lying on Back	Up to 30 min							

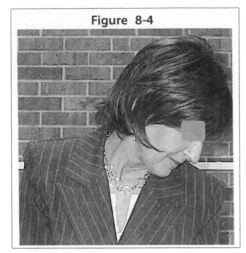

Figure 8-4

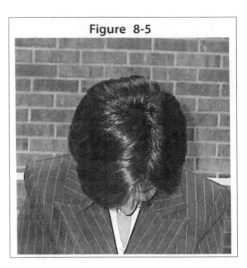

Figure 8-5

Forward Head Rolls

See Figure 8-4 and Figure 8-5.

<u>Purpose:</u> To increase lymph flow through the neck and shoulders.

<u>Start Position:</u> Sitting facing forward, with good posture and relaxed shoulders. <u>Alternative Position:</u> Standing.

<u>Exercise:</u> The patient tilts their head to the right, and then slowly rolls the head forward and to the left, finishing with the head tilted to the left. Return to the start position.

Note: The patient should not roll their head back, since this may irritate the neck joints and nerves and cause pain.

Shoulder Shrugs and Presses

See Figure 8-6.

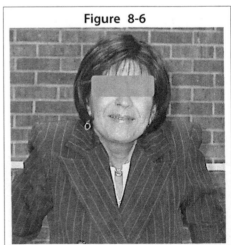

Figure 8-6

<u>Purpose:</u> To increase lymph flow through the neck and shoulders.

<u>Start Position:</u> Sitting facing forward, with good posture and relaxed shoulders. <u>Alternative Positions:</u> Standing or lying on back.

Exercise: The patient lifts their shoulders (shoulder blades) up as high as possible toward the ears. The patient slowly lowers the shoulders to the start position and then presses the shoulders firmly down past the start position. Return to the start position.

Shoulder Points and Squeezes

See Figure 8-7 and Figure 8-8.

Purpose: To increase lymph flow through the neck and shoulders.

Start Position: Sitting facing forward, with good posture and relaxed shoulders. Alternative Positions: Standing or lying on back.

Exercise: The patient moves their shoulders (shoulder blades) forward, and then squeezes the shoulders back as much as possible. Hold the squeeze for up to 5 seconds. Return to the start position.

Bent Elbow Shoulder Squeezes

See Figure 8-9 and Figure 8-10 on page 160.

Purpose: To increase lymph flow through the neck and shoulders.

Start Position: Sitting facing forward, with good posture and the arms raised overhead with the hands resting at the back (or side) of the head. The patient should be cautioned not to pull the head forward during this exercise. Alternative Positions: Standing or lying on back.

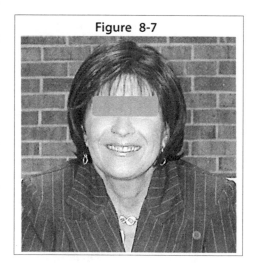

Figure 8-7

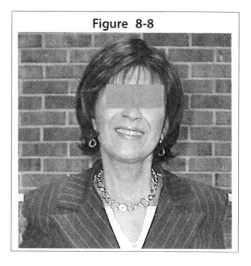

Figure 8-8

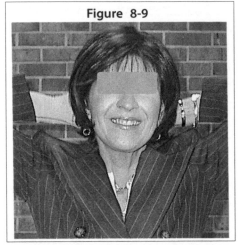

Figure 8-9

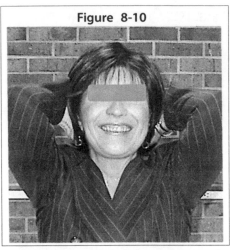

Figure 8-10

Exercise: The patient moves their elbows forward and holds 1-2 seconds, then moves the elbows back as they squeeze the shoulder blades together. Hold the squeeze for up to 5 seconds. Return to the start position.

Shoulder Rolls

See Figure 8-11.

Purpose: To increase lymph flow through the neck and shoulders.

Start Position: Sitting facing forward, with good posture and relaxed shoulders. Alternative Position: Standing.

Exercise: The patient lifts their shoulders (shoulder blades) forward and up as high as possible toward the ears, then squeezes the shoulders back and down, lowering them to the start position. Now change directions, squeezing the shoulders (shoulder blades) backwards and lifting up as high as possible toward the ears, then moving the shoulders forward and down, lowering them to the start position.

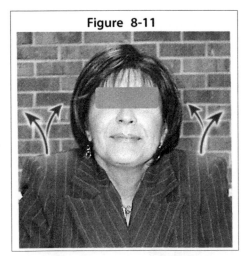

Figure 8-11

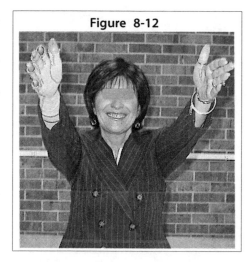

Figure 8-12

Forward Arm Raises

See Figure 8-12.

<u>Purpose:</u> To increase lymph flow through the shoulders and arms.

<u>Start Position:</u> Sitting facing forward, with good posture and relaxed shoulders. The patient's arms should be straight, with the thumbs pointed up. <u>Alternative Positions:</u> Standing or lying on back.

<u>Exercise:</u> The patient moves their arms forward and up over their head as high as possible, holds 1-2 seconds, then slowly lowers their arms to the start position.

Side Arm Raises

See Figure 8-13.

<u>Purpose:</u> To increase lymph flow through the shoulders and arms.

<u>Start Position:</u> Sitting facing forward, with good posture and relaxed shoulders. The patient's arms should be straight out to the sides, with the palms of the hands turned forward and thumbs pointed up. <u>Alternative Position:</u> Standing.

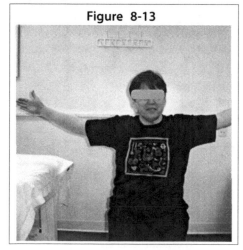

Figure 8-13

<u>Exercise:</u> The patient moves their arms sideways and up over their head as high as possible, holds 1-2 seconds, then slowly lowers their arms to the start position.

Deep or Diaphragmatic Breathing

<u>Purpose:</u> To increase lymph flow through the trunk.

<u>Start Position:</u> Sitting facing forward, with good posture and relaxed shoulders. <u>Alternative Positions:</u> Standing or lying on back.

<u>Exercise:</u> The patient takes a full deep breath in through the nose, and then slowly breathes out through the mouth. The lower abdomen should inflate and deflate with each breath, see page 71.

Body Side Bends

See Figure 8-14.

<u>Purpose:</u> Increase lymph flow along the upper and lower body and the side pathways.

<u>Start Position:</u> Sitting facing forward, with good posture and relaxed shoulders. The patient's arms should be straight, with the palms of the hands turned forward and thumbs pointed up. <u>Alternative Position:</u> Standing.

<u>Exercise:</u> The patient raises one arm up to the side and reaches overhead toward the opposite side allowing the body to bend with the reach. The

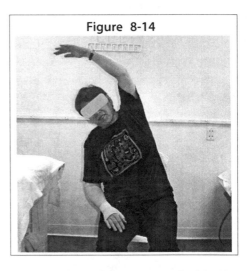

Figure 8-14

patient may feel a stretch along the side of the body. The patient holds the stretch for 3-5 seconds, and then slowly lowers the arm to the start position. Next, the patient raises the other arm up and reaches overhead to the opposite side, holds 3-5 seconds, and returns to start position.

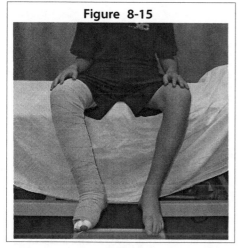

Figure 8-15

Bent Knee Hip Rotation

See Figure 8-15.

<u>Purpose:</u> To increase lymph flow through the hips and legs.

<u>Start Position:</u> Sitting at the edge of the chair, facing forward, with good posture and relaxed shoulders. The patient's feet should be flat on the floor about shoulder width apart. <u>Alternative Positions:</u> Standing or lying on back.

<u>Exercise:</u> The patient turns one or both knees out and away from the other as far as possible, holds the stretched position 3-5 seconds, and then slowly returns to the start position. The patient may allow their feet to move slightly off the floor during this exercise.

Head and Neck Exercises

Neck Back Bends

See Figure 8-16.

<u>Purpose:</u> Increase lymph flow through the neck. Stretch to the front of the neck.

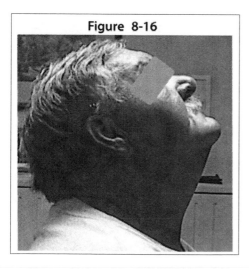

Figure 8-16

<u>Start Position:</u> Sitting facing forward, with good posture and relaxed shoulders. <u>Alternative Position:</u> Standing.

<u>Exercise:</u> The patient tilts their head back, keeping the mouth closed and looking up toward the ceiling, holds 1-2 seconds (increase the stretch time to 5-10 seconds if the patient has neck stiffness due to surgery). Return to the start position. The patient may support their head and neck with their hands during this exercise.

Chin Tucks

See Figure 8-17.

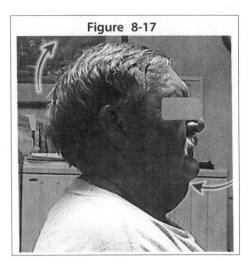
Figure 8-17

Purpose: Increase lymph flow at the back of the neck. Improve head posture.

Start Position: Sitting facing forward, with good posture and relaxed shoulders. Alternative Position: Standing.

Exercise: The patient moves their head back, keeping the chin tucked in (slightly nodded down), then holds 1-2 seconds. Return to the start position. When done correctly, the patient will have flattened the back of the neck and will appear to have a "double chin."

Jaw Open and Clench

Purpose: Increase lymph flow around the ears and mouth.[4]

Start Position: Sitting facing forward, with good posture and relaxed shoulders. This exercise may be done facing a mirror. Alternative Position: Standing.

Exercise: With the tip of the tongue on the roof of the mouth, the patient opens the mouth fully, holds 1-2 seconds, and then closes the mouth, holds a light clench 1-2 seconds and relaxes. Soft cotton rolls may be placed on the bottom back teeth prior to closure to help prevent excessive clench pressure.

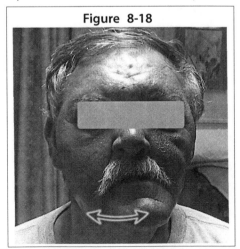
Figure 8-18

Lateral Jaw Relaxer

See Figure 8-18.

Purpose: Increase lymph flow around the ears and mouth.[5]

Start Position: Sitting facing forward, with good posture and relaxed shoulders. Alternative Position: Standing.

Exercise: With relaxed jaw, the patient moves the jaw slowly from side to side.

Mouth Exercises

Purpose: Increase lymph flow through the face. [6]

Start Position: Sitting facing forward, with good posture and relaxed shoulders. Alternative Position: Standing.

Exercise: The patient moves the mouth making various faces (smile up and to side, frown, pucker, sneer, pout, "Oops") or sound motions ("A – E – I – O – U").

Face Exercises

Purpose: Increase lymph flow around the eyes. [7]

Start Position: Sitting facing forward, with good posture and relaxed shoulders. Alternative Position: Standing.

Exercise: The patient moves the eyebrows, eyes, and nose to make various expressions: surprise or question, concern or anger, sneer, "funny" smell, wink.

Upper Body and Arm Exercises

Elevated Arm Circles

See Figure 8-19.

<u>Purpose:</u> Increase lymph flow through the arms and shoulders.

<u>Start Position:</u> Sitting facing forward, with good posture and relaxed shoulders. The patient's arms should be straight, with the thumbs pointed up. <u>Alternative Positions:</u> Standing or lying on back.

<u>Exercise:</u> The patient raises their arms up over their head, and then makes small circles with their arms, first clockwise, then counter-clockwise. After completing the circles, the patient lowers the arms to the start position.

Arm Press-ups ("Picking Apples")

See Figure 8-20 and Figure 8-21.

<u>Purpose:</u> To increase lymph flow through the hands and arms.

<u>Start Position:</u> Sitting facing forward, with good posture and relaxed shoulders. <u>Alternative Positions:</u> Standing or lying on back.

<u>Exercise:</u> The patient raises one arm up above their head with an open hand. Next, the patient closes the hand and lowers the arm down, allowing the

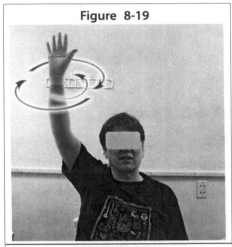

Figure 8-19

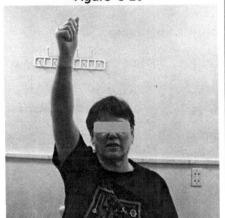

Figure 8-20

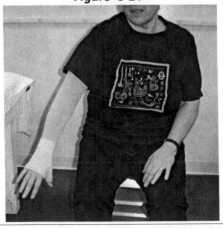

Figure 8-21

elbow to naturally bend and straighten with this exercise. The patient may visualize reaching up and grabbing an apple off a tree, then placing the apple in a basket on the floor.

Arm Twists (Rotating the Arm)

See Figure 8-22.

Purpose: To increase lymph flow through the arms.

Start Position: Sitting facing forward, with good posture and relaxed shoulders. Alternative Positions: Standing, lying on back, or sitting with arm supported by pillows.

Figure 8-22

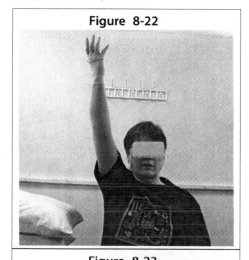

Exercise: With the swollen arm elevated and the elbow straight, the patient twists the arm fully in one direction beginning with the hand, then the forearm and shoulder; the patient holds the full twist for 1-2 seconds. Next, the patient releases the twist and relaxes the arm fully. The patient twists the arm fully in the opposite direction, holds 1-2 seconds, releases the twist, and relaxes.

Elbow Bends

Figure 8-23

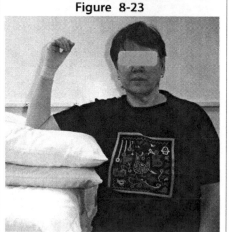

See Figure 8-23.

Purpose: To increase lymph flow through the elbows and arms.

Start Position: Sitting facing forward, with good posture and relaxed shoulders. Elbow may be elevated on pillows to enhance lymph flow. Alternative Positions: Standing or lying on back.

Exercise: The patient bends their elbow fully and holds 1-2 seconds, and then straightens the arm fully and holds 1-2 seconds.

Wrist Bends
(Palm up and Palm down)

Figure 8-24 shows a patient demonstrating this exercise using a one pound weight.

Purpose: To increase lymph flow through the hands and forearms.

Start Position: Sitting facing forward, with good posture and relaxed shoulders. Alternative Positions: Standing or lying on back.

Exercise: With forearm supported and wrist over the edge of a pillow or table, the patient bends the wrist up. Have the patient repeat the exercise first with the palm up, then with the palm down.

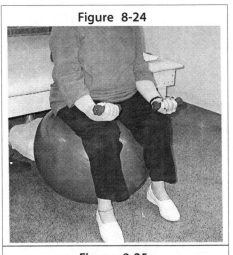

Figure 8-24

Wrist Circles

See Figure 8-25.

Purpose: To increase lymph flow through the hands and forearms.

Start Position: Sitting facing forward, with good posture and relaxed shoulders. Alternative Positions: Standing or lying on back.

Exercise: With forearm supported and wrist over the edge of a pillow or table, the patient moves the hand and wrist in a circle, first clockwise, then counter-clockwise.

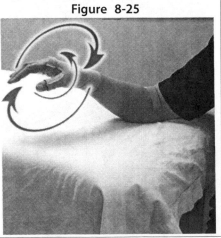

Figure 8-25

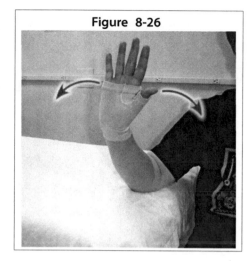

Figure 8-26

Hand Waves (Ulnar and Radial Deviation)

See Figure 8-26.

<u>Purpose:</u> To increase lymph flow through the hands and forearms.

<u>Start Position:</u> Sitting facing forward, with good posture and relaxed shoulders. <u>Alternative Positions:</u> Standing or lying on back.

<u>Exercise:</u> The patient bends the wrist toward the thumb and then toward the pinky finger as if waving to someone.

Hand Grips and Opens

See Figure 8-27.

<u>Purpose:</u> To increase lymph flow through the hands and forearms.

<u>Start Position:</u> Sitting facing forward, with good posture and relaxed shoulders. <u>Alternative Positions:</u> Standing or lying on back.

<u>Exercise:</u> The patient grips the fingers fully into a fist, holds 1-2 seconds, then opens the hand fully, and holds 1-2 seconds.

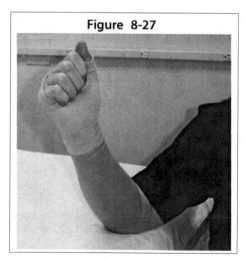

Figure 8-27

Finger Curls (Claw)

See Figure 8-28.

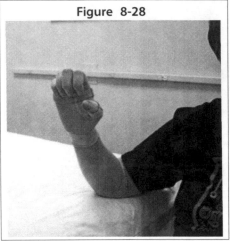

Figure 8-28

Purpose: To increase lymph flow through the hands and forearms.

Start Position: Sitting facing forward, with good posture and relaxed shoulders. Alternative Positions: Standing or lying on back.

Exercise: The patient closes the fingers and thumb moving the finger tips toward the palm side of the knuckles, holds 1-2 seconds, then opens fingers and thumbs fully and holds 1-2 seconds.

Hand Puppet

See Figure 8-29.

Purpose: To increase lymph flow through the hands and forearms.

Start Position: Sitting facing forward, with good posture and relaxed shoulders. Alternative Positions: Standing or lying on back.

Exercise: The patient bends the fingers and thumb at the knuckles as if making a puppet face, holds 1-2 seconds, then opens fingers and thumb fully and holds 1-2 seconds.

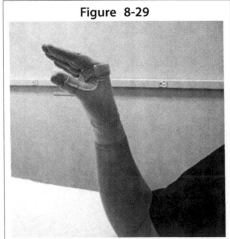

Figure 8-29

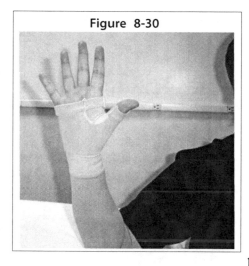

Figure 8-30

Finger Spread and Squeezes

See Figure 8-30.

<u>Purpose:</u> To increase lymph flow through the hands and forearms.

<u>Start Position:</u> Sitting facing forward, with good posture and relaxed shoulders. <u>Alternative Positions:</u> Standing or lying on back.

<u>Exercise:</u> The patient spreads the fingers and thumb out away from the other fingers as far as possible and holds 1-2 seconds, and then closes fingers and thumb fully and holds 1-2 seconds.

Post-Mastectomy Stretches

Forward Wall Walking

See Figure 8-31.

<u>Purpose:</u> To increase the flexibility of the shoulder joint muscles and tissues.

<u>Start Position:</u> The patient stands facing a wall from about two steps away with their back straight, shoulders relaxed, and one foot a step forward for balance.

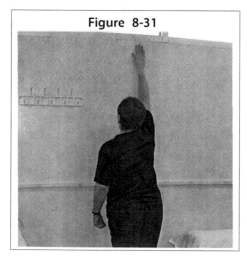

Figure 8-31

<u>Exercise:</u> The patient raises their affected arm up over their head as high as possible allowing the hand to slide up the wall. Using the fingers, the patient attempts to reach higher by walking the fingers up the wall. The patient holds a comfortable stretch for up to 30 seconds, and then slowly lowers their arms to the start position. If it is too painful to hold the maximum position for 30 seconds, have the patient lower their arm 1-3 inches

to a position that is more comfortable for them to hold and stretch. Repeat with the other arm if necessary.

Sideways Wall Walking

See Figure 8-32.

<u>Purpose:</u> To increase the flexibility of the shoulder joint muscles and tissues.

<u>Start Position:</u> The patient stands slightly less than an arm's length away from a wall facing sideways. Their posture is straight with relaxed shoulders and feet wide apart for balance.

<u>Exercise:</u> The patient raises the arm closer to the wall over their head as high as possible allowing the hand to slide up the wall. Using the fingers, the patient attempts to reach up further by walking the fingers up the wall. The patient holds a comfortable stretch for up to 30 seconds, and then slowly lowers their arm to the start position. If it is too painful to hold the maximum position for 30 seconds, have the patient lower their arm 1-3 inches to a position that is more comfortable for them to hold and stretch. Turn and repeat with the other arm if necessary.

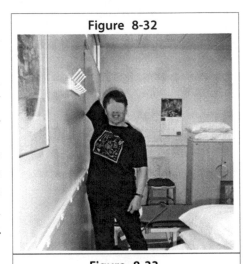

Figure 8-32

Figure 8-33

Corner Wall Stretch

See Figure 8-33.

<u>Purpose:</u> To increase the flexibility of the chest wall muscles and tissues.

<u>Start Position:</u> The patient stands about two steps away from the corner of a wall, with one hand on each wall at shoulder height. Their posture is straight with relaxed shoulders.

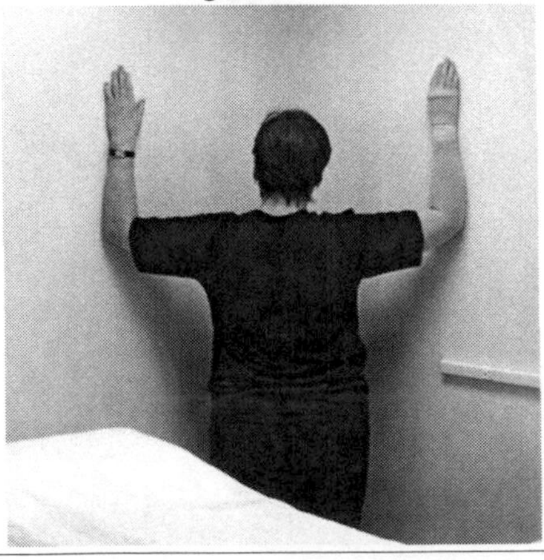

Exercise: The patient leans forward into the corner. The patient holds a comfortable stretch for up to 30 seconds, and then pushes into the wall to return to the start position.

Lower Body and Leg Exercises

Seat Squeezes

Purpose: To increase lymph flow through the lower back, buttocks, and hips.

Start Position: The patient is lying on their back.
Alternative Position: Standing

Exercise: The patient tightens or "squeezes" the buttock muscles slowly (to a 3 count), holds for 3 seconds, slowly releases the buttock squeeze (to a 3 count), and relaxes. To assist with the count, the caregiver may instruct the patient to "Tighten-2-3, hold-2-3, release-2-3, and relax-2-3."

Marching in Place

See Figure 8-34.

Purpose: To increase lymph flow through the legs and hips.

Start Position: Sitting at the edge of their chair, facing forward, with good posture and relaxed shoulders. The patient's feet should be flat on the floor and about shoulder width apart. Alternative Position: Standing.

Exercise: The patient raises one leg up toward their chest, then back down; the patient then raises their other leg up toward the chest, then back down.

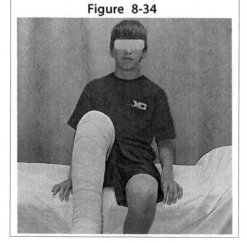

Figure 8-34

Heel Slide/Single Knee to Chest

See Figure 8-35.

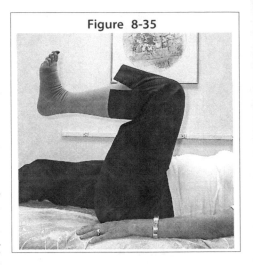

Figure 8-35

Purpose: To increase lymph flow through the legs and hips.

Start Position: The patient is lying on their back.

Exercise: The patient bends one leg up, sliding the foot on the bed and raising the knee toward the chest, then slowly lowers the leg down extending the knee fully; next, the patient bends their other knee up and slowly lowers it back down.

Knee Extensions

See Figure 8-36.

Purpose: To increase lymph flow through the legs and hips.

Start Position: Sitting facing forward, with good posture and relaxed shoulders. The thighs should be fully supported by the chair seat, with the patient's feet on the floor about shoulder width apart. Alternative Positions: Standing or lying on back with a large blanket roll under the patient's knees.

Exercise: The patient straightens one knee raising the foot up, holds the straight knee 3-5 seconds, then slowly bends the knee and lowers the foot to the floor or bed; the patient then straightens their other knee, holds 3-5 seconds, and then lowers leg.

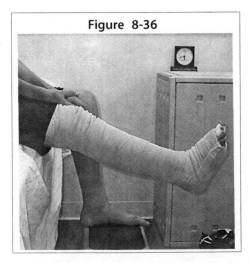

Figure 8-36

Figure 8-37	Figure 8-38
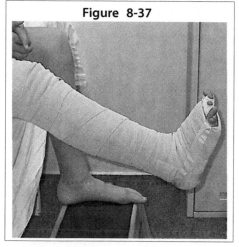	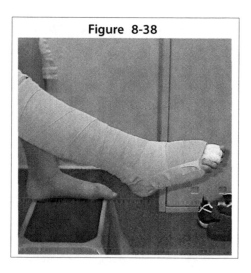

Ankle Pumps

See Figure 8-37 and Figure 8-38.

Purpose: To increase lymph flow through the ankles and lower legs.

Start Position: Sitting facing forward, with good posture and relaxed shoulders. The thighs should be fully supported by the chair seat. Alternative Positions: Standing or lying on back with legs on bed, elevated overhead, or propped against wall.

Exercise: With one foot lifted up off the floor, the patient points the foot down and holds 1-2 seconds, then flexes the ankle up and holds 1-2 seconds. The same is done with the other foot.

Ankle Waves

See Figure 8-39 and Figure 8-40 on page 176.

Purpose: To increase lymph flow through the ankles and lower legs.

Start Position: Sitting facing forward, with good posture and relaxed shoulders. The thighs should be fully supported by the chair seat. Alternative Positions: Standing or lying on back with legs on bed, elevated overhead, or propped against wall.

Figure 8-39	Figure 8-40
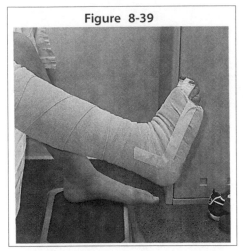	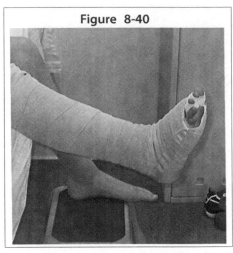

Exercise: With one foot off the floor, the patient turns the ankle in and holds 1-2 seconds, then turns the ankle out and holds 1-2 seconds. The same is done with the other foot.

Ankle Circles

Purpose: To increase lymph flow through the ankles and lower legs.

Start Position: Sitting facing forward, with good posture and relaxed shoulders. The thighs should be fully supported by the chair seat. Alternative Positions: Standing or lying on back with legs on bed, elevated overhead, or propped against wall.

Exercise: The patient raises one foot off the floor and circles the ankle, first clockwise, then counter-clockwise.

Toe Curls and Wiggles

Purpose: To increase lymph flow through the foot and toes.

Start Position: Sitting facing forward, with good posture and relaxed shoulders. The thighs should be fully supported by the chair seat. Alternative Positions: Standing or lying on back with legs on bed, elevated overhead, or propped against wall.

Exercise: The patient raises one foot off the floor, then curls and flexes their toes. Next, the patient wiggles their toes.

Advanced Exercises

Most of the following advanced exercises were designed by Drs. Casley-Smith for upper and lower body, arm and leg lymphedema. Many of the advanced leg exercises are difficult, and may be stressful to the lower back.[8] These exercises should only be done when specifically recommended by a certified lymphedema therapist for a patient who is well-conditioned.

Relaxation

Purpose: Relax muscles prior to and after exercise.

Start Position: Lying on their back on the bed or floor.

Exercise: Speaking slowly, ask the patient to begin by relaxing their stomach and hips (pelvis) so that they feel heavy and sink into the bed or floor. Then have them relax their thighs, knees, lower legs, feet, and toes. Next, ask the patient to relax their whole lower body and legs. Continue with relaxing the waist, the upper back, the chest, and the shoulders. Have the patient relax their upper arms, forearms, hands and fingers. Now, relax both arms completely. Finally, ask the patient to relax their neck, back, the sides of their head, ears, forehead, eyebrows, eyelids, nose, cheeks, mouth, and chin. Finish by having the patient relax their whole body.

Relax: At least one minute before exercise and up to 30 minutes post exercise.

Deep Breathing with Partial Sit-ups/Body Curls

See Figure 8-41 on page 178. This movement is a sit-up when the patient is on their back or a body curl if the patient is standing or sitting.

Purpose: Increase lymph flow through the trunk.

Start Position: Lying on their back with their knees bent up and feet on the bed or floor. Alternative Positions: Standing or sitting (for body curls).

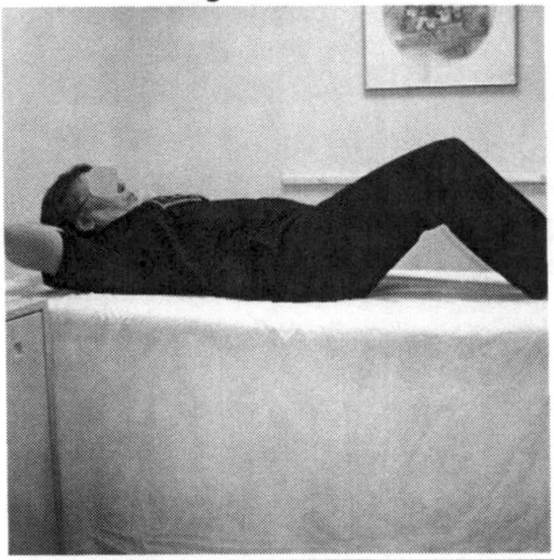

Exercise: The patient takes a full, deep breath in through their nose. Next, the patient raises their head and shoulders off of the bed or floor, reaching their hands toward their bent knees as they breathe out through the mouth strongly and fully to a 3-5 count. The patient slowly lowers their head and shoulders back down as they take in the next full breath. If the patient is sitting or standing, the patient bends the head and shoulders forward as they breathe out.

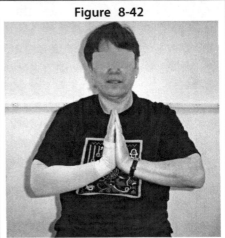

Figure 8-41

Figure 8-42

Pressing Hands Together

See Figure 8-42.

Purpose: Increase lymph flow through the chest wall and upper body.

Start Position: Sitting facing forward, with good posture and relaxed shoulders. Alternative Positions: Standing or lying on back.

Exercise: With the elbows bent, the patient places the palms of their hands together in front of their chest and presses the palms together, holds 3 seconds as they take a breath in, and then relaxes the pressure at the hands as they breathe out 3 seconds.

Broomstick Arm Raises

See Figure 8-43 on page 179.

Purpose: Increase lymph flow through the shoulders and arms.

Start Position: Sitting facing forward, with good posture and relaxed shoulders. The patient begins with arms extended at shoulder height, holding the stick with palms up. Alternative Positions: Standing.

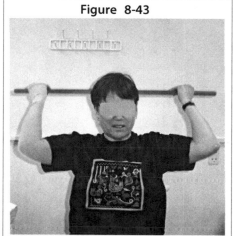

Figure 8-43

Exercise: The patient lifts the broomstick up and over their head fully and holds 1-2 seconds, then lowers the broomstick behind their head to shoulder height and holds 1-2 seconds. Next, the patient lifts the broomstick back up over their head, holds 1-2 seconds and then lowers the broomstick down to the start position at the front of their chest at shoulder height.

Bracing Against Wall with Hands

See Figure 8-44.

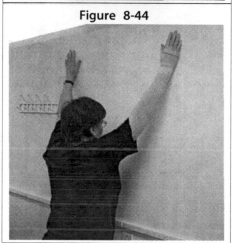

Figure 8-44

Purpose: Increase lymph flow through the chest and upper body.

Start Position: The patient stands facing a wall with their arms raised overhead and hands resting on the wall.

Exercise: The patient pushes their hands against the wall (without their body moving from the start position), holds 3 seconds, and then releases the pressure, relaxing for 3 seconds.

Playing the Piano

See Figure 8-45 on page 180.

Purpose: Increase lymph flow through the arm and hand.

Start Position: The patient stands facing a wall and raises their affected arm overhead with the fingertips resting on the wall. The heel of hand and wrist should be held away from the wall and in a neutral position.

Exercise: The patient taps the fingertips one at a time on the wall as if playing the piano, one second per fingertip.

Bouncing Knee to Chest

See Figure 8-46.

Purpose: To increase lymph flow through the upper thighs.

Start Position: The patient is lying on their back with legs straight.

Exercise: The patient bends one leg up raising the knee toward the chest and holds the knee with their hands; next, the patient gently and slowly bounces the bent knee against the body. After completing all bounces, the patient slowly lowers the foot to the bed and slides it down until the leg is straight. The patient relaxes briefly, and then does the same with the other leg.

Bouncing Both Knees to Chest

See Figure 8-47.

Purpose: To increase lymph flow through the upper thighs.

Start Position: The patient is lying on their back with legs straight.

Exercise: The patient bends both legs up raising the knees toward the chest and holds the knees with the hands; next, the patient gently and slowly bounces the bent knees against the body. After completing all bounces, the patient slowly lowers one foot at a time to the bed and slides it down until the leg is straight.

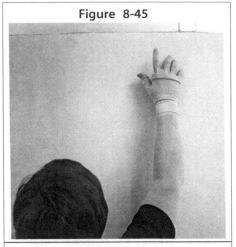

Figure 8-45

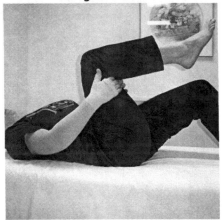

Figure 8-46

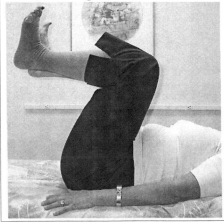

Figure 8-47

Bent Knee Seat Squeezes

<u>Purpose:</u> Increase lymph flow through the lower back, buttocks, and hips.

<u>Start Position:</u> The patient is lying on their back with the swollen leg bent. The foot of the bent leg should be even with the opposite knee.

<u>Exercise:</u> The patient tightens or "squeezes" the buttock muscles of the bent knee slowly and holds for 2 seconds, then slowly releases the buttock squeeze and relaxes. The patient may allow the body to slightly turn as if rolling toward the opposite side. The patient does the same with the other leg if it is also swollen.

Lower Back Contractions

See Figure 8-48.

<u>Purpose:</u> Increase lymph flow through the lower back, buttocks, and hips.

<u>Start Position:</u> The patient is lying on their back with the swollen leg bent and turned out to the side. The foot of the bent leg should be even with the opposite knee, and the outer thigh should rest near the bed or floor. <u>Alternative Position:</u> Standing.

<u>Exercise:</u> The patient tenses or "squeezes" the buttock muscles and slowly tilts the pelvis up toward the shoulder on the same side. This will use the muscles of the low back and trunk. The shoulder should remain relaxed during this exercise. If standing, the foot (on the same side as the contraction) will rise up off the floor about 1-2 inches.

Figure 8-48

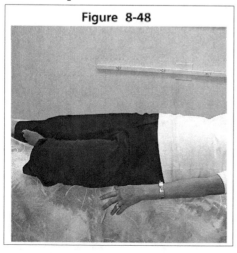

Bouncing Bent Knee Sideways

See Figure 8-49.

<u>Purpose:</u> To increase lymph flow through the upper thighs.

<u>Start Position:</u> The patient is lying on their back with legs straight.

<u>Exercise:</u> The patient bends one leg up with the knee turned sideways; next, the patient gently and slowly bounces the bent knee. After completing all bounces, the patient slowly lowers the foot to the bed and slides it down until the leg is straight. The patient relaxes briefly, and then does the same with the other leg.

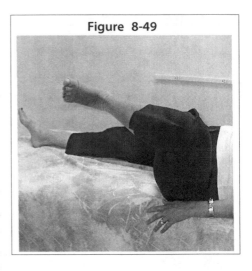

Figure 8-49

Leg Twists

See Figure 8-50 and Figure 8-51.

<u>Purpose:</u> To increase lymph flow through the hips and legs.

<u>Start Position:</u> The patient is lying on their back with their legs straight on the bed, elevated overhead, or with feet propped up against a wall.

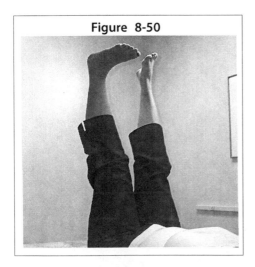

Figure 8-50

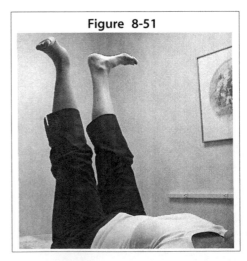

Figure 8-51

<u>Exercise:</u> The patient tightens (squeezes) one or both sides of the buttocks, causing the leg (not just the foot) to rotate out; holds the position for 3 seconds; and then slowly returns to the start position. Next, the patient twists the legs, causing the feet and knees to turn inwards, holds briefly, and then relaxes.

Bouncing Knee

See Figure 8-52.

<u>Purpose:</u> To increase lymph flow through the knee.

<u>Start Position:</u> The patient is lying on their back with legs straight.

<u>Exercise:</u> The patient lifts one knee up, raising the foot slightly off the bed; next, the patient gently and slowly bounces or flexes the bent knee. After completing all bounces, the patient slowly lowers the foot to the bed and slides it down until the leg is straight. The patient relaxes briefly, and then does the same with the other leg.

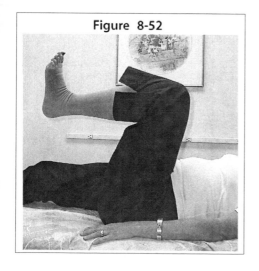

Figure 8-52

Elevated Leg Stretches

See Figure 8-53 and Figure 8-54.

<u>Purpose:</u> To increase lymph flow through the legs.

<u>Start Position:</u> The patient is lying on their back with their legs straight, elevated overhead, or with feet propped up against a wall.

<u>Exercise:</u> The patient stretches their legs, pointing their toes toward the ceiling, holds the position 1-2 seconds, and then relaxes briefly. Next, the patient flexes the feet and stretches the heels toward the ceiling, holds 1-2 seconds, and then relaxes.

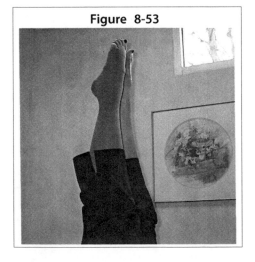

Figure 8-53

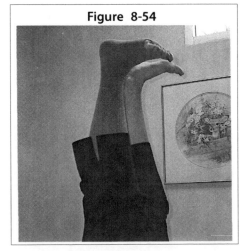

Figure 8-54

Elevated Knee Bends Sideways

See Figure 8-55 and Figure 8-56.

<u>Purpose:</u> To increase lymph flow through the legs.

<u>Start Position:</u> The patient is lying on their back with legs elevated overhead or with feet propped up against a wall; knees are straight.

<u>Exercise:</u> While keeping the heels together, the patient bends both legs as the knee turns sideways similar to a "frog leg" position. Next, the patient pushes their feet up straightening the legs fully.

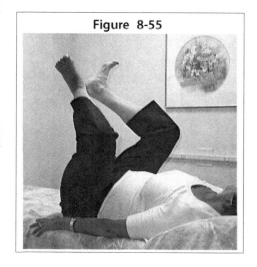

Figure 8-55

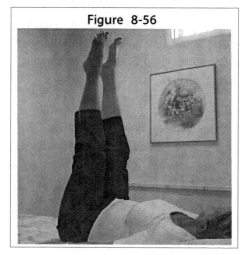

Figure 8-56

Elevated Legs Walking, Scissors, and Bicycles

See Figure 8-57, Figure 8-58, and Figure 8-59.

Purpose: To increase lymph flow through the legs.

Start Position: The patient is lying on their back with legs elevated overhead or with feet propped up against a wall; knees are relatively straight (patient may bend their knees as necessary for comfort).

Exercise: While keeping the legs elevated, the patient moves their feet forward and back as if walking; apart, together, and crossed for scissoring; and (if not propped against a wall), moves the feet in circles as if pedaling a bicycle.

Bent Knee Side to Side

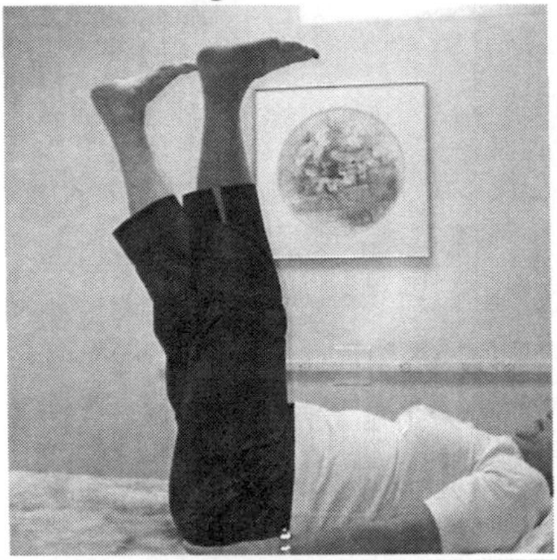

Purpose: To increase lymph flow through the buttocks and hips.

Start Position: The patient is lying on their back with the swollen leg bent. The foot of the bent leg should be even with the opposite knee.

Exercise: The patient rocks the knee from one side to the other side as far as they can without allowing the back to rise up off the floor. The patient does the same with the other leg if it is also swollen.

Figure 8-57

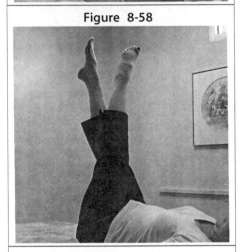
Figure 8-58

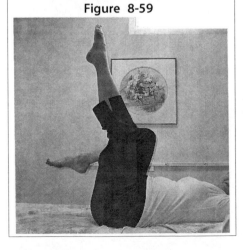
Figure 8-59

Frequently Asked Questions

Why do neck exercises for lower extremity lymphedema?

Lymph from all parts of the body flows though the neck area where it is returned to the venous circulation. Exercise and simple lymph drainage (SLD) start by stimulating the neck region to create space for lymph that will be moved by the exercises.

Why exercise with compression?

Decongestive exercises are designed to promote the flow of lymph and compression garments or bandages enhance the action of the muscle pumps in helping to move the lymph.

Can a patient with arthritis do these exercises safely?

Most of the basic exercises are easy to do and are beneficial for a variety of health-related issues. Review the exercise program with the patient's doctor or therapist to determine what exercises are safe for the patient. You may also want to explore alternative exercises. For example, aquatic exercises can be performed with a minimum of stress on the joints. What is important is finding the right combination of exercises for your patient.

Notes

1   Position Statement of the National Lymphedema Network Topic: Exercise NLN Medical Advisory Committee, 2005.

2   **The American Physical Therapy Association Book of Body Maintenance and Repair** by Marilyn Moffat and Steve Vickery. Henry Holt & Company, 1999.

3   **Modern Treatment for Lymphoedema** by Judith R. Casley-Smith and J. R. Casley-Smith. The Lymphoedema Association of Australia, Inc. 1997.

4   **The American Physical Therapy Association Book of Body Maintenance and Repair** by Marilyn Moffat and Steve Vickery. Henry Holt & Company, 1999.

5   **The American Physical Therapy Association Book of Body Maintenance and Repair** by Marilyn Moffat and Steve Vickery. Henry Holt & Company, New York, 1999.

6   **Muscles, Testing and Function Fourth Edition with Posture and Pain** by Florence Peterson Kendall, Elizabeth Kendall McCreary, and Patricia Geise Provance. Williams & Wilkins, 1993.

7   **Muscles, Testing and Function Fourth Edition with Posture and Pain** by Florence Peterson Kendall, Elizabeth Kendall McCreary, and Patricia Geise Provance. Williams & Wilkins, 1993.

8   **Modern Treatment for Lymphoedema** by Judith R. Casley-Smith and J. R. Casley-Smith. The Lymphoedema Association of Australia, Inc. 1997.

Chapter 9

Emotional Care and Support

Emotional care is an essential part of care giving. The goal is to help the patient achieve the best possible quality of life; this includes helping the patient feel better emotionally, as well as physically.

This chapter covers:

- Common emotional reactions to lymphedema and ways that you can help your patient overcome them.

- Motivation and issues that can interfere with self-care.

- The process of change and ways to help patients modify their behavior.

In addition, there is related information in the "Communicating Effectively" chapter (page 205) and the chapter on "Roles, Goals, and Relationships" (page 395).

Common Emotional Reactions

You will be a better caregiver if you understand the common emotional reactions to lymphedema and support the patient's efforts to overcome them. It is natural for patients with lymphedema to feel overwhelmed, sad, anxious, or even angry. Another common reaction is not doing self-care for a variety of reasons. This section explains each emotion and suggests ways that you can help your patient.

Feeling Overwhelmed

Many patients feel overwhelmed when they are first diagnosed with lymph-edema—especially if the lymphedema resulted from medical treatment—and again (or further) as they learn about home-care and monitoring. Sometimes it can all seem too much.

You can help someone who feels overwhelmed by lymphedema care by breaking tasks down into small pieces. Making changes in small manage-able steps helps a person feel that they are in control. Your guiding principle should be "One step at a time."

Make exercise and home-care as much fun and easy as possible. Listening to music, audio books, podcasts, or the patient's favorite television or radio programs during care activities may help.

Encourage the patient to write down questions and concerns and discuss them with the lymphedema therapist or medical team. Keep these questions in the Patient Notebook and take them to the next appointment (see page 372). It may help the patient to take notes during their appointments, or to have someone take notes for them.

Be supportive and encouraging. Discuss information until it is understood. Keep asking questions until treatment recommendations are clear.

A patient (or caregiver) will feel less overwhelmed if they ask for help and support and recognize that they have options. Encourage the patient to make a list of people who might be willing to help, and then make specific requests of these people.

Feeling Sad

Feeling sad about having lymphedema is understandable. Most people need time to grieve and come to terms with how their life has changed after being diagnosed with a chronic condition. At the same time, you do not want temporary sadness to change into chronic self-pity or to interfere with active self-care.

Here are ways you can help as a caregiver:

- When the patient feels discouraged or down, let them talk. Offer sympathy, but remain encouraging and optimistic.

- Take a positive approach. Focus on problem-solving.

- Read stories from **Voices of Lymphedema**[1] where other people with lymphedema share their inspiring, uplifting personal experiences of success and coping along with practical tips and helpful hints. Hearing people with the same condition describe, in their own words, how they lead satisfying lives despite lymphedema can be encouraging and reassuring. It is possible to control lymphedema and lead an active, fulfilling, happy life.

- Urge the patient to do things they normally enjoy and to spend time with people they like. Help them identify activities that they think are important, meaningful, or uplifting, as well as activities that are pleasurable.

- Encourage physical activity for emotional reasons. Exercise is a natural antidepressant, lifting one's spirits as well as helping to move lymph and build strength.

- Doing something enjoyable or distracting can lift a person's mood.

- During SLD and bandaging, some patients watch a favorite television show, listen to music, meditate, or follow some form of spiritual practice such as prayer or mindfulness.

- For patients who prefer to be actively involved during physical care, ask questions about their life, hobbies, interests, activities, family members, and other topics of interest to them. Notice what gets them excited and talking, and engage their attention to make lymphedema care and exercise more pleasant.

Depression

Feeling sad and sorry for oneself at times is perfectly natural. Being discouraged about dealing with a chronic condition like lymphedema is normal. But sometimes these feelings of sadness stop being mild, temporary, or occasional, and turn into depression.

Depression is a much more serious problem than brief normal sadness. Psychotherapy and/or medication may be needed if the patient shows several signs of depression. Treatment for depression can be very helpful, even life-saving. Untreated depression impairs quality of life and may interfere with immune system functioning.

Depression Warning Signs

- Feeling sad, anxious or "empty" most of the day for two weeks or longer

- Hopelessness or pessimism

- Feelings of guilt, worthlessness, or helplessness

- Irritability, restlessness, or agitation

- Loss of interest in activities or hobbies that used to be pleasurable

- Fatigue or decreased energy

- Trouble concentrating, remembering details, or making decisions

- Trouble getting to sleep or staying asleep, waking too early, or sleeping too much

- Overeating or appetite loss

- Persistent aches or pains, headaches, cramps or digestive problems that do not ease with treatment

- Wanting to die, talking about suicide, suicide plans, or suicide attempts

If the patient says they are planning to commit suicide, contact someone immediately and take emergency action to make sure the patient remains safe.

Warning signs of possible depression are shown in the box above. If you notice these signs, share your observations with the appropriate members of the patient's family, the person or agency arranging care, and the patient's health care team.

Feeling Anxious

A patient with lymphedema may feel anxious for several reasons. First, they may worry about everyday actions that can put them at risk for infection. Second, they may become self-conscious, or worry about other people's reactions, because swelling and bandages or compression garments are often visible to others. Third, just the fact of having a chronic condition that requires daily care can be scary.

Patients may be uncomfortable about needing assistance or losing their independence, and the resulting changes in their relationships with family and friends. Patients and caregivers may be embarrassed and uncomfortable with the physical aspects of care including nudity and touching.

As a caregiver you can help reduce anxiety, worry, or self-consciousness in these ways:

- Listen. Let them talk. Often just listening can be the most helpful thing you do.

- Help them identify all their fears. Encourage them to tell you everything they are afraid may happen, even those fears they think may be silly. The act of putting worries into words often helps.

- Encourage them to get facts about their worries. Find accurate information about whether fears are justified. As a general principle, the more we know, the less afraid we are. Help them plan how to discover or test out how likely or realistic their worries are.

- Help them make a plan of action based on the facts. We can cope with most anything—if we don't let anxiety talk us out of trying. A caregiver can be a coach and cheerleader.

- You can practice with them what they will say if others ask about their swelling or the compression. Rehearse until they feel comfortable and sound confident.

- Often we worry needlessly. When fears are unlikely to come true and the facts are reassuring, review the facts together. You may need to do this over and over; but with time the person should become calmer and more confident. Help them face their fears.

- If the patient is appropriately anxious because of a **real** or likely problem, encourage them to plan ways to either avoid **the problem** or cope with it.

- Offer support, encouragement, and sympathy. Encourage reaching out to people who can comfort and support them.

After you have identified specific fears or concerns, you can find ways to change the care routine to address these fears or minimize embarrassment. For example:

- Allowing the patient to wash themselves and do skin inspection in private.

- Teaching the patient self-massage for areas where they are uncomfortable being touched for SLD.

Getting Angry

Anger is a common response to uncomfortable feelings (like those discussed above) or to finding ourselves in a situation we do not like. Therefore, it is understandable that people with lymphedema may feel angry.

Even though the patient is really angry about the lymphedema, they may direct their anger at you. People who need care may lash out at those who are trying to help them and they may even get angry at people they love. When you are the target of an angry outburst, it helps to remember that other things are triggering the anger and other feelings underlie the anger. See the chapter on Emotional Demands page 395 for suggestions about coping with an angry patient.

Anger is not a feeling that happens on its own. No matter how quickly anger occurs, it is not actually the first feeling a person has. People get angry in response to some *other* feeling, such as feeling hurt, threatened, or fearful. The purpose of anger is to energize us to either solve a problem or protect ourselves from a threat.

Try to identify the problem or threat that is causing the anger. When the person you are helping is angry at you, listen sympathetically. This may be difficult, especially when the patient says things that 'push your buttons' and upset you. Take a few deep breaths and remind yourself to focus on what is underneath their anger. See "Communicating Effectively" (page 205) for tips on diffusing anger and communicating with an angry patient.

When they are calmer, ask them to tell you more about how they are feeling. In particular, ask them about anything that could be making them feel sad, hurt, threatened, overwhelmed, stressed, disrespected, or uncomfortable.

Anger is a signal of some other upsetting feeling or unresolved problem. Find out what is triggering the anger. Increased irritability can be a sign of depression, so review the signs of depression on page 191. Is the patient angry because they are depressed? Worried? Overwhelmed? Lonely?

Become partners with the patient. The two of you can become detectives, working to uncover the real, underlying problem—and solve it.

Not Doing Self-Care

Sometimes it feels easier to "run away" from problems. A patient may be trying to run away from lymphedema by giving up, by denying the need for care, by being inactive or uncooperative, or by seeking comfort through overeating. How can you respond as a caregiver?

First, you can make self-care less intimidating. Make it as easy and enjoyable as possible to do what is healthy. Encourage small changes. Praise the patient. Point out every sign of progress.

Second, you can help the patient feel more confident and able to cope. You want the patient to see himself or herself as an effective, worthwhile person. Have them talk about what they take pride in about themselves, their lives, their work, or their relationships. Ask about accomplishments and achievements. Ask about other challenges they have faced and overcome in life. Focus on their strengths and successes. Encourage them to talk about the positives they see in themselves. Remind them of these positives.

Third, you can help increase motivation to do self-care. Read on to learn how.

Motivation and Self-Care

Effective self-care takes time, thought, and energy. Changes have to be made in the patient's daily routine. Good lymphedema care means making a series of day-to-day choices and changes. Making and sustaining these changes takes motivation.

As caregiver, part of your job is to help motivate the person with lymphedema. The more motivated the patient is, the more likely they are to succeed at self-care.

In this section, we give you knowledge and tools to successfully increase and support the lymphedema patient's motivation for self-care.

First, we cover some reasons why a person might *not* be motivated to make changes that can keep them healthier. Gaining a deeper understanding of the reasons behind the problem will help you be a better caregiver. You will learn specific tips and techniques for increasing motivation.

Second, we review the steps a person goes through in the process of making the types of changes required for good lymphedema self-care. Understanding the process of change, and where the patient is in this process, will allow you adapt what you say to be appropriate for where they are in the change process and to help them move ahead to the next step.

Third, if the patient has trouble maintaining new behaviors and relapses into old patterns, we have practical suggestions for helping the patent get back on track and maintain healthy changes over time.

Some patients will not change, no matter how hard the caregiver works. Caregivers must recognize this, not blame themselves, and protect themselves. We discuss this further in the chapter on "Emotional Demands" (page 395).

The principles of motivation and the process of change are not specific to lymphedema care. You can even use these ideas whenever you want to change your own behavior.

Reasons for Lack of Motivation

Let's begin by exploring possible reasons for lack of motivation. As a caregiver, it can be frustrating and upsetting when the patient does not follow self-care recommendations. Why would someone with a chronic condition like lymphedema *not* do everything possible to take care of themselves?

It can feel as if the other person is fighting your efforts to help them. It can be hard to understand why a person would not be motivated to act in ways that can improve and protect their health. Here are some reasons people behave this way.

"Why bother?"

Some people lack motivation because they don't see how self-care will make their lives better. To want to change, a person has to believe that changing will lead to real, actual improvements in important areas of their life.

Here are some ways to address this problem:

- Point out every sign of progress that occurs as a result of your care or their actions.

- Urge them to ask their lymphedema therapist or doctor about the reasons behind self-care recommendations and what benefits they can expect.

- Encourage them to talk about how their life can improve if self-care is effective and what improvements or goals would be more important or satisfying to them. What would improve their quality of life the most?

- Share stories of other people with lymphedema whose lives improved because of good self-care. The book **Voices of Lymphedema**[2] is full of such encouraging stories.

- Search online for stories of people with lymphedema who are inspiring examples of improvement.

"Self-care is boring"

Frankly, self-care *is* boring. It can be time-consuming, repetitive, and feel restrictive. The more restricted people's lives feel, the more bored they become. People who are bored with their daily lives can be negative, sad, lonely, irritable, inactive, passive, hopeless, and unmotivated. This is a vicious cycle you want to help break.

Get the patient involved in something interesting. The antidote to boredom is having things to look forward to, being physically and mentally active, and doing things that make the person feel needed and valued.

Ask what they used to do for enjoyment. Ask about what they are good at and what is important to them. How can they make such things part of their daily life? In what ways can they use their talents—especially in ways that make them feel valued and useful? Everyone wants to feel part of something larger than ourselves.

Exercise and interesting conversation help decrease boredom. Encourage the patient to get out of the house and to walk or do some other physical activity. Encourage them to go places and talk to people they like. Encourage them to explore new activities and hobbies.

The patient's quality of life will improve. Plus, motivation for good self-management can increase because an interesting life full of valued activities is worth living to the fullest.

"I'm afraid that getting better will make things worse"

Some patients lack motivation because they think lymphedema self-management will make life harder in some way. Some worry that self-care will be too hard and demanding. Others fear that if they improve they will lose love, support, and attention from others. They may worry that if they improve, they will be expected to do too much, or to do things they can't or don't want to do.

If you think about it, it makes perfect sense that a patient would not do something they think will make life worse for them. As a caregiver, if you believe this is an issue, explore with the patient through gentle, nonjudgmental questions, what they think life will be like if they comply with self-care recommendations. What will be worse? What will be better? What will change?

Listen. This can be one of the most helpful things you can do in providing emotional care. Ask questions and listen carefully. Don't jump in right away with suggestions or even encouragement.

Help the patient talk out their worries. Ask questions and repeat back things they have said. Be caring, concerned, and curious.

Act as a sounding board. Encourage them to think about ways to handle or avoid the problems that concern them. Express your belief that they can improve their lymphedema self-care, while avoiding or coping with potential problems.

"It's no use" or "I can't"

When your patient makes statements like these, you need to take the initiative as the caregiver. Start doing care giving for the patient. Involve them one small step at a time. Use lots and lots of praise. Be supportive. Use all of the earlier tips for increasing motivation, especially the ideas suggested for boredom.

If things do not improve, talk to the patient's family, lymphedema therapist, doctor and/or to your supervisor. Maybe another problem, physical or emotional, is interfering.

Some people lack motivation because they are depressed. Depression takes away motivation to do self-care because it takes away hope. Depression can make a person feel pessimistic, negative, hopeless, helpless, and like a failure. It can make them feel overwhelmed and like giving up. It can even make patients feel they don't deserve to get better. In "Depression" on page 191, you learned some of the signs of depression.

The Process of Change

People think of making a change as something that either happens or not; you either follow the recommendations or you don't—open and shut. Researchers found that people actually go through five predictable steps (or 'stages') and have to work up to making a change. They named the five stages: Precontemplation, Contemplation, Preparation, Action, and Maintenance.

Some patients lack motivation because they are too early in the change process. Knowing where the patient is in the change process will help you understand how they are thinking and feeling, and why they act the way they do. This allows you to more successfully motivate them because different actions are needed at each step.

Precontemplation: "What problem? I don't have a problem."

What is it? This is the very earliest step in the change process. A person at this step does not think lymphedema swelling is a problem. Naturally, they are not ready to change their normal behavior and follow self-care recommendations. They see no reason to do so.

What to do? Information is needed about lymphedema, and the effects of doing (or not doing) self-care. The patient needs reasons to believe that changing their daily routine and normal behavior in order to do self-care will really make a difference.

- Encourage them to tell you what they know about lymphedema.

- Ask them what they think will happen if they do follow lymphedema care recommendations. What do they think will happen if they do not?

- Ask the patient to explain to you what doctors, nurses, or lymphedema therapists have told them. How much of this information do they understand or believe? What questions they have?

- Encourage them to ask questions and look for informed, understandable answers.

- Gently urge them to be honest with the people who treat their lymphedema.

- Share stories with them about other people's experiences with lymphedema. Sometimes before and after pictures of limbs can help a person see what a difference good self-care can make.

At this stage, you will be probably be doing all the work of care. The most you should expect from your patient is grudging, passive, reluctant cooperation. Do not expect enthusiasm or to active participation. They don't see the point.

Try to make it fun. Use praise and rewards. Bring to their attention any specific positive changes that occur because of your care. Also gently point out negative changes that occur because of lack of good self-care.

If the patient is hostile, see "Getting Angry" on page 194 and the chapter on communication skills" (page 205).

Contemplation:
"Okay, I see that lymphedema may be a problem—but I'm not sure I'm ready to do anything differently."

What is it? This is the next step closer to being ready to change. At this step, the person is aware that not following lymphedema care recommendations can be a problem, but has very mixed feelings and is not yet ready to change.

What to do? Actively encourage the patient to think about the pros—and the cons—of changing their behavior. Help them think about their current situation, the available options, and the consequences of different choices.

At this stage, your job is not to tell them why they should change. Your job is to help them tell *you* why they might want to change.

You want them to think about why they are dissatisfied with their present condition, and to talk about why and how changing might help them. Their reasons are what will motivate them—and their reasons may differ from your reasons.

- Ask what bothers them most about their lymphedema. Encourage the patient to talk about any problems caused by swelling. In what ways does their condition interfere with their life? How does lymphedema make them dissatisfied, frustrated, or unhappy?

- Have them talk to you about the benefits they expect if swelling were better controlled. How might better home care help? What improvements would they expect? What is important to them? Help them explore reasons to cooperate more actively in their home care. How would they gain from becoming more active or changing their daily life to move lymph fluid or lose weight?

- If the patient says they know self-care activities are important, but still doesn't do them, ask what stops them. Instead of telling them the benefits of change, ask them about the problems of change. How do they feel about the idea of changing? What are the obstacles or downsides? What problems do they think will arise? What might they lose if they follow self-care recommendations?

- Ask and listen with acceptance.

- Repeat back why they are dissatisfied with their present situation. This increases their personal motivation to change.

- Empathize with their dilemma.

- Encourage them to problem solve. How can they avoid any problems change might bring?

- What are their feelings about change and what would make them feel better?

- Ask them to tell you how they think things will be in six months, or in a few years, if they change—or if they don't. How will they feel physically and emotionally?

Remember, they need to convince themselves. You can't make this decision for them. At this stage, ask a lot of questions. Encourage them to talk. Listen without judging. Repeat back to them *their* words, *their* reasons to change, and *their* feelings about their plans.

Preparation: "Lymphedema is a problem and I'm getting ready to do something about it."

What is it? This is the step right before actually changing. The person has not changed yet, but is gathering information and getting ready to change soon.

What to do? At this stage, practical help from a caregiver is welcomed. Specific advice from you that would have been rejected at earlier steps is likely to be accepted now. The patient is preparing to take a more active role in activities like skin care, SLD or self-massage, and compression. They may ask more questions and want you to explain and teach.

- Help the patient plan, prepare, and organize whatever they need to take over more self-care or to make changes in daily lifestyle.

- Encourage the patient to find people who support their self-care and lifestyle changes, and to tell these people about plans to change.

This is the step when it helps for the patient to share their plans and to publicly make a commitment to putting their plans in action.

Action: "Look, I'm doing it!"

What is it? This is the step when visible, outside change takes place. The thing to remember is that all the other steps happen first and are part of the process of getting here.

What to do? This is the most exciting and satisfying stage of the change process. At this stage, the patient actively cooperates with you. They effectively carry out self-management even when you are not there.

Occasionally the patient will want your advice or help solving a problem. Most of the time your job as caregiver is to offer praise, be a cheerleader, and help with anything the patient physically cannot do for themselves.

- Encourage the patient's independence.
- Point out benefits and positive changes.

- Offer encouragement and support them if the patient becomes discouraged.

Maintenance:
"I have to keep doing this day after day, after day....?!?"

What is it? Since lymphedema self-care is a lifelong process, this step lasts the rest of the patient's life. When a patient falls back to an earlier step in the change process and stops some part of self-care, the caregiver's job is to help them return to this step.

Caregiver goals at this stage are preventing burnout and making self-management a habitual, accepted part of daily routine that can be maintained over the long haul.

What to do? Be a source of long-term, ongoing encouragement, praise, and support.

Help arrange rewards for doing self-care. The patients need reasons to sustain lifestyle changes over time.

- Help record and track changes in swelling, limb or body weight, exercise, and anything else important to the patient's quality of life and health.

- Encourage the patient to stay in touch with people who support good self-care.

- At this stage, some patients reach out to others with lymphedema and serve as a peer role model.

- Ask about what might interfere with good lymphedema care, and then encourage the patient to plan in advance for solving these problems. For example, how will they care for their lymphedema when traveling?

- Encourage the patient (and the patient's family if appropriate) to arrange rewards for continuing good self-care actions.

Read on to discover what to do if the patient stops recommended self-care. This is called having a relapse. It means the patient has temporarily gone back to an earlier step in the change process.

Dealing with a Relapse

It is common to slip back temporarily from the Maintenance step to an earlier step in the change process. If the person you are helping stops self-care, help them work their way back to the Action and Maintenance steps as follows:

- Figure out what step in the process of change the patient is on now.

- Do the suggested actions for that step.

- Treat relapses as temporary. Do not be discouraged or surprised. Help the patient restart self-care and lifestyle changes as soon as possible.

- Be hopeful, encouraging, sympathetic, and upbeat.

Relapses are valuable learning opportunities. They are chances to solve problems and to strengthen the daily routine so self-care is easier and can be continued, even when situations change or problems arise.

Notes

1 **Voices of Lymphedema** edited by Ann Ehrlich and Elizabeth McMahon. Lymph Notes, 2007.

2 **Voices of Lymphedema** edited by Ann Ehrlich and Elizabeth McMahon. Lymph Notes, 2007.

Chapter **10:**
Communicating Effectively

Good communication makes everything else possible. Bad communication can ruin a good caregiving relationship.

The following tips on effective communication will help you handle issues that arise in the course of care giving. Using them strengthens your relationship with your patient and their (or your) family members, improves your ability to care for them emotionally, and increases the other person's willingness to cooperate and communicate with you so that you are an effective care giving team.

If you want to further improve your communications skills, look for courses in effective communication at a local community college or other agency.

Respect Emotional Needs

A good caregiver meets the patient's physical and emotional care needs and increases their ability to function independently. Achieving these goals requires that you respect the patient's emotional needs.

As discussed previously in "Emotional Care and Support," lymphedema has an emotional impact. A person with lymphedema may struggle with feeling overwhelmed, sad, helpless, angry, resentful, scared, worried, uncertain, self-conscious, ashamed, guilty, stressed—or all of the above at different times! Sometimes issues from their past resurface.

Some people respond to lymphedema by becoming overly cautious; others react by ignoring appropriate precautions. Some patients ask for too much help and refuse to take appropriate responsibility for self-care; others have trouble asking for help even when it is needed and appropriate.

As a caregiver, sometimes you may need to push patients to do more; sometimes, you may need to encourage them to ask for help. Because you want to create a care giving team, you and your patient need to communicate and give feedback to each other. As their caregiver, you want the patient to feel respected, supported, and encouraged.

These books are good resources: **Living Well with Lymphedema**[1] discusses common emotional challenges of lymphedema in Chapter 8; **Overcoming the Emotional Challenges of Lymphedema**[2] covers this topic in much more detail and has many practical suggestions for family members, friends, and medical professionals.

Need for Independence

Encourage patient independence. Allow and encourage the patient to do as much for themselves as possible. Don't immediately take over if there are problems.

Help the patient find ways to do self-care. Discuss what could help them be more independent. The patient's lymphedema therapist may have some helpful suggestions.

Be prepared to give repeated encouragement and lots of praise and support. Be patient. Break down the tasks of self-care into small steps. Teach one step at a time. (See "Learning Styles" on page 211 for ideas about helping someone learn.) Have them take over self-care one step at a time. Gradually do less and less.

Need for Help

Some people need to be encouraged to ask for less help, but others need to be encouraged to ask for *more* help. Some people feel timid about asking for help because they fear that they are being a burden.

Encourage the patient to speak up and to let you know when they need assistance. Respond positively to their requests or comments. Thank them for their feedback or questions. When you help them speak up, you become a more effective caregiver. Both you and the patient are members of the care

Story: Grace and Latoya

Latoya did everything for Grace. She cleaned Grace's skin and put lotion on it, and looked for signs of infection. She measured the affected limb, wrote down the measurements. She did SLD and put on the compression garment, doing all of the work herself. She did all the chores. At first Grace was grateful and cooperative, and Latoya felt good about being helpful.

But as time passed things began to change—and not for the better. Grace became less cooperative and sullen. Latoya began to feel overworked and taken for granted. Both felt disrespected. One Friday afternoon at the end of Latoya's shift, it all came to a head.

Grace started crying and yelling, "*I feel like I'm useless. You're just taking over everything!*" Latoya was astounded and insulted. She shot back, "What are you talking about? I'm just doing what I'm supposed to. And you make me work too hard!" It was clear that things needed to be talked about.

Over the weekend, each thought about what the other had said. Since they really did like each other and wanted their relationship to continue, they talked about what could change. They realized they both would feel better if Grace was more involved in her own self-care. But Latoya tended to get impatient and take over, while Grace tended to give up and withdraw when she didn't know how to do something.

They redefined Latoya's job as teaching Grace, not just doing for her. And they redefined Grace's job as asking questions, not simply holding still. Latoya slowed down the pace of her care. She explained more to Grace and had Grace repeat the explanations. Latoya put Grace's hands on top of hers when massaging. Over time, Grace began to do SLD with Latoya's hands guiding her. Gradually Grace took over while Latoya advised and praised.

Grace's family told Latoya they couldn't believe how much happier Grace was. Grace's lymphedema was better controlled, which pleased everyone. Latoya felt better about doing the tasks that Grace was unable to do and Grace felt better about herself and being more active.

giving team and have important roles to play and information to share. Take pride in working together.

Need for Feedback

Accurate feedback makes it possible to resolve problems. Fast, accurate feedback motivates patients and caregivers to improve and guides our efforts toward success.

You need to know when compression is too tight or too loose so you can adjust it. The patient may need to tell you if they have pain or other problems. You may need to tell the patient if you see changes in swelling, skin health, signs of infection, or other problems.

Sometimes feedback is needed about other aspects of care giving such as feelings about receiving or giving care. A respectful, honest discussion can help you and your patient understand each other better and avoid or solve conflicts.

When problems arise in the care relationship, discuss them early when they are easier to resolve. Encourage the other person to do the same with you.

Need for Respect and Support

Everyone wants to feel respected. This may be one reason nearly everyone reacts better to praise and support than criticism. But people differ in their styles and personalities.

Encourage the other person to tell you when something you do or say seems respectful or disrespectful to them. Does the person you are helping respond better to warm enthusiasm or to a more matter-of-fact manner? Do they appreciate physical expressions of encouragement, like hugs, or not?

Ask them what make them feel encouraged and supported. Notice what works. See "Learning Styles" on page 211 and "Cultural Differences" on page 213.

Listening and Communicating

Good communication creates good work relationships. A good work relationship with your patient and any family members involved makes care giving more enjoyable and successful.

The 5 to 1 Rule

Good communicating means being able to disagree without hurting your relationship. Effective communication skills can make you a better, and happier, caregiver.

A secret of good enduring relationships is to have at least five positives to every one negative in your interactions. Think of it as the "5 to 1" rule.

Follow this rule—especially in the middle of a difficult discussion or a disagreement. It lets you honestly state your opinions, and still protect your relationship.

Research psychologists, such as Dr. John Gottman, found that this rule predicted whether couples would remain happily married. They watched couples during disagreements and discovered that most of the couples where the partners had at least five positive interactions to every one negative interaction remained happily married, while most of the couples with fewer positives to each negative did not.

How people communicated during disagreements predicted with nearly 90% accuracy the future of their relationship. Use what these researchers learned to strengthen your care giving relationships.

What are positives?

Here are some of the positive actions that researchers found improved communication. Do as many of these as possible. They should strengthen your relationship and help you handle disagreements more successfully.

- Pay attention to what the other person is saying.

- Lean toward the speaker with open arms and a relaxed body posture.

- Show by your facial expression that you understand and care.

- Nod your head when you understand or agree.

- Smile gently and naturally.

- Use a concerned, caring, warm, empathic, or affectionate tone of voice.

- Make eye contact, if appropriate. Most European-based cultures use eye contact to show interest, but this is considered rude in some Asian and Native American cultures (see "Cultural Differences" on page 213 for more information).

What are negatives?

These are some of the negative actions that researchers found increased unhappiness, harmed relationships, and interfered with successful problem solving:

- Sit tensely with arms folded or fists clenched and a rigid body posture.

- Turn away physically.

- Use sarcasm.

- Belittle or criticize the other person.

- Dismiss or ignore what the other person has said.

- Yell or use an angry tone of voice.

- Avoid eye contact (as mentioned above, this may vary with the person's cultural background).

Work hard to avoid doing these. Replace them with the positive behaviors described earlier.

Listening

You might think that listening and communicating are easy. Just say what you mean, right? What could be hard about that? Well, actually, a lot!

The problem is that when we speak, our listeners only hear what we say—they don't hear what we mean. In our heads, we know what our words mean; but outside, heard by someone else, those words may mean something very different.

When we listen, our problem is that we have to translate what the other person's words mean. We know what *we* think they mean. We forget that this may not be what they actually meant.

The solution to these problems is to listen in two steps:

*   **First:** pay attention to the other person. Listen as best you can to what they are saying. Try to imagine how they are feeling. Stop and really listen to their point of view, especially if it is surprising, upsetting, or different from your own.

*   **Second:** check what you heard with the other person. Before jumping to conclusions and reacting, say what you think they mean and how you think they are feeling. What you heard, or even what they said, may not actually be what they are trying to communicate.

Learning Styles

The "5 to 1" rule and good listening skills will help you, as a caregiver, communicate and teach more successfully. These are useful skills in care giving and in other relationships.

Other factors also affect learning and communication. The two we will discuss are different learning styles and cultural differences.

You and your patient are unique individuals. People learn in different ways. As the caregiver, you can help the patient learn by adapting the way you teach a skill to the patient's preferred learning style.

You can identify a patient's learning style by asking them how they learn best or by listening carefully to the words they use to describe skills. Here are some examples:

- Doing or kinesthetic learning through movement. People who learn by doing may talk about things in terms of what feels right or use other action oriented phrases.

- Listening or auditory learners learn by hearing. Auditory learners may talk about things that sound right or say that they hear you.

- Reading written information or taking notes. People who learn by reading may want to see things in writing or refer to something on paper.

- Visual or pictorial learning by seeing or visualizing. Visual learners will talk about things that look right or say that they see what you are saying.

We also discuss the use of stories with all learning styles.

Doing

Some people learn best through doing. When this is the case, get the patient physically involved in self-care, SLD, compression, and so on. For example, you could have them put their hands on yours as you do each step of the care routine. As they learn and become more skilled, alternate between you doing part of the step and having them repeat it. Next have the patient to take over midway. With your guidance, they learn as they do.

Listening

Other people learn best through listening. Being told what to do works for these patients. When care giving, the more you explain what, why, and how you are doing each step of the lymphedema care, they better they will learn. They may want to tape-record care giving sessions or recommendations.

Reading

Some people prefer to follow written directions. These patients learn best when they have instructions and information in written form to read and review. Encourage them to write notes to themselves as they learn self-management from you. Write instructions for them.

Encourage them to ask their therapist for written material and for the names of recommended books or websites.

Visual

Some people are particularly visual and tend to think in pictures. And, of course, some people cannot read. These patients learn best through seeing pictures of the skills, or seeing skills demonstrated. Illustrating the process of home care with pictures, photographs, or drawings may be particularly effective. Watching you do the home care routine is a good approach. You may want to help them videotape a care giving session.

Describing lymphedema care in terms of something visual may also help. For example, you might have them visualize the lymphatic system as the branches of a tree and SLD as moving the sap from tiny branches to bigger branches and finally into the main trunk. Or they might picture self-massage as moving water from the soggy ground into tiny streams that eventually join the river.

Stories

This last teaching approach will be most useful to you as a caregiver: telling stories. Stories help everyone learn and remember. Share stories about your own training or experiences, or encouraging stories about people who have learned to manage lymphedema successfully and live active, fulfilling lives. If you don't have stories like these, encourage the patient to ask their lymphedema therapist or to look at books (like **Voices of Lymphedema**[3]) and websites (like www.LymphNotes.com) for these stories.

Cultural Differences

We all have different personalities, backgrounds, and life experiences. You and the patient may have grown up speaking different languages or speaking the same language but using somewhat different words for certain things. Different accents can make it hard to understand what the other person is saying. These are examples of cultural differences.

If the patient uses an expression you don't understand, ask what they said or what they mean. Sometimes fear of embarrassment keeps us silent, which creates confusion. Encourage the patient to speak up and ask you if they don't understand anything you say.

Even when you share a common language, you may come from different ethnic or cultural backgrounds. You may use some words in different ways, have different views on what words are or are not acceptable, or phrase things differently. You and the patient may have different expectations about how much personal information to share, or about how much physical closeness and touching is comfortable.

People from different generations or different regions of the same country have different ways of interacting. People have different preferences about how fast or how loud to talk. What one person considers animated conversation can sound intimidating or angry to another. Different people vary in how long they pause and wait after one person has spoken, how much talking is comfortable, and how much noise or silence they prefer generally.

Ask about the patient's culture, their background, and their experiences. Ask about their preferences and expectations. Encourage them to be honest with you about what is comfortable to them, and what is not. You might talk about your own past experiences and upbringing.

Ask family members about how the patient likes to interact with others. Ask if there are any "hot button" topics that should be avoided. Be respectful of differences in religious and political beliefs. Emphasize what you and the person you are helping have in common. Look for ways you can both be enriched by your differences.

Problem Resolution

Problems crop up occasionally in even the smoothest relationships. They are just part of life. As a caregiver, you should anticipate the possibility of problems in the course of providing care.

When the patient, family member, or supervisor tells you about a problem, be grateful, even though it is uncomfortable. Why? Because talking about problems opens the door to solutions, and resolving problems strengthens relationships.

Use these five steps to help resolve problems:

1. Ask the other person how they feel and what they want. Listen carefully. Check your understanding of what they said and how they feel. Keep listening and checking until the other person confirms that you understand their point of view.

2. Find something you can agree with. If you don't agree with everything they said, maybe you can agree with part of it. Or perhaps you can agree with the goal of honest communication and solving the problem. Sometimes you can agree that you can understand how they feel even if you don't agree with what they think the problem or the solution is.

3. Be honest about any way in which you may contribute to the problem. This lets the other person know that you are listening to them and being honest, which makes them more ready and able to listen to you.

4. State your feelings and your point of view. Sometimes you have to repeat the steps above and let the other person talk some more before they are ready to listen. If you repeat the listening, agreeing, and admitting steps, eventually get back to stating your side. Your feelings and wishes are important.

5. Try to find a solution that is acceptable to both you and the other person. You want a solution that works for everyone. Solutions that leave either person unhappy are not likely to last, and can cause problems in the future.

Resolving a problem is like planning a car trip with two or more drivers. Everyone has to agree on where they're going and how to get there. Otherwise, the different drivers will drive in different directions; the car will go in circles; and no one will get anywhere!

You, the patient, and anyone else involved in planning care giving want to agree on who will do what, when, why, and how.

Notes

1   **Living Well With Lymphedema** by Ann Ehrlich, Alma Vinjé-Harrewijn, and Elizabeth McMahon. Lymph Notes 2005.

2   **Overcoming the Emotional Challenges of Lymphedema** by Elizabeth McMahon. Lymph Notes 2005.

3   **Voices of Lymphedema** edited by Ann Ehrlich and Elizabeth McMahon. Lymph Notes 2007.

Chapter 11:
Infant and Child Care

The goals of home care for an infant or child with primary lymphedema include containing the swelling to develop a better fluid balance within the child's body and maintaining healthy skin that is free of serious infections. Complete swelling reduction may not be achievable given the child's lymphatic system deficiencies.

As the child grows older, the care goals expand to include training the child to manage their own care and to minimize their risks during activities of daily living.

Successful lymphedema management requires a lifelong combination of professional treatment and home care. Swelling and care needs change as the child grows, goes through puberty, and becomes an independent adult.

An infant or child's first intensive treatment series should start as soon as possible after the time of diagnosis. An intensive is a series of daily professional treatments designed to reduce swelling. At certain ages (or stages of development) the child may benefit from additional intensive treatments that also provide an opportunity for the therapist to help the child learn, or review, self care skills.

During the first intensive there will also be a focus on establishing a home care routine. Depending on the age of the infant or child this may include:

- Helping the caregiver(s) learn the home care routine, including bandaging. Ideally all caregivers should be trained by the child's therapist.

- Teaching the child to manage their swelling according to their age and abilities.

Regular professional monitoring and care is required throughout childhood (and beyond). Here is a sample schedule:

- After the first intensive: continuation appointments once or twice a week, or as needed, to adjust the home care program as the child grows and develops.

- During childhood: follow-up appointments every three to six months to further advance the home care program. The child progressively takes on more responsibility for home care with monitoring and assistance by caregivers.

- During puberty and the teenage years: additional intensive treatments may be scheduled every year, or every other year, (usually during the school vacations) to transition the child to independent self-care. The caregiver continues to monitor and provide assistance with lymphedema management until the child is fully self-sufficient.

- Follow-up appointments continue every six months between each intensive phase, according to the patient's needs.

More frequent professional monitoring is recommended during periods of rapid growth or changes in swelling. Compression garments and aids may have to be replaced if the size of the affected area is changing.

Lymphedema care for an infant or child uses the same techniques as caring for other patients—skin care, simple lymph drainage (SLD), compression, decongestive exercises, emotional care and support, and risk reduction in activities of daily living—but adapted to suit the patient's size and abilities.

The subsections that follow cover care planning, adapting care activities, and tips for working with children.

Care Planning

Care planning for an infant or child is similar to planning for other patients; see page 331. As explained below there are additional considerations in preparing a safe care location and in scheduling care and other activities.

Care Location

These issues should be considered before treating an infant or young child:

- Find a good location for treatment such as a small bedroom where the door can be closed to confine the child to the area. A wide bed, or a comfortable carpet or mat on the floor, may be the safest place for treating a toddler.

- Child-proof the area by removing any potentially harmful items and covering any electrical outlets that are within reach.

- Find age-appropriate toys, music, or videos to hold the child's attention during care.

Care Schedule

Scheduling care for an infant or young child involves two related issues:

- Breaking care activities into smaller chunks of time.

- Giving the child some play time without bandages.

Adjust the care schedule to fit the child's limited attention span and their desire to be active. For example, the caregiver may perform 5-10 minutes of SLD with a toddler, and then allow the child to exercise or play (or both) for a short while, before completing 5-10 more minutes of SLD.

Provide some playtime without bandages to ensure development of normal feeling and movement (sensory-motor control) in the involved limb for an infant or child under the age of two who wears bandages during the day. The schedule will vary according to the child's swelling issues and caregiver time constraints. Many therapists suggest starting with bandages on for two hours, followed by bandages off for two hours, alternated throughout the day. This schedule is adjusted as the child gets older to include more time with bandages on and less time with bandages off.

Children age three and older can typically wear compression garments during the day and bandages throughout the night

Adapting Care Activities

This subsection explains how care activities can be adapted for an infant or child.

Skin Care

Maintaining good skin care can be a challenge with a child who is very active, even with appropriate guidance from parents and other caregivers. Good skin care and risk reduction techniques should be emphasized, while still allowing the child to live an active life.

Although it may seem necessary to restrict a child's activities in order to minimize the risks of injury, swelling, and infection, a better solution is to combine proactive and reactive skin care and lymphedema management with an active lifestyle. See "Skin Care" (page 45) and "Risk Reduction (page 247) for more information.

Simple Lymph Drainage

SLD sequences of strokes and circles for adults explained in "Simple Lymph Drainage" (page 67) are very similar to the techniques for infants and young children. The main differences are that the caregiver may only need their finger pads, instead of the full hand, to perform the circles and that SLD takes less time, due to children's smaller size and limited attention span.

During SLD with infants, only one or two finger pads are needed to perform the circles at the tiny lymph node clusters. See Figure 11-1, Figure 11-2, and Figure 11-3 for examples of circles at the sides of the neck, elbow, and upper thigh. When a child is in diapers, keep the diaper on during SLD. Un-tape one side of the diaper at a time to access the upper thigh and buttock area during strokes and circles.

With older infants and very young children, the pressure of the strokes and circles should be *very light and gentle.* The caregiver may only need two to

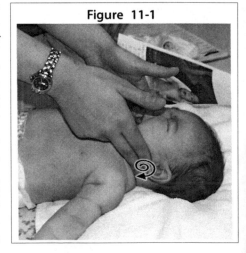

Figure 11-1

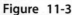

Figure 11-2

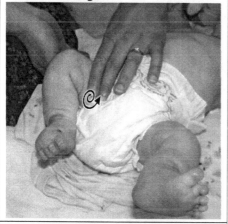

Figure 11-3

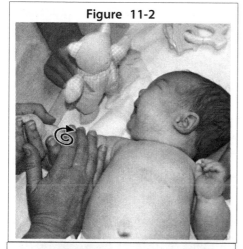

Figure 11-4

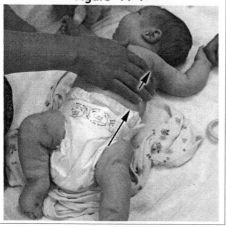

three fingers to manipulate the skin over the tiny lymph node clusters.

Circles performed along alternative pathways of the body or along stroking routes of the arms or legs may require only a few different hand placements to cover the whole limb or body pathway. Figure 11-4 shows stroking along the side pathways.

The child may not understand how to take deep breaths; however, this is a very important component of SLD with swelling due to primary lymphedema. See "Decongestive Exercises" on page 223 for ways to encourage deep breathing with young children.

Caregivers may begin teaching the child SLD in the same way one would teach a child other self-care activities such as brushing their teeth, bathing, dressing, and tying their shoes. The level of caregiver instruction should be appropriate to the child's age and ability to learn. The toddler of 1-3 years of age can be encouraged to perform simple stroking techniques on their swollen limbs. By age 4 to 5, the child can learn more advanced techniques, such as circles at the appropriate lymph node clusters, by imitating the adult.

As the child grows older, they can learn to do SLD independently based on visual cues, such as a video of SLD instruction. Older children (ages 13-18) should be able to perform a complete program based on written materials. After initial instruction, teenagers may only require verbal reminders to perform their SLD on a daily basis.

Compression Bandaging

An infant or child can use compression bandages day and night, until they grow large enough to obtain well-fitting compression garments.

Compression bandaging an infant or child offers some unique challenges. The small body size, fragility of the skin, and inability of the child to explain personal discomfort are among the issues that may arise. Basic techniques are provided in the chapter on compression bandaging (page 95). A few additional suggestions are provided below.

Because of the size of a child, smaller bandages are used to wrap the arm or leg. Also, given the fragility of the skin, especially with children under 5 years of age, soft textured bandages and extra padding should be used. For example:

- For infants under 12 months of age, use Velfoam padding and one to two-inch (2.5-5 cm) wide soft-textured bandages, such as Transelast or Mollelast, on the arm or leg (see Figure 11-5 and Figure 11-6). Toes are usually not wrapped until the child has grown larger in size.

- Between 12 and 24 months of age, soft-textured bandages can be replaced with 4 cm wide short-stretch bandages, as directed by the child's therapist.

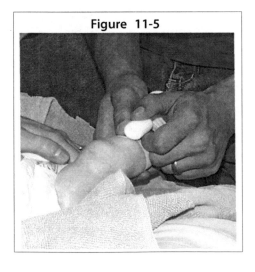

Figure 11-5

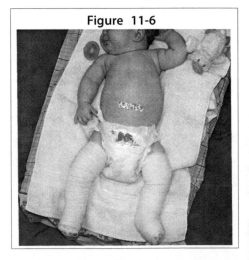

Figure 11-6

- From 2-5 years old and depending on the child's size, the child may progress to bandages that are 4 and 6 cm wide. Toe bandages may be included if the child has toe swelling.

Apply the bandage using very light tension to protect the delicate lymph structures in the child's skin. After bandages have been applied, monitor the child for any signs of excessive pressure. A young child may only be able to express their discomfort through unusual behaviors such as persistent crying or irritability. See "After Bandaging" on page 120 for instructions on checking and adjusting bandage tension.

Compression Garments

Compression garments are not typically ordered for children until they reach 1-2 years of age. Smaller garments do not to fit infants and toddlers well and children outgrow them rapidly.

Panty length garments for toddlers are available with Velcro closures that make diaper changing easier. A child who is being potty-trained will need multiple pairs of leg garments to allow for more frequent changes.

Most children will need custom-made compression garments for optimal fit and effectiveness. Even teenagers may require custom-made garments, because garments designed for adults may not fit them correctly in both circumference and length.

Decongestive Exercises

The best way to incorporate exercises into the child's routine is to be creative and playful, possibly making up funny names for the exercises. The exercise sequence should follow the lymph system beginning with the neck and shoulders, progressing to arm or leg exercises, and include deep breathing. Whenever possible, the swollen limb should be elevated during exercise, see Figure 11-7 on page 224.

For example:

- *Head turns:* the caregiver may move an infant's head or use a baby rattle positioned to the right or the left of the child to encourage him or her to turn towards the rattle.

- *Arm raises:* the caregiver can use a ball to have the child reach their arms up overhead as shown in Figure 11-8.

- *Elevated leg bicycling:* can be renamed "a bug on their back" to create a game where the child lies on his or her back and moves their arms and legs as if they were a ladybug that has gotten stuck in this position and is trying to turn over. See "Elevated Legs Walking, Scissors, and Bicycles" on page 186.

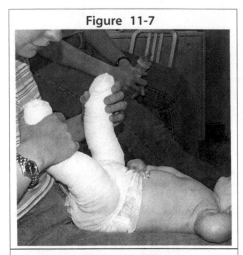

Figure 11-7

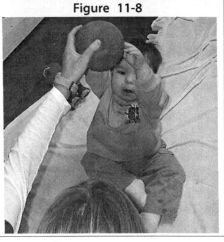

Figure 11-8

Infants naturally breathe deeply so the caregiver does not have to worry about achieving deep breathing at such an early age.

Toddlers can be encouraged to breathe deeply, by making the child laugh, or playing peek-a-boo, having them blow bubbles, or encourage them to sing.

Older children often love musical instruments, and a harmonica or another wind instrument (even whistling) can be an excellent way to encourage deep breathing. These activities can become enjoyable lifelong habits.

Most children with lymphedema are able to participate in a variety of activities. When a child plays sports, encourage them to wear proper compression and maintain good hygiene. Plan to perform SLD with the affected limb elevated after the activity or game. When appropriate, guide the child toward those sports that are less strenuous for the affected limb.

Lastly, the caregiver should be mindful of the outdoor temperature, since weather conditions can impact the child's swelling. For more information see "Sports and Exercise" on page 254.

Diet

Some children with primary lymphedema experience abdominal swelling and problems with fat digestion caused by impaired lymphatic vessels around the small intestine, a condition known as *lymphostatic protein-losing enteropathy.* The child's diet can be modified to replace long-chain fats (long-chain triglycerides) with medium-chain triglycerides (MCT), typically in the form of oil. Medium-chain triglycerides are more easily absorbed by the blood capillaries in the gut, reducing the lymphatic load from the long-chain fats and decreasing swelling in the intestinal wall.[1]

Discuss concerns about abdominal swelling and digestive problems with the child's physician. A complete medical work-up is necessary before using MCT oil.

Working with Children

Working with children offers special rewards—and special challenges. Here are suggestions for adapting your care giving for children.

You want to make lymphedema care an accepted part of the daily routine and avoid ongoing battles. Be matter-of-fact and calm. Do not skip daily care just because the child doesn't want to do it. If you skip daily care because the child objects, the child is rewarded for objecting and will resist more strongly.

Praise the child for cooperating. You may even praise each step along the way. Reward the child as soon as daily care is completed.

Find ways to make care fun and interesting or find ways to keep the child distracted. Examples of rewards and ways to interest or distract a child are found later in this section.

The younger the child is, the more you will do as caregiver. However, even with young children, teach the child about lymphedema and find ways for them to help. You are preparing them to be able to care for themselves in the future. Help them by having them do more and more over time.

Teach the child what to do as early as possible. Find ways for the child to help. Explain the reasons for daily care actions. Show them pictures of the lymphatic system. Have them draw their ideas about what they think compression does. Tell them stories (or ask them to tell you stories) about the lymphatic system and about other children with lymphedema who control their condition and do fun, exciting activities.

Point out the benefits of self-care. Talk about any improvements in their condition. Encourage them to tell you what they can do as a result of lymphedema care.

When the child complains, listen sympathetically. Letting off steam can be helpful, as long as it doesn't interfere with the actual care.

Younger children may enjoy making up stories about scientists finding a treatment where lymphedema magically goes away. With older children, you may be able to ask for their ideas about what they'd like to be different and perhaps problem-solve together.

Praise works better than criticism or punishment. Praise helps children feel competent, confident, and good about themselves. Praise builds a positive relationship with you. When children like us, they are more apt to do what we ask and to believe the things we say.

An important goal of caregiving is to help the child become as independent as possible. You are preparing them to care for themselves. As an adolescent and young adult, the child with lymphedema will want to leave home for camp or college and to travel, live, and work independently.

If you are the parent of a child with lymphedema, you not only need to educate your child, you need to educate those who are responsible for your child at day care or school. You may want to have basic written instructions for baby sitters, day care workers, teachers or school nurses. If your child is active in sports, talk with your child and the lymphedema therapist about guidelines for activities and share that information with their coaches. When your child begins to stay overnight with friends, or goes away for camp or school, work out a plan for how your child can continue lymphedema self-care away from home or explain to the adults in charge what assistance is needed. Depending on the child's age and other factors, you may want to provide written instructions for the adults in charge.

Many of these tips were contributed by Judith Sedlak, PT, CLT and Ruthi Peleg, BPt, BS, CLT.[2]

Involve the child in lymphedema care as soon as possible. They can participate by: holding materials until needed, handing you materials, helping hold down bandages, rubbing lotion, tearing tape for wrappings, or rolling bandages. Put all the steps in writing (or in pictures for a younger child) and have the child tell you what step you are on and what to do next. As soon as possible, let them help wrap. Let them measure their own limbs, or have them measure the limbs of their dolls or stuffed animals.

Distract the child with absorbing activities. Keep a box of toys that are played with only during lymphedema care. Rotate the toys and add new toys to maintain interest. Make a long list of activities they really enjoy and alternate activities. Here are some ideas: watching favorite TV shows or DVDs, listening to music, playing video games, playing with coloring books or sticker books, drawing, singing, playing word games (the kind you might use during a long car ride), looking at picture books, being read to, reading, telling favorite stories, recalling special times or happy memories, planning fun activities for afterward, and playing pretend from favorite stories, shows, movies, etc.

Use rewards. Rewards can be verbal such as praise. Praise the child during and after compression. Comment on their cooperative behavior, how big they are getting, how helpful they are being, and how proud you are of them. Be specific in your praise. Tell them exactly what they did. Praise them to others in their hearing.

Rewards can be: hugs, special time with you doing a favorite activity, time with a special toy or game, TV/DVD/videogame/Internet time, money, outings, treats, putting stickers on their bandages, or putting stickers on the calendar and earning rewards with their stickers. Point out how much faster compression goes when they cooperate. Use the "extra saved" time to play a game of their choice with them.

Notes

1   **Textbook of Lymphology for Physicians and Lymphedema Therapists** by M. Földi, E. Földi, and S. Kubik (eds.). Urban & Fischer, 2003. p. 310.

2   **Voices of Lymphedema** edited by Ann Ehrlich and Elizabeth McMahon. Lymph Notes 2007.

Chapter **12:**

Special Situations

This chapter provides tips for lymphedema care in these special situations:

- Working with elderly patients (below).

- Patients who are obese (page 235) or wheelchair-bound (page 236).

- Palliative care for terminal patients (page 237).

- Treating weeping lymphedema (page 238.

- Using a sequential compression pump (page 240).

- Kinesio taping for lymphedema (page 241).

Tips for Working with Elders

Just as working with children offers certain rewards and challenges, so does working with elders. Older people have the benefits of more life experience. They often bring more wisdom, more problem-solving skills, and more perspective to the task of lymphedema care than many other patients.

On the other hand, they may also have multiple medical problems. They may be physically weaker. They may be less able to learn and remember new information than they were in the past. However, it is important to recognize that knowing a person's age does not predict their level of mental or physical functioning.

People age at different rates. The person is more important than the birth date. Some people at eighty years old are as mentally and physically active as others are at fifty.

General Tips

Everyone wants respect. Treat an older person with the same interest and respect that you would treat a younger adult.

An older person may have more medical problems than a younger person. Ask if medical problems affect their ability to perform lymphedema self-care activities. They may have less flexibility, less strength, or poor balance. Have the patient do those activities that are within their abilities and help them maintain a level of independence. For example, if the patient can transfer in and out of bed, don't automatically pull them into a standing position or lift their legs onto the bed. Allowing the patient to move on their own may take longer but it provides both psychological and physical benefits.

Older patients are also more likely to be taking multiple medications. Medicines can have side effects as well as benefits. You may want to know if their medications are causing sleepiness, dizziness, anxiety, irritability, or other side effects that could affect your work with the patient.

Hearing lessens as we age. You may need to speak more loudly, more clearly, or more slowly than usual to be understood.

Eyesight worsens with age. You may need to write things in larger print. You may need to read instructions if the print is too small for the patient to read. Lots of light, and perhaps a magnifying glass, can help an older person see better and read better.

In general, learning new skills and remembering new information become harder with age. Be prepared to repeat information and to remind the patient what they are about to do and why they are doing it. If possible, write down information that you want an older person to remember. For example, if your patient wants to take off their bandages earlier than scheduled, you can write a note on a piece of tape and stick it on the bandage saying 'Do not remove your wraps' or put a sign on the bathroom mirror with the daily schedule 'Morning: remove bandages and put garment on, Evening: take garment off.'

What is Normal?

Some changes are normal with aging and are not causes for concern. For example, it is normal for an older person to occasionally forget names or appointments. It is normal to occasionally forget what we were about to say and to have trouble finding the right word. As we get older, we can forget the day of the week, where we were going, or why we came into a room. It is normal to temporarily misplace items like keys or a wallet. It can become more difficult to balance a checkbook.

Sometimes people's personalities do change with age. They can become more rigid, irritable, or suspicious and less adaptable to changes. It is perfectly normal to feel occasionally sad, moody, or weary of work or social demands.

Some changes are not normal and may be cause for concern. Age, even advanced age, does not mean that a person is no longer mentally active or interested in things. Aging is not a reason to become depressed, hopeless, and unable to enjoy things.

Signs of Trouble

Certain changes are not normal signs of aging and may be signs of trouble. Sudden onset of the following symptoms may indicate a stroke; treat this as a medical emergency and call 911, or your local emergency services number, and get medical help:[1]

- Trouble walking, sudden dizziness, changes in balance or loss of coordination.

- Difficulty speaking, slurred speech, or word finding problems.

- Paralysis, weakness, or numbness on one side of the body.

- Impaired, blurred or blackened vision, or seeing double.

- Headache that is severe or unusual and may be accompanied by a stiff neck, facial pain, vomiting or altered consciousness.

The following changes may be signs of physical or emotional problems. Immediately alert your employer, supervisor, family members, or the doctor in charge if the person you care for is:

- Suddenly much sleepier or unable to sleep.

- Suddenly behaving inappropriately or acting very different from their normal self.

- Persistently tearful or anxious, feeling sad, hopeless, or worthless, or talking about wanting to die.

- Getting more and more forgetful, confused, or difficult to understand, or becoming less and less interested in anything.

Alzheimer's Disease or Dementia

Alzheimer's disease or other conditions may cause dementia. Dementia is different from normal age-related memory changes as explained in "Alzheimer's vs. Normal Aging" on page 233.

If your patient has been diagnosed with Alzheimer's disease or dementia, you should remain aware of their condition in order to protect yourself and the patient. You can adapt the way you interact with your patient, as explained below, to minimize frustration.

Alzheimer's is a progressive illness where the patient's ability to think and remember declines over time. For more information, see the Alzheimer's Association website (www.alz.org).

Tell someone in charge if you notice that the patient is doing things that could result in harm to themselves or others. This may include wandering outside and getting lost, becoming agitated and violent, or forgetting things on the stove that could start fires.

Alzheimer's and dementia can affect lymphedema care in many ways:

- People with dementia forget more often and find it very hard to remember new information. It can be hard for them to plan or complete everyday tasks. They may lose track of the steps involved in lymphedema self-care. Be prepared to explain things over and over and to answer the same questions repeatedly.

Alzheimer's vs. Normal Aging

Someone with Alzheimer's disease symptoms	Someone with age related memory changes
Forgets entire experiences	Forgets part of an experience
Rarely remembers later	Often remembers later
Is gradually unable to follow written/spoken directions	Is usually able to follow written/spoken directions
Is gradually unable to use notes as reminders	Is usually able to use notes as reminders
Is gradually unable to care for themselves	Is usually able to care for themselves

- A person with dementia may forget simple words or substitute unusual words. This makes it hard to understand what they are saying. For example, they may want the bandage winder but ask you for "that thing that goes around."

- People with dementia can become lost in their own neighborhood, forget where they are and how they got there, and not know how to get back home. As a caregiver, you may need to stay closer to them than you did in the past or than you would with other patients. You may need to lock doors so they can't wander outside or into dangerous areas.

- Patients with Alzheimer's may show poor judgment or dress inappropriately. They may put garments on inside out, put compression garments over other clothing, or forget to wear compression. Rather than arguing with them, try distracting them for a few minutes; then continue with lymphedema care.

- Someone with dementia may have difficulty with complex mental tasks. For example, they may forget how to use numbers. They are more likely to remember simpler tasks, things they have done many times, and things they learned long ago. Try to find simple, repetitive tasks for them to do when helping with lymphedema care. Someone with Alzheimer's who has cared for their own lymphedema for many years may be able to do more self-care than someone who developed lymphedema recently. Keep explanations simple. Notice what the person can actually do and adjust your expectations to match.

- A person with Alzheimer's disease may put things in unusual places that make no sense, like putting a wristwatch in the sugar bowl. You may need to take responsibility for storing lymphedema supplies. You may even need to lock up supplies so the patient can't move them to unexpected places.

- Someone with Alzheimer's disease may show rapid mood swings—from calm to tears to anger—for no apparent reason, and their personality can change dramatically so they become extremely confused, suspicious, fearful, or dependent. Be prepared to be very patient and remember that this is the disease, not the person. Be soothing and calm. Do not argue with them about things they say that aren't true, such as saying they don't have lymphedema or that a deceased spouse is alive. Use distraction, soothing, and good general communication skills. Talk to your employer, supervisor, or the doctor in charge if this begins to happen or is getting worse.

- Alzheimer's disease can make a person become very passive, for example sitting in front of the TV for hours (when they did not do this before), sleeping more than usual, or not wanting to do usual activities. This can interfere with exercise or self-care. Sometimes gentle encouragement is helpful in getting the patient to cooperate with care. In the early stages of Alzheimer's, reminders such as a written schedule can help. Follow a routine. Tell the person what you are going to do. Remind them a few minutes before starting care. Give them time to get ready.

Obese Patients

Obesity combined with lymphedema can be difficult to treat and frustrating for the caregiver and patient. There are success stories demonstrating that a supportive team can help a bedridden patient reduce their swelling, lose weight, and be able to walk again (see "AZ Goes to Wal-Mart" in **Voices of Lymphedema**[2]).

Lymphedema and obesity are linked together and treatment of both conditions must be approached in a frank and supportive way. Some patients may be in denial about their obesity and want to focus on just treating edema, but this is not realistic. In general, patients who are able to maintain their weight, or lose weight, benefit from lymphedema treatment while those who continue to gain weight respond poorly.[3] Patients should ask their health care providers if they have a medical condition that may contribute to obesity (such as thyroid or endocrine disorders) or lipedema (see page 26), and about medical options for obesity treatment.

Daily lymphedema care for obese patients may be modified in several ways:

- Skin care is especially important because obese patients have an increased risk of skin infections, especially if they are also have diabetes. Good hygiene and moisture control are important for preventing skin infections.

- Foot care and foot infections may be an issue because the feet (and other areas) can be hard for the patient to reach or see. Long-handled tools for bathing, dressing, or skin inspection are available at medical supply companies.

- SLD, the use of compression, and decongestive exercise may be limited by the patient's mobility constraints and other health issues.

- Compression bandaging is often used instead of compression garments or aids. If garments or aids are used, they are more likely to be custom-made.

- Depending on the size of the patient, more bandages may be required for each limb, it may take two or three people to apply the bandages, and bandaging will take more time (up to an hour per limb).

If your responsibilities as a caregiver include managing the patient's diet, ask the doctor for help with weight control. The doctor may be able to recommend a specific diet or refer the patient a dietitian or weight management program. If you are not responsible for the patient's diet, please try not do anything that would undermine weight control efforts.

Caregivers working with obese patients need to protect themselves:

- Physically from lifting injuries and stress, see "Body Mechanics" (page 383). Depending on the patient's size and mobility, care may require multiple people and special equipment for lifting, transfers, weighing, and position changes.

- Psychologically from burnout, see "Emotional Demands" (page 395). Both obesity and lymphedema can be treated but they are chronic conditions and the treatments take time; manage your expectations and celebrate small victories.

Wheelchair-Bound Patients

When caring for a patient who spends most of their time in a wheelchair or power chair:

- Feet and legs affected by lymphedema should be elevated as often as possible.

- Hands and feet that are bandaged may need modified bandages (see below) to avoid slipping during transfers.

- Encourage the patient to stand up or walk as much as they can safely throughout the day. Simply standing helps improve circulation.

- Have the patient exercise from the wheelchair as much as they are able. See "Basic Exercise Routine for Lower Body and Leg Swelling" on page 151.

If the patient is not able to exercise on their own, the caregiver may perform the exercises by moving the patient's legs through the specified motions. This may be through:

- Active Assist exercises where the patient does part of the exercise but is not strong enough to perform the complete motion on their own.

- Passive Range of Motion, where the caregiver moves a paralyzed limb.

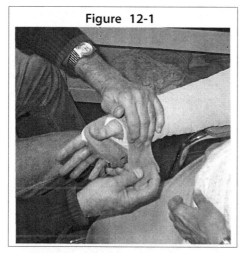

Figure 12-1

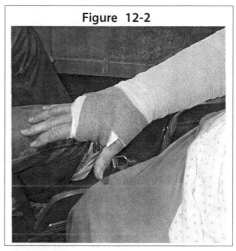

Figure 12-2

Hand and Foot Bandage Modifications

Figure 12-1 and Figure 12-2 show the caregiver applying a self-adhering elastic bandage over the patient's hand bandages to provide extra grip so that the patient may safely transfer in and out of her wheelchair and use crutches without slipping.

Self-adhering bandages can also be used over the bandages around the foot for extra grip, although shoes or anti-slip socks better protect the patient from slipping and help keep the bandages clean. Self-adhering bandages include Coban and Colastic.

Be careful not to pull the bandage too tightly or apply additional pressure when applying an extra elastic wrap over the short-stretch bandage.

Palliative Care

The goal of palliative or hospice care is to keep the patient as comfortable as possible, given their situation. Simple lymph drainage can minimize swelling, decrease symptoms of pain, and aid relaxation and sleep. SLD has the added benefit of creating an opportunity for connection with the dying patient.

Patients who are near the end of life may not be able to tolerate parts of lymphedema care for varying reasons. For example, exercising or even having someone passively move the limbs, may be too painful, too fatiguing, or cause oxygen depletion that triggers physical and psychological distress.

Putting on or removing a compression garment can be too fatiguing or painful. It can also damage the skin, which may become very fragile.

Check with the patient's doctor and lymphedema therapist to see what care is appropriate and allow the patient to select the aspects of care that they find comfortable, comforting, or beneficial. Anticipate that the patient's needs and desires may change over time.

At some point, all care for lymphedema and other disease conditions may need to stop. Families and patients often need to be given permission by healthcare providers to stop care when the risks outweigh the benefits. Usually the frequency of care will have already been reduced before care is totally discontinued.

Changes to the care routine may include:

- Skin care: to maintain skin integrity and comfort. Continue skin inspections to be aware of any developing problems.

- Lymph drainage: self massage, SLD, or MLD as desired and available.

- Compression: reduced pressure bandaging, compression garments or aids as desired for comfort and pain control.

- Exercise: gentle passive or active exercises to maintain mobility and limb function, if comfortable.

- Elevate swollen limbs and provide support to relieve joint pressure.

Weeping Lymphedema

Sometimes, excess lymph will seep through the skin of a swollen limb; this is called *weeping lymphedema* or *lymphorrhea*. The first appearance of weeping lymphedema may frighten the patient or caregiver. If weeping lymphedema develops in an affected area that has not had this condition in the past, contact the patient's therapist for care instructions.

Weeping lymphedema indicates there are multiple tiny openings in the skin, and is considered to be an open wound even though there is no bleeding. Follow the instructions provided by the patient's lymphedema therapist and doctor for wound care and infection control.

Typically, weeping lymphedema is treated by compression bandaging with gauze, ABD pads (also known as abdominal pads or absorbent wound dressing pads), or diapers under the bandages to absorb the moisture.

Use clean technique to minimize the risk of infection when wrapping a weeping area:

- Wash your hands with soap and water before working with the wound.

- Wear clean disposable medical gloves when working on the affected area.

- Remove old wound dressing materials, double bag and seal the soiled dressings for disposal.

- Clean the limb as directed.

- Apply wound dressings directly from the package to the skin. Do not let the dressing contact any unclean surface; throw away any contaminated dressings.

- Wash your hand with soap and water after working with the patient's wounds.

Depending on the amount of fluid produced, padding and bandages may have to be changed several times a day. Weeping typically responds quickly to compression bandaging and dries up within 7-10 days. Consult the patient's therapist if the condition does not respond to treatment as expected.

If the patient has a history of weeping lymphedema, the presence or absence of weeping should be noted in the Weekly Care Plan record.

A significant increase in the amount of weeping, a change in the color of the fluid, or an unpleasant odor may indicate that the area is becoming infected; notify the patient's medical care provider and therapist.

Sequential Compression Pump

Sequential compression pumps are FDA-approved lymphedema treatment devices that simulate the effects of lymphatic drainage through the action of special garments with multiple air chambers. A device controller inflates and deflates chambers in sequences that are designed to promote lymphatic drainage. Examples include the Flexitouch system from Tactile Systems Technology, Inc. (www.flexitouch.com) and Lympha Press from Mego Afek (www.lympha-press.com).

Keep in mind:

- Pneumatic devices are not appropriate for all patients. The patient's doctor is responsible for evaluating suitability and prescribing a treatment device in cooperation with the patient's therapist.

- A device can assist with some aspects of lymphatic drainage, but the patient should continue with the other elements of daily lymphedema treatment including skin care, lymphatic drainage (MLD or SLD), compression, and exercise (see "Complete Decongestive Therapy" on page 30).

- A mechanical device is only beneficial if it is used regularly and correctly. Just having the device but not using it will not help.

- Devices that are not properly fitted or used can be harmful. If the patient has multiple garments, such as a sleeve and a jacket, it is important that both parts be used as directed.

One concern is that a pneumatic device can move excess fluid out of the areas covered by the garments and into other parts of the body. Proper device usage can involve simple lymph drainage (SLD) before using the device to make space for displaced fluid and SLD again after using the device to remove displaced fluid. If this has been recommended, it is important that the caregiver follow these instructions. If swelling develops in other areas—such as the trunk, breast, or genitals—discontinue device use and contact the patient's therapist.

If the patient uses a pneumatic device for lymphedema treatment:

- Device use should be included as one of the activities in the Weekly Care Plan (see page 333) developed in cooperation with the patient's therapist. The Care Activity Form should describe the steps required for preparing the patient and using the device.

- The Equipment Form (see page 315) for the device should include information on the device company contacts in the customer service department and the local representative or trainer.

- Caregivers should be trained by the patient's therapist or a trainer from the device company on the proper setup and operation of the device.

- Entertainment, such as television or watching a DVD, may make using the device more acceptable to the patient.

Each device is different and caregivers should be trained by the manufacturer on the correct usage of the device. In general, caregiver responsibilities will include:

- Preparing the patient to use the device. Typically, this will involve removing bandages or compression garments, performing skin care, and some preparatory SLD.

- Setting up the device correctly with all connections and settings.

- Helping the patient into the garments and assuring proper fit and placement.

- Connecting the garments to the control unit, setting, and starting the device.

- Monitoring usage and operation during the treatment period, typically an hour.

- Removing the garments from the patient and storing the equipment.

- Post- usage SLD, if recommended, followed by the remainder of the daily care routine including compression and exercise.

Kinesio Taping

Kinesio Tex Tape is a specialized elastic therapeutic tape that has proven to be useful in some aspects of lymphedema treatment. This tape can be used to direct lymph flow away from an affected area or to stabilize joints affected by lymphedema. It is particularly helpful on the trunk and in other areas where it is difficult to apply compression.

Kinesio tape will stretch in one direction and comes pre-stretched on a paper backing. When Kinesio tape is used to guide lymph flow, it may be shaped into two parts: an anchor and one or more tails. The anchor or base is a full-width area of tape with no tension. The tails or fingers are narrower working strips of tape that are applied with some tension.

Kinesio tape is comfortable to wear and an average application will stay in place for 3-5 days. The patient may shower or bathe with the tape on. Tape should be protected from hair dryers or other heat sources because the adhesive is heat activated.

Tape should be carefully removed within five days by pressing the patient's skin away from the tape as the tape is gently lifted. If necessary, baby oil, olive oil, or medical adhesive remover (available from medical supply stores) can be used to make the adhesive easier to remove. The skin should be allowed to rest for 24 hours (or more) before tape is reapplied. Although the tape is latex free, some patients may be allergic to the adhesive or other components; test in a small area if your patient has a history of allergies.[4]

The patient's lymphedema therapist will decide if Kinesio tape is appropriate for a patient, what type and size tape to use, and how the tape should be applied. Do not substitute other types of tape, change products, or change tape usage without checking with the patient's therapist.

The therapist should demonstrate how to cut the tape into the desired shape and size or provide pre-cut pieces. Typically, tape is cut to the length of the area to be treated and partial lengthwise cuts are made to form the anchor and the tails. You may want to save the paper backing as a template.

The therapist should teach the caregiver how to apply and remove the tape and give the caregiver a chance to practice.

If you are using Kinesio tape:

- Do not apply the tape if the skin is irritated or there are signs of an infection.

- If there is an indication of a rash or allergic reaction, remove the tape immediately. If the reaction is severe, contact the patient's therapist or doctor.

- Skin should be clean and free of oils or lotions prior to tape application. This may mean changing the daily care routine so that tape is applied after SLD and not immediately after applying moisturizer.

- Skin prep pads may be used to clean and prepare the skin before taping.

- If the patient has a lot of body hair, trimming the hair or shaving the area to be taped may help the tape stick and to make tape removal more comfortable.

- Tape removal is easier when the patient has just bathed and the tape is moist.

In Figure 12-3, Kinesio tape has been applied to the patient's back. The narrow tails, or fingers, encourage the flow of lymph from the swollen area toward the anchor or base. The wider base acts like a funnel to help the lymph flow across the midline to the unaffected area of the back where it will return to the normal lymph flow.

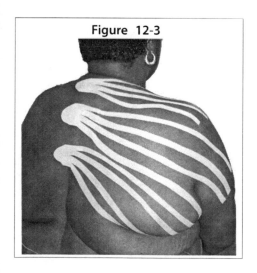

Figure 12-3

Notes

1   "Stroke" by the Mayo Clinic Staff. Available at
     www.mayoclinic.com/health/stroke/DS00150, accessed 2008-07-28.

2   **Voices of Lymphedema** edited by Ann Ehrlich and Elizabeth
     McMahon. Lymph Notes, 2007.

3   "Morbid Obesity and Lymphedema Management" by Caroline Fife,
     Susan Benevides, and Gordon Otto. *Lymph Link*, July-September
     2007.

4   **Kinesio Taping for Lymphoedema and Chronic Swelling** by K. Kase
     and K. R. Stockheimer. Kinesio USA, 2006.

Section **III**:

Activities of Daily Living

Sometimes caregivers assist with, or participate in, activities of daily living with a person with lymphedema. For those who are involved in these activities, we provide suggestions for:

- Risk reduction tips for protecting the skin and adapting activities, including sports and exercise, travel, and sleep comfort.

- First aid for areas affected by lymphedema.

- Diet and nutrition for lymphedema patients (and caregivers).

For more suggestions about activities of daily living, travel tips, and stories of how people have adapted their activities for lymphedema, see Voices of Lymphedema[1].

Notes

1   **Voices of Lymphedema** edited by Ann Ehrlich and Elizabeth McMahon. Lymph Notes, 2007.

Chapter **13:**
Risk Reduction

Life involves activities that can cause the patient's lymphedema to fluctuate. The caregiver's goal is to help the patient make informed decisions about their activities, and—in some cases—modify activities to reduce their risk of increased swelling.

This chapter provides specific suggestions for:

- Understanding factors that may contribute to fluctuations in swelling.

- Protecting the skin.

- Balancing beneficial and high risk activities, and ways to minimize swelling.

- Sports and exercise programs.

- Traveling.

- Sleep comfort.

Understanding Fluctuations

Lymphedema-related swelling is affected by a variety of factors including changes in activity (see below), temperature, and barometric pressure. Understanding the triggers that increase swelling will help the caregiver and patient manage the patient's condition.

Temperature

The body responds to heat by increasing blood circulation to the skin, which helps cool the body and maintain a consistent core body temperature. As blood circulation to the skin increases, a greater amount of fluid (blood plasma) leaves the blood vessels and enters the tissue spaces. With normal lymphatics, the lymph vessels carry the extra fluid away quickly once the person cools off. When the lymphatic system is impaired, the extra fluid is removed more slowly, which can result in an increase in swelling.

Normal room temperatures generally do not affect the swollen limb. Relatively cool temperatures (that make the body shiver) can slow the flow of lymph. Even colder temperatures (such as an ice pack) can lead to a rebound effect where blood flow to the cold limb is enhanced after the cold stimulus is removed, causing an increase in swelling.

Because extremes of temperature may increase swelling from a patient's lymphedema, the caregiver should encourage the patient to keep shower, hot tub, and Jacuzzi water temperatures below 102° F (38.9°C); and limit exposure to heat, including heating pads, to less than 15 minutes.[1] Swimming pool temperatures should range from 68-94°F (20-34°C).[2] Extreme temperatures can also damage the integrity of the skin; resulting in sunburns in the hot sun or dry chapped skin in cold wintry weather. Have the patient use protective clothing and lotions, and limit the time they spend outdoors under these conditions.

Pressure

Air pressure and water pressure influence lymphedema-related swelling by increasing or decreasing tissue pressures and lymph production. Fluctuations due to barometric pressure and weather patterns are unavoidable and the best response is to manage the swelling through SLD, exercise, and increased compression if necessary. Increased swelling when flying or at high altitudes can be minimized by modifying the patient's travel routine as explained in "Travel Tips" on page 255.

Protect the Skin

It is important to avoid skin damage or injury in lymphedema affected tissues because of the increased risk of infection and slow healing. The caregiver should advise the patient to take specific steps to protect their skin and lymphatic system.

Cover Affected Areas

Protect the skin from cuts, scratches, irritation, or burns. Coverings may include hats, long-sleeved shirts, long pants, and sunscreen (SPF 15+). Gloves are important when skin is exposed to harmful detergents (such as bleach and bathroom cleansers), when working outdoors, cleaning fish, or doing anything that may involve contact with feces. Oven mitts (not pads) are recommended for grasping hot items from the stove or oven.

Careful with Sharps

Be extra careful with sharp objects:

- In the kitchen, prevent cuts by taking extra time to concentrate fully when using knives, graters, or vegetable peelers.

- When using nail clippers, cuticle removers, or disposable shavers, try to avoid cutting the skin and consider sanitizing tools with alcohol between uses.

- When shaving, be particularly careful in areas where there is poor sensation due to lymph node removal or neuropathy.

- When working in the yard or shop, be especially careful with tools and other equipment.

Use Insect Repellent

Use insect repellent or bug spray during seasons when bugs are more prevalent. DEET-based insect repellents provide the most effective protection and are recommended by the Center for Disease Control.[3] Apply bug spray according to the manufacturer's instructions. For children, repellent with less than 10% DEET is best. Bug bites can be quite itchy and may tempt the patient to scratch, leaving small breaks in the skin and providing an opportunity for bacteria to enter the body.

No Needles

Request that blood work and injections be done in an uninvolved limb. Even though health care providers use sterile technique, needle sticks or injections still pierce the skin.[4] For individuals with thigh swelling and diabetes, insulin injections are best done in the upper part of the stomach. Patients should not get tattoos or body piercings in affected areas.

No Blood Pressure

Avoid having blood pressure readings taken on the affected limb. A blood pressure cuff can alter or damage lymphatic function.

Clothing and Accessories

Clean clothes, including socks, should be worn each day, since soiled clothing can increase the risk of skin infections. Avoid tight or restrictive clothing. Tight bras, underwear, socks, and jewelry can cause swelling by constricting lymph flow; a heavy purse or backpack resting on the patient's shoulders can have the same effect. The caregiver should make sure the patient's clothing and accessories are loose and comfortable, never leaving indentations in the patient's skin.

Shoes and Socks

Make sure the patient's shoes fit properly, are supportive and comfortable, and have sufficient foot and toe space. Shoes that are too tight may increase skin irritation when the foot is swollen. Patients should wear clean socks every day and alternate shoes every other day. Anti-fungal powders may also be used inside shoes. Consider socks or liners containing silver which protects against fungus and bacteria; be sure and follow the specific care instructions for silver garments.

Socks and shoes are particularly important for protecting feet from microorganisms and unseen objects on the floor or outdoors, such as pins, tacks, broken glass, or small pebbles which may cause injury. When traveling, make sure the patient wears slippers or socks in hotel rooms and water shoes in public showers and pools where fungal infections are common. It is best to avoid bare feet in any public area, including dressing rooms, shoe stores, and treatment areas at medical facilities.

Posture

Other activities that patients should avoid due to potential lymph constriction include: sleeping with the swollen arm under the body (see "Sleep Comfort" on page 256), crossing one's legs for an extended period of time, and allowing the involved arm or leg to dangle without support.

Dental Care

Good dental care is recommended for patients—especially patients with head or neck lymphedema— to minimize the risk of bacteria entering the bloodstream through bleeding gums. Encourage the patient to:

- Gently and regularly brush (with a soft-bristled toothbrush) and floss their teeth.

- Gargle with an antiseptic mouthwash (such as Listerine) to reduce the amount of bacteria in the mouth if the gums bleed after brushing or flossing.

- Inform the dentist that they have lymphedema and reduced immune system effectiveness in the affected areas. The dentist will determine the need for prophylactic antibiotics based on the risk factors and planned procedures.

Massage

Massage of the affected area, or areas at risk for lymphedema, by anyone other than a lymphedema therapist should be avoided, especially aggressive or deep muscle massage. Any rubbing of swollen areas should be gentle to prevent excessive blood flow to affected skin.

Activities

Bathing, dressing, cooking, cleaning, doing yard work, performing job duties, exercising, and traveling all necessitate the use of our arms and legs. While some activities are easy and not stressful to the body, other activities are more difficult and may place strain on a limb or increase the heart rate (and lymph formation). Swollen limbs respond to activity with either a decrease or increase in swelling.

Activities that are more likely to decrease swelling are referred to as beneficial activities, whereas activities that are more likely to increase swelling are known as high risk activities.[5] Although the patient's lifestyle may provide a relative balance of light and heavy activities, rarely does swelling stay the same.

Beneficial Activities for the Arm and Upper Body

The patient should be encouraged to do these activities frequently throughout the day:

*   Elevate the arm, raising the arm towards the ceiling or the sky

*   Light exercises for the head and neck and the upper body and arms, see "Decongestive Exercises" (page 143).

*   Deep breathing

*   Stretching

*   Walking, with periodic arm elevation (wave to your neighbors)

*   Swimming

*   Water aerobics

High Risk Activities for Upper Extremity

These activities may cause an increase in the patient's swelling and require modifications to control:

*   Lifting and carrying heavy items such as purses, briefcases, backpacks, groceries, luggage, children, or grandchildren.

*   Repetitive arm movements that involve straining the arm. For example, reaching a high shelf.

*   Cleaning and household chores

*   Moving furniture

*   Leaning on the swollen arm for a long time

*   Intense gripping activities (white-knuckled driving, horseback riding)

*   Gardening and yard work

*   Playing intense sports such as tennis, golf, or gymnastics

Beneficial Activities for Lower Extremity

The patient should be encouraged to do these activities frequently throughout the day:

- Elevate the legs, raising the foot and leg above the heart

- Light exercises for the head and neck, upper and lower body and legs, see "Decongestive Exercises" (page 143).

- Deep breathing

- Stretching

- Walking, biking, or swimming

- Water aerobics

High Risk Activities for Lower Extremity

These activities may cause an increase in the patient's swelling:

- Sitting, standing, or squatting in one position for long periods of time

- Heavy lifting and carrying (boxes, luggage)

- Cleaning and household chores

- Moving furniture

- Yard work

- Running and playing intense sports, such as soccer or basketball

Modifications for High Risk Activities

High risk activities do not have to be avoided, but discretion should be used to minimize risks. The caregiver may offer guidance as follows:

- Have the patient pace themselves, take frequent breaks, and stop when tired.

- Encourage the patient to balance high risk activities with beneficial activities.

- Add extra compression for activities that are known to increase the patient's swelling.

- Suggest cooler times of the day for activities that might increase swelling.

- Perform SLD and/or decongestive exercises before, during, or after high risk activities to help remove any excess swelling.

- Monitor the affected arm or leg and stop the activity if increased swelling is observed.

Sports and Exercise

Patients who participated in sports or group exercise programs before developing lymphedema may wish to resume these activities. Other patients may want to take up a sport or start an exercise program. Sports like walking, swimming, bicycling, running, hiking, soccer, tennis, golf, or bowling, and exercises like Yoga, Pilates, Water Aerobics, Tai Chi, circuit training, or dancing can be beneficial.

The Lebed Method, Focus on Healing Through Movement and Dance is a therapeutic exercise and movement program specifically designed for people with lymphedema and cancer survivors.[6] This program is available in many communities, see www.lebedmethod.com for more information.

Many programs include exercises similar to those described in the chapter on decongestive exercise (page 143), and substitutions can be easily made. Additional exercises to enhance the lymphatic system can be incorporated before, during, or after participating in a sport or an exercise group.

Follow the risk reduction guidelines provided in "Modifications for High Risk Activities" on page 253 with any conditioning program.

Gradually build up an exercise regimen, instead of jumping right in at maximum intensity. If the patient is returning to a previous exercise routine, they should start out by doing only 25-50% of the previous number of repetitions or weight; when resuming an exercise class, the patient can begin with every second or third repetition of arm or leg lifts. Every 1-2 weeks, the patient can increase the number of repetitions or amount of weight. For golf, start with 15-30 minutes at the driving range for a few weeks, then a 9-18 hole par 3 course, prior to a regular course. With swimming, biking, walking, running, or hiking, the patient may initially scale back the time by 50% or more, and then gradually increase over several weeks or months to their previous level.

Travel Tips

Many individuals with lymphedema are still active travelers. These tips include their suggestions for trip planning and precautions associated with lymphedema. For more information, see the *National Lymphedema Network Position Statement on Air Travel* at www.lymphnet.org.

Before You Leave

- Plan your travels (and time before and after your trip) for a more relaxed pace to minimize stress and to allow for extra rest as necessary.

- Have the patient wear a "Medic Alert" bracelet or necklace to make emergency medical personnel aware of their lymphedema. (This should be an everyday routine!)

- Ask the patient's health care provider to prescribe standby antibiotics in case of infection. Have the prescription filled and carry the pills in the labeled container from the pharmacy.

- Ask the patient's healthcare provider for a "note" that explains the patient's lymphedema. This may be useful if airport security has questions about bandages or compression garments or if the patient requires medical treatment during the trip.

- Pack a mini-first aid kit that includes disinfectant wipes, antibiotic cream, and band-aids. If you plan to do a lot of walking, pack padding, such as Artiflex, for use on tender spots that might become blisters.

- Pack wisely to minimize the amount of baggage and make each item manageable. Wrestling heavy luggage places a strain on the entire body! Duffle bags are available for bulky compression garments.

- Consider taking a back-up form of compression such as bandages, in addition to a compression aid. If something happens to the patient's compression aid, you may not be able to obtain a replacement.

- If traveling in a dry climate, take extra lotion to keep the skin of the affected limb well moisturized. If traveling to a hot and humid climate, take powder to help control moisture.

- Take soap powder to wash compression garments and two skirt hangers to hang them out to dry.

During the Trip

- Have the patient wear appropriate compression when traveling by plane. Some travelers wear their compression aids to save suitcase space. As part of your planning, particularly for longer trips, consult with the lymphedema therapist for guidance on how much compression would be best.

- Encourage your patient to drink lots of water! Have them avoid alcohol, coffee, and soft drinks containing caffeine since these beverages increase the amount of fluid excreted. Keep a bottle or other water container handy, if possible.

- If the patient's legs are affected, have them keep their shoes on while flying. Low air pressure can cause the feet to swell and they might not be able to get their shoes back on at the end of the flight.

- While staying at higher altitudes, have the patient wear compression as they would on an airplane. After arrival, allow some time for the patient's body to adjust to the altitude change before exercising.

- Use SPF 15 or higher sunscreen, even under compression garments. Wear insect repellent, long sleeves or trousers to protect the affected area. If sunscreen and insect repellent are used together, use a higher SPF sunscreen and reapply it more frequently.

After the Trip

After you return, review which ideas worked, and which didn't. Add these notes and the packing list to the Caregiver Handbook (see page 375) for use in planning future trips.

Sleep Comfort

Restful sleep is important for both patients and caregivers. Habitual sleep positions may have to be changed for comfortable rest and to recover from the day's activities. Sleeping positions may also have to be adjusted if compression aids are worn at night.

Patients with upper extremity lymphedema need support for the affected arm(s) and should not sleep on an affected arm. If the shoulder is affected, use a pillow under the arm to keep the shoulder in a neutral position. Patients with lower extremity lymphedema need support for the leg(s).

Sleep positions can be modified to keep the spine supported in a neutral position:

- **Side lying**: head pillow should hold the head so the neck is not tilted up or down. Place thick pillows between the legs, hug thick pillows to support the arm and hand, and an optional towel roll at the waist, see Figure 13-1.

- **Back lying**: small pillow under the head, thick pillows under the legs and a thick pillow under each arm and shoulder; optionally, add a small roll under the lower back.

- **Stomach lying**: two or more pillows under hips and lower chest, pillow under the feet; optional small soft pillow under upper chest and front of neck or towel roll under forehead. Avoid long periods on the stomach to minimize excessive neck rotation or pain.

- **Partial stomach lying**: pillows under the lower chest and one knee, with the knee bent (drawn up); thick pillows under upper arm and chest.

Figure 13-1

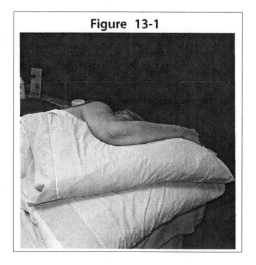

Notes

1 NLN Position Paper: Lymphedema Risk Reduction Practices, NLN Medical Advisory Committee, National Lymphedema Network (NLN), 2008.

2 "Water Exercises for Lymphedema" www.lymphnotes.com, 2007.

3 www.bam.gov/sub_yoursafety/playitsafe_hiking.html

4 **Lymphedema Risk Reduction Practices.** National Lymphedema Network, 2008.

5 **Lymphedema Certification Course**, Academy of Lymphatic Studies, Sebastian, FL, 2000.

6 **Thriving after Breast Cancer** by Sherry Lebed Davis with Stephanie Gunning. Broadway Books, 2002.

Chapter 14

First Aid

This chapter provides lymphedema-specific first aid tips for minor injuries including cuts and scratches, itchy rash, itching without rash, insect or spider bite, animal bites, burns, and bumps, bruises, and falls.

This guide is not a substitute for professional medical advice or formal first aid training. If you have a medical emergency, or if you are not sure if an injury is serious, call 911, or your local emergency medical assistance number, and let them evaluate the injury.

Cut and Scratches

Cuts and scratches are an inevitable part of life. If the patient gets a cut or scratch, first wash the area thoroughly with soap and water. If the cut or scratch is large, deep, or dirty, apply a thin coating of an antibacterial ointment (such as Neosporin, Polysporin, Bacitracin or a triple antibiotic) to the injury several times a day for the next few days until the area has scabbed over. Cover the area with a band-aid or a gauze dressing to protect the injured area as it heals.

Keep a close eye on the area for signs of infection— such as redness, warmth, and tenderness of the wound, a yellowish-white fluid (pus) that may have a foul smell, or if the patient develops a fever (see "Body Temperature" on page 65)—and contact the patient's health care provider, or an emergency department physician, as soon as an infection is suspected. See also "Recognizing Infections and Irritation" on page 49.

Itchy Rash

Warning: itching or a rash without any obvious cause may be a symptom of infection and require prompt medical treatment, see page 49. If the patient develops a widespread rash, or a rash that starts in a location that is not being treated for lymphedema, contact the patient's health care provider for advice.

A rash is a change in skin color and texture that indicates an allergic reaction (histamine response) in the skin; a rash is frequently but not always, itchy.[1] Rash may be caused by:

- Increased skin temperature, especially under bandages, compression garments or aids.

- Pressure (or excess pressure) from bandages, compression garments, or aids.

- Contact between the skin and an irritant or allergen. For example, poison ivy or poison oak, soap, certain metals, latex, moisturizing lotion, padding, bandaging materials, etc.

- Reaction to food or drugs.

- Diseases such as chickenpox, eczema, psoriasis, shingles, etc.

The location and extent of a rash is frequently an important clue to the cause of the rash and should be noted on the Weekly Care Plan and (optionally) documented with photos. A rash that is related to bandaging, or other lymphedema treatment, typically starts in the area being treated, although it may spread.

Treatment for a rash involves providing symptom relief and trying to identify and remove the cause, as explained below.

Symptom Relief

First, ask the patient not to scratch the area, then treat the rash with one or more of these solutions:

- Clean the area with cool water and rinse thoroughly. If blisters are present, do not break them.

- Try relieving the itch with over-the-counter anti-itch ointments containing hydrocortisone or Benadryl.

- Have the patient take an over-the-counter antihistamine pill (such as Benadryl) to relieve severe itching. Check with the patient's physician prior to starting any new medication.

- Apply a cold pack on the outside of the bandages (not to the skin directly) to cool the patient's skin.

- Remove the bandages until the rash clears (as a last resort).

Watch for trouble! The irritants that are producing the rash may cause increased swelling in the affected area and there is always the possibility of an infection. Contact the patient's health care provider if the rash has not improved within 24-48 hours after attempting to manage it, or sooner, if the rash becomes severe or spreads.

Cause Removal

A rash related to compression and lymphedema care may be caused by temperature, excess pressure, or contact with an irritant or allergen.

Rash caused by temperature, or heat rash, can be aided by keeping the patient as cool as possible and keeping the skin in the affected area dry.

If the patient is wearing bandages, excess pressure can be corrected by adjusting bandage pressure, see "Adjusting Bandage Tension" on page 122. If the patient is using a compression garment or aid, check for proper fit (see "How can I tell if a garment doesn't fit?" on page 140) or have the therapist or fitter check.

A rash may be caused by contact with an irritant or an allergen, and some materials are both. Long term exposure to an irritant may cause a rash. Once a person is sensitized to an allergen, even a brief exposure can cause a reaction. Patients can develop allergies to materials they have used for years without any problems and once an allergy develops, it remains for life.

Identifying and removing the cause of a rash caused by contact takes some detective work. If there have been any recent changes in lotion, soaps, or materials in direct contact with the patient's skin, consider these as possible allergens.

Here are some general things you can try:

- Changing the moisturizing lotion used before bandage application.

- Washing all bandages or compression garments thoroughly.

- Replacing synthetic padding used under bandages (cotton-like padding rolls) with 100% cotton or foam rolls such as Rosidal Soft.

- Changing the soap used for washing bandages to ensure that the patient is not allergic to the laundry detergent.

Itching without Rash

Sometimes one gets an itch, but just doesn't know why. When there is no sign of a scratch, rash, or infection, first try applying lotion to treat any possible dry skin. If the itch persists, try hydrocortisone cream such as Cortaid or Benadryl cream.

Persistent itchiness that does not abate within a few days should be evaluated by the patient's medical care provider, as there may be some unknown underlying cause, such as an allergic reaction (*dermatitis*) to a medication, lotion, or bandaging material.

Insect or Spider Bites

Seek emergency medical help immediately if the patient has a history of severe allergic reactions, difficulty breathing, facial swelling, abdominal pain, if you think the insect or spider might be poisonous, if there are multiple bites on an affected limb, or if there is a sudden increase in swelling.

Skin or tissue infections, including MRSA, generally start as small red bumps that resemble spider bites. Seek treatment for the patient if they develop signs of infection such as redness, warmth, and tenderness of the wound, a yellowish-white fluid (pus) that may have a foul smell, or a fever.

Instruct the patient not to scratch. Apply an anti-itch hydrocortisone cream, such as Cortaid or Benadryl cream, and a cool pack to the area. Repeat applications of anti-itch cream several times a day until the itch goes away. Seek treatment if the bite does not improve within 2-3 days.

Animal Bites

Bites from dogs, cats, or other animals can cause serious infections and should be evaluated immediately by a physician for appropriate care.

Burns

When a burn happens, evaluate the extent of the burn and act accordingly:[2]

- **Third degree burns**, also known as *full-thickness burns*, destroy all layers of the skin and the underlying fat, muscles, bones, and nerves; this can be a life-threatening medical emergency. Call 911 or your local medical emergency number and perform CPR if needed; cover the burn with a cool moist sterile bandage or clean cloth.

- **Second degree burns**, also known as *partial thickness burns, cause blisters and damage the outer layer of skin.* If the burn is on lymphedema-affected tissue (even if the area is small), or if the burned area is more than 2 inches (5 cm) in diameter, seek medical care immediately; otherwise follow the minor burn procedure below.

- **First degree burns**, *also known as superficial burns, cause redness but not blisters or breaks in the skin.* Follow the minor burn procedure below.

Minor burns can be treated by:

- Cooling the burned area under running water or by applying a cold, wet cloth. Do not use ice, ice water, butter, or oil.

- Continuing to apply cold water or a wet cloth for 20 minutes and then remove it for 20 minutes, until the area is pain-free.

- Examining the burned area for blistering or breaks in the skin. If these are present, seek medical care promptly.

- Applying an antibiotic cream, aloe vera lotion, or a low pH moisturizer over the burn to prevent the tissue from drying out.

- Covering the burn area loosely with a sterile gauze bandage.

- Giving the patient an anti-inflammatory drug such as aspirin, ibuprofen (Advil, Motrin), naproxen (Aleve), or acetaminophen (Tylenol), unless this is contraindicated or the patient is already taking a similar medication.

Extra caution should be taken when dealing with a burn on lymphedema-affected tissues and all burns should be monitored several times daily for signs of infection.

Bumps, Bruises, and Falls

Following a patient injury, first determine if medical attention is needed. If necessary, or if you are not sure, call 911 or your local medical emergency number.

If the injury is minor, apply a cold pack, a plastic bag filled with ice and water, or a bag of frozen peas. Cover the bag with a warm wet towel and apply to the injured area. The warmth of the wet towel will make the initial application easier to bear, but will quickly turn cool. Cold packs should not be applied directly to the skin, but only over a towel, and they should not be used for more than 15 minutes at a time. This can be repeated several times during the first 24-48 hours.

Acetaminophen (Tylenol) may help relieve the pain, unless contraindicated or the patient is already taking a similar medication. If you have any questions, check with the patient's medical care provider.

Hot packs and heating pads are discouraged, especially during the first 1-2 days after an injury, since these increase blood flow to the area and can increase swelling.

Notes

1   www.netdoctor.co.uk/diseases/facts/nettlerash.htm.

2   **American Red Cross Emergency Response**. Staywell, 2001. p 249-256.

Chapter 15:
Diet and Nutrition

Proper nutrition and weight control are essential for optimum health and may help minimize the swelling of lymphedema. Current recommendations for a well-balanced diet include:

- Focusing on fruits, vegetables, and whole grains.

- Moderate amounts of low-fat, or fat-free, milk and milk products, lean meats, poultry, fish, beans, eggs, and nuts.

- Minimizing quantities of saturated fats, trans-fats, cholesterol, salt (sodium), and processed sugars.

If your caregiver duties include meal planning, you will need to balance what is currently considered to be a healthy diet, what is comfortable, comforting, and appropriate for the patient, and what is available and affordable. Many people have foods that they find comforting. Find out what your patient likes and try to incorporate their favorite foods within the constraints of the recommended diet.

Any problems with food choices, eating patterns (including not eating or overeating), or weight changes (up or down) should be brought to the attention of the patient's family and doctor. See "Weight" on page 66 for more information.

Patients may benefit from pineapple, yogurt, moderate amounts of protein and salt, and lots of water, as explained below.

Fresh Pineapple

Fresh pineapple contains bromelain enzymes that appear to have an anti-inflammatory and diuretic effect that may have a beneficial impact on lymphedema.[1] To benefit from this enzyme, pineapple must be eaten raw and between meals:

- When pineapple is eaten with meals the bromelain is consumed in digesting the other foods and its beneficial actions do not reach other areas of the bodies.

- Bromelain is deactivated by heat, as in cooking or canning, so pineapple juice and canned pineapple are not good sources of bromelain.

Yogurt

Patients with lymphedema may be taking preventative antibiotics long term or antibiotics to treat an infection. Diarrhea or yeast infections (skin rash, thrush, or vaginitis) may develop as a side effect because antibiotics also kill helpful bacteria that normally control the yeast. Yogurt, and other foods containing live acidophilus cultures, may help re-establish the helpful bacteria in the body, especially if eaten two to four hours before, or after, taking oral antibiotics.

Dietary Protein

Because lymphedema is associated with the presence of protein-rich lymphatic fluid, the question often arises, *"Should I stop eating protein so there will be less protein in this fluid?"* The answer to this question is, *"No, do not stop eating protein. Less protein will not improve the situation."* In fact, not eating enough protein, or problems digesting protein, can cause swelling that weakens muscles and other tissues.

When there is not enough protein in the diet to meet the needs of the body, protein will be diverted from the tissues and muscles. A severe shortage of dietary protein leads to muscle wasting and generalized swelling from leaking cell membranes. This is known as *hunger edema* or nutritional edema, and can be seen in the swollen bellies of starving children.

Dietary proteins are essential nutrients found in meat, fish, dairy and soy products, beans, eggs, nuts, seeds and grains. The goal for each individual should be to eat the appropriate amount of protein to meet their daily needs, including protein from a variety of sources (not just meat), and with a minimal amount of fat.

The average American diet includes 70-100 grams of protein per day, 70% of which comes from animal sources. This is roughly twice the recommended daily allowance for protein (46 grams for women and 56 grams for men) and a major source of excess calories and cholesterol that contribute to obesity and cardiac disease. There is also research showing health benefits from a diet with lower protein levels (below the recommended daily allowance) and little or no animal protein.[2]

Low Salt Diet

Salt, or sodium, is an essential nutrient and saltiness enhances the enjoyment of certain foods. Excess salt in the diet contributes to fluid retention and is associated with high blood pressure and some heart problems. Patients with these conditions are frequently put on a low-salt diet. If a patient is on a low-salt diet for medical conditions other than lymphedema, they should continue to follow the recommended diet.[3]

There has been very little research on the relationship between salt and swelling associated with lymphedema, or the role of a low-salt diet in lymphedema care. Many patients have reported that meals that are high in salt make their lymphedema worse and that they feel better when they limit their salt intake.

Since the goal is to eat a diet that provides the best possible health, it is reasonable to keep salt intake within the recommended dietary guidelines. The current recommended daily value for sodium is less than 2,300 milligrams per day. This is about one teaspoon of table salt and includes ALL sodium consumed, including that used in cooking, added at the table, in snacks and beverages. For people with high blood pressure, African-Americans, and everyone who is middle-aged (or older), the recommended daily value is only 1,500 milligrams.

Information about sodium content can be found on food labels and in nutrition databases. The amount of salt quickly adds up to surprisingly high levels particularly in processed foods. For better health, it is a good idea to substitute fresh fruit for salty snacks, such as chips and pretzels, which contribute only salt, fat and empty calories to the diet.

Water Intake

The term *hydrated* describes the state of having adequate fluids in the body; maintaining this balance is essential to good health. The generally accepted guidelines are to drink at least six to eight 8-ounce glasses of fluid a day. This fluid intake can be in the form of juice, milk, soup, or other beverages; however, it should include at least two glasses of water.

Drinking adequate fluids to keep the body properly hydrated is extremely important for those with lymphedema. Reducing fluid intake in an attempt to reduce the swelling of lymphedema is not effective. If a patient becomes partially dehydrated, fluid will migrate into the affected areas.

Some patients may have fluid restrictions because of other health issues, such as kidney disease. If your patient has been told to restrict fluid intake, they should be sure to follow that advice.

Drinking plenty of water is particularly important before and after MLD, SLD, or exercise to help the body flush out waste. Caregivers can help their patients (and themselves) stay hydrated by making water available and encouraging the patient to drink. Flavored waters (sugar free), make an interesting variation.

Coffee, tea, chocolate, soft drinks, energy drinks, and some alcoholic beverages contain caffeine and should be consumed in moderation, because caffeine is a mild diuretic and may interfere with sleep. Many juices and juice drinks, sweetened teas, sodas, smoothies and blended drinks are high in calories, and should be avoided unless the patient is trying to gain weight.

Notes

1   NLN Position Paper: Lymphedema Treatment, National Lymphedema Network, 2006.

2   **The China Study** by T. Colin Campbell and Thomas M. Campbell II. Benbella Books 2006.

3   **Dietary Guidelines for Americans** by the Department of Health and Human Services and USDA. US Government Printing Office, 2005.

Managing
Supplies and Equipment

Lymphedema care requires a variety of supplies, bandages, compression garments and aids, other equipment, and medications. The goal of this section is to help you understand what is needed, make informed purchasing decisions, and have a process for managing replenishment and replacement. This process also provides budgeting information (see "Develop a Budget" on page 350) and documentation for tax deductions, if applicable.

Management can be less formal if only one person provides or arranges care, especially if supplies can be obtained quickly. Careful management becomes more important when there are multiple caregivers, budgets are tight, or it takes time to obtain supplies.

The next chapter describes a process for managing orders and reimbursement for all types of purchases. This is followed by chapters with specific instructions for managing each of these categories:

- Supplies—such as lotion, tape, or gloves—that are used up during the course of care.

- Bandages and bandaging materials.

- Compression garments and compression aids.

- Equipment used in providing care.

- Medications including prescription and over-the-counter medications.

See also "Finding and Paying for Care" (page 347) for more information on budgeting, sources of financial support, and situations where care expenses are tax deductible.

Chapter 16

Managing Orders

The term 'order' is used to cover all types of purchasing including in-store shopping, online orders, telephone orders, orders placed through the patient's doctor or therapist, rented or leased equipment, etc. The goal of the order management process is to make sure that the caregiver and patient have what they need without spending any more than necessary on purchases, shipping charges, or shopping trips. One order may include items from multiple categories.

The process described here assumes that a caregiver or care arranger (who may be the patient) is responsible for figuring out what is needed and placing orders. You may need to modify this process to fit your care situation in terms of:

- Reviewing and approving orders before they are placed to make sure they are within the available budget and insurance reimbursement program limits.

- Tracking orders that are placed on behalf of the patient by a therapist or other medical care provider.

- Requesting and tracking reimbursement from Medicare or other health benefit provider.

- Accounting for money that is being paid by a caregiver or care arranger that will be reimbursed by the patient or their family.

- Documenting medical expenses for tax deductions that can be claimed by the patient or by someone who can claim the patient as their dependent.

Order management includes placing orders, checking in orders that are received, resolving any errors or missing orders, reimbursing caregivers for purchases they pay for, and obtaining insurance reimbursement for covered expenses.

Before going into details of order management, we explain reimbursement issues. This section can be skipped if you are not concerned with reimbursement or if you are already familiar with reimbursement rules and processes.

Reimbursement Issues

Medicare, Medigap (Medicare supplemental insurance), or other medical insurance plans may pay for certain home care supplies, equipment, and medication based on specific definitions of covered items and services contained in their contract and any relevant laws. Coverage may be subject to certain limits or deductibles and may not cover 100% of the cost. The patient—or their family—may be expected to pay the portion of the cost that is not reimbursed.

Reimbursement is based on what is 'medically necessary' for the diagnosis or treatment of the patient's medical condition and that meets accepted standards of medical practice. In most cases, a prescription, letter, or other document signed by a doctor is required to show medical necessity.

If there is any desire to offset the cost of care items by reimbursement from Medicare or other insurance provider, understand the reimbursement issues before placing the order. Reimbursement issues may impact what is ordered, who places the order, the choice of vendor, what documentation is required in advance, etc.

Just because something is covered, or eligible for reimbursement, does not mean that it is free. There may be significant costs involved for co-payment, co-insurance, deductibles, or costs that exceed coverage limits.

If money is an issue, be sure you know—and are comfortable with—the answers to the following questions before you order anything assuming that the expense will be covered:

- What is the total cost, how much will be reimbursed, and how much will the patient (or their family) have to pay?

- Do you have the documentation and approvals required for reimbursement?

- Will the patient (or their family) be expected to pay the total and then be reimbursed later?

- How long will it take to receive the payment for reimbursement?

Coverage Categories

The rules for reimbursement by Medicare and other insurance providers vary based on the type of coverage or benefit that applies (if any) for each expense or purchase. Each coverage or benefit type may have a different process for ordering and reimbursement, different deductibles or co-payments, and different coverage limits.

The common coverage categories are:

- Covered Items and Services such as diabetes testing supplies or surgical dressings.

- Durable Medical Equipment (DME) such as wheelchairs and walkers.

- Drug Benefits for medications, typically prescription medications.

Commonly Covered Items

Coverage for lymphedema care items varies between insurance providers and, in some cases, by location for the same provider. Although Medicare is a national program, there are state and regional differences in coverage rules. Rules also change over time and there are efforts underway to expand coverage for lymphedema care, see page 353.

Currently, most insurance programs cover only some of the items needed for lymphedema care. For example:

- Supplies are generally not reimbursable. It may be possible to pay for supplies using a tax-advantaged Health Savings Account.

- Bandages are frequently not covered but some programs consider them to be durable medical equipment.

- Compression Garments and Aids are covered by some programs as durable medical equipment.

- Care equipment classified as durable medical equipment and medically necessary is typically covered. Other care equipment may not be covered.

- Medications are covered subject to the specific terms of the patient's drug plan. See the discussion in Managing Medications (page 321).

Ask Before Ordering

If you plan to seek reimbursement for a purchase you should verify coverage, terms or charges, the required process, the expected documentation, and acceptable vendors before placing an order. The patient's therapist or an insurance specialist at the treatment facility may be familiar with the rules and procedures that Medicare and other insurance plans in your area apply to lymphedema care items.

Health insurance plans are required to provide documents that explain their coverage rules for each diagnosis. You may want to obtain and review these documents. Look for titles like Summary Plan Description, Summary of Material Modifications, or Summary Annual Report. Once you find out what is covered, you should also research the rules for obtaining reimbursement. For example, an insurance provider may require that the patient's doctor or therapist order medical equipment, and some insurance plans will only pay for equipment supplied by their approved vendors.

Appealing a Denial

If your claim for reimbursement is denied, the patient has the right to appeal or the patient's doctor may be able to appeal. The appeals process and rules vary based on the insurer. For an example appeal letter and other information, see the chapter on insurance issues in **Living Well With Lymphedema**[1] or contact Bob Weiss, NLN Patient Advocate, at LymphActivist@aol.com.

Forms and Records

This subsection explains the forms and records used to manage supplies, equipment, and medications.

Forms

The following forms are used to track and manage supplies, equipment, and medications, and to order or reorder them as needed:

- Supply Form (page 430) tracks usage and purchases of a consumable supply.

- Equipment Form (page 431) is used to track bandages, compression garments, compression aids, medical equipment and other equipment.

- Medication Form (page 432) is used to manage pills and topical medications.

- Vendor Form (page 433) has the information on a vendor or supplier.

- Item Needed Form (page 434 is used to identify what should be ordered.

- Order Form (page 435) is used to create and track an order.

Blank forms can be copied from Appendix C. Electronic versions of these forms are available on the book website (www.Lymphedema-Caregiver.com).

Any supply or equipment item mentioned on a Care Activity Form (see page 338) should have a Supply or Equipment Form. Medication forms should cover each of the items on the list of medications in the Patient Notebook (see page 372), and any medications mentioned on a Care Activity Form.

Records and Files

Management records can be maintained by setting up and keeping files with one folder for each applicable category of tracking form: Supplies, Bandages, Compression Garments and Aids, Equipment, and Medications plus a file for Vendors.

You may also want files for Inactive Supplies, Inactive Bandages, Inactive Compression Garments and Aids, Inactive Equipment and Inactive Medications. This is where you would keep information on things that are not currently being used but might be reused; these records might also be needed for tax purposes.

The following files will be used for managing orders and related information:

- Pending Requests: Item Needed Forms with information about things that may be ordered.

- Pending Orders: Order Forms and supporting information for orders that have been placed but not yet received.

- Completed Orders: information on orders that have been received including Order Forms and other receipts.

- Prescriptions: one file for all prescriptions or separate files for medication prescriptions and equipment prescriptions.

- Product Information: one file for all product information or separate files for medications and equipment.

These files can be organized chronologically with the newest information added at the back of the folder.

Getting Started

When you first start managing supplies and equipment, you will have to go through the steps outlined below to create the necessary records. Typically, this is only done once but you may have to repeat this process if there have been major changes in the care routine or care environment.

Start by reading and working through the Getting Started subsection in the chapter on managing each category that applies for this patient. Categories include:

- ☐ Supplies (page 281),

- ☐ Bandages (page 287),

- ☐ Compression garments and aids (page 299),

- ☐ Equipment (page 315), and

- ☐ Medications (page 321).

Each of these chapters also includes instructions for adding or discontinuing an item. The chapters on supplies, equipment, and medications also include suggested lists of items that may be needed for patient care.

After working through "Getting Started" you should know:

- What supplies, equipment, and medication are needed for care, and you will have created the appropriate tracking forms.

- What is available, and you should have Item Needed forms listing anything that needs to be ordered.

Once you have that information, follow the order management processes described below.

Order Management Processes

There are a couple of steps or processes involved in managing orders. The first two should be done as needed:

- Track Needs by filling out an Item Needed Form any time additional supplies, equipment or medication are needed, and put the forms in the Pending Requests file. If something important is needed urgently, bring this to the attention of the person who handles Review Needs and Place Orders (see page 278).

- Check-in Received Orders should be done any time an order is received or someone returns from shopping for tracked items.

The other two processes should be done about once a week. Although it may seem backwards, we recommend doing the processes in this sequence:

- Follow-up on Pending Orders, to see if any orders or items have not been received. By checking this first, you'll know if anything should be reordered.

- Review Needs and Place Orders, if any orders are needed.

Instructions for each of these processes are provided below.

Track Needs

The Item Needed Form can be used to track requests for things. The caregiver, care arranger, or patient can fill out this form and add it to the Pending Request file at any time.

The need for additional or different items can be identified based on:

- Changes in the lymphedema care routine that require different supplies or equipment.

- Change in prescriptions or care that require new or different medications.

- The management processes for supplies, bandages, compression garments and aids, or medications identifies something to be ordered.

Review Needs and Place Orders

The person responsible for ordering should review the pending requests and determine what orders, if any, should be placed. Orders should be placed often enough that all necessary equipment and supplies are available, but not so often that ordering or shopping requires too much time or expense.

This process includes:

- Reviewing the Item Needed Forms in the Pending Request file to see what has been requested.

- Decide what should be ordered at this time—and in what quantity or size—taking into account the importance of each item, the urgency of the need, the quantity on-hand (if any), reimbursement issues, and any budget constraints.

- Decide which vendors to order from and what to order from each vendor. Fill out a separate Order Form with the list of items for each vendor.

- Locate the appropriate Supply, Equipment, or Medication form for each item being ordered and update the form with the order information.

- Place the order(s). This may mean placing an online or telephone order, deciding that someone should go shopping, or contacting the patient's therapist or doctor if they have to order something. Check-off each item in the Ordered column as it is ordered.

- Put a copy of each order in the Pending Order file.

Supplies and equipment for lymphedema care are ordered from a variety of sources including drug stores, medical supply companies, and specialty suppliers like the companies listed in Appendix B (page 418). The patient's therapist may be able to suggest where to purchase specific care items. Create a Vendor Form to help track each source, keep these in the Vendors file.

Prescription medications are typically purchased from a pharmacy. The health insurance program that covers the patient may impose specific requirements on medication purchases that will be reimbursed.

Check-in Received Orders

When an order is received it should be checked and processed as follows:

- Find the original order in the Pending Order file and fill in the Received Date.

- Check what was received against the order and deal with any differences as follows:

  - Wrong item: contact the vendor to arrange the return and replacement. After you finish with the rest of the order, put the order information in the Pending Orders file, if you will need to follow up on the return.

  - Damaged or defective items: contact the vendor to correct the situation; put the order information in the Pending Orders file until the credit is received.

- For each item received that was ordered:

  - Check off the item in the Received column of the Order Form.

  - Find the matching Supply, Equipment, or Medication form and update the information on the form with the purchase information.

- If the item includes new instructions, add these to the Product Information File.

• If there are items on the order that were not received:

  - If the item was back-ordered, or the order was shipped in multiple parts, add a note to the order and put it in the Pending Order file.

  - If the vendor cannot provide the item, add it to an Item Needed Form with a note so the item can be ordered from a different supplier or a substitute item can be ordered.

  - Check that the charges reflect only what was received.

• File the completed order in the Completed Orders and Receipts file.

Follow-up Pending Orders

Review the contents of the Pending Order file about once a week and take appropriate actions as follows:

• If there are orders that have not been received within the expected time period, follow-up with the vendor to have the situation corrected. Document your actions and put the order back in the Pending Orders File. If you cancel an order, move the order information into the Completed Orders file.

• If there are orders with returns or adjustments, check to see if the credit has been received or the account has been adjusted. If the return has been completed, move the information in the Completed Orders file; if it is not complete, document your actions and put the information back in the Pending Orders File.

Notes

1 **Living Well With Lymphedema** by Ann Ehrlich, Alma Vinjé-Harrewijn, and Elizabeth McMahon. Lymph Notes 2005.

Chapter **17:**
Managing Supplies

Consumable supplies include anything that gets used up in the course of providing care. Care Activity Forms (see page 338) should list the supplies needed for each activity. Supply usage is tracked using Supply Forms (see page 430).

This chapter includes:

- Getting started managing supplies and identifying what supplies will be needed.

- Changing supply requirements.

- Reordering supplies.

- Suggested supplies for each care activity and recommendations for selecting certain supplies.

Getting Started

This subsection describes how to get started managing supplies. Since most supplies are listed on at least one Care Activity Form, you can identify supplies while you document care activities.

The process of figuring out what supplies are needed will be different in a situation where lymphedema care is starting, or restarting—compared to a situation where care (or self care) is ongoing and most supplies are available.

The steps to getting started managing supplies include:

- Identify what supplies will be used in home care by reviewing the list of recommended supplies (see page 284) with the patient (if they have been doing their own care) and the patient's therapist. If Care Activity Forms have been created, check these forms for the supplies needed for each activity.

- For each supply item that will be used in home care, fill out a Supply Form.

- For each Supply Form, check if the supply item is available and take the appropriate action:

  - If a supply is available, update the Supply Form with the quantity on hand so usage can be tracked. Estimate how long the current supply will last, and consider ordering more if there is less than a two week supply on hand.

  - If a supply item is not available, add it to an Item Needed Form so that it can be ordered.

Perform the Review Needs and Place Orders process (see page 278) after you have completed the Getting Started process for all supplies, equipment, and medications.

Changing Supply Requirements

As the care routine changes, supply items may be added or the use of a supply may be discontinued.

Adding a Supply Item

If a supply item is added it may be new or it might be something that had been used previously and discontinued. Separate instructions are provided below.

If a new supply is added:

- Create a new Supply Form with the information about the item.

- Fill out an Item Needed Form if the item has to be ordered.

- Update the Care Activity Forms to show where the supply is used, if applicable.

If a supply is added that had been used previously:

- Look for a Supply Form with the information about the item in the Inactive Supplies folder. Create a new form if you do not find one.

- Check if there is a sufficient and usable quantity on hand.

- If the supply has to be ordered, add it to an Item Needed Form.

- Update the Care Activity Forms to indicate when and how the supply is used, if applicable.

Discontinuing a Supply Item

If the use of a supply item is discontinued:

- Locate any remaining supply. If you think this item might be used again in the future, store it separately from other supplies; otherwise dispose of it properly.

- Remove the Supply Form and mark it as discontinued. If you think the item might be used again, put the form in the Inactive Supplies folder.

- Update the Care Activity Forms to remove any reference to the item.

Reordering Supplies

There are two ways to track consumable supplies and decide when to reorder:

- Periodically check the quantities on hand and reorder any supplies that are running low by listing the item on the Item Needed form.

- Keep a spare package of each supply on hand; when the current package is used up, open the spare package and add the supply to the Item Needed Form for ordering.

The first method works well for tapes and lotions where one container lasts several weeks and you can estimate how much remains. The second method is best for supplies that are used up quickly. If several packages are used per week, re-order when there is less than a two week supply on hand.

Recommended Supplies

These lists show supplies that may be used for each home care activity. Use this as a starting point for figuring out what supplies are required. Many patients will not need all of them.

Supplies for Skin Care

- Soap for washing skin, see page 286.

- Medical gloves, see page 285.

- Moisturizing lotion or cream, see page 285.

- Disposable washcloths or towels.

- Vinegar, if a vinegar wash is used.

- Powder, or baby powder.

- Cotton swabs such as Q-tips.

Supplies for Taking Measurements

- A washable marker, ballpoint pen, or eyebrow pencil for marking measurement positions.

- Thermometer covers for digital thermometers.

Supplies for Bandaging

- Padding, stockinette, etc. See page 294.

- Tape, see page 286.

- Soap for washing bandages, see page 292.

- Fabric marking pen for labeling bandages.

Supplies for Compression Garments and Aids

- Lubricant for donning compression garments, see page 312.

- Soap for washing compression garments (see page 305) or aids (see page 307).

* Fabric marking pen for labeling garments and aids.

Supplies for Decongestive Exercise

No supplies needed.

Other Supplies

* Kinesio Tape if used, see "Kinesio Taping" on page 242.

* First aid kit, or equivalent supplies, including band aids, gauze dressings, surgical tape for securing dressings, antibiotic cream, anti-itch cream, etc.

The subsections that follow discuss some specific types of supplies.

Medical Gloves

Disposable medical gloves, or examination gloves, are used to prevent contamination between the patient and caregiver. Use these gloves any time your hands may touch someone else's body fluids (such as blood, respiratory secretions, vomit, urine or feces) or hazardous drugs.

Latex-based gloves should not be used if either the patient or the caregiver has any sensitivity to natural rubber latex. Instead, choose gloves made from synthetic materials, such as polyvinyl chloride (PVC), nitrile rubber, or polyurethane. After removing gloves, wash your hands thoroughly with soap and water or an alcohol-based hand rub. Never reuse medical gloves.

Moisturizing Lotion or Cream

When selecting a moisturizer, look for:

* Fragrance-free or unscented products.

* Water as the first item in the ingredient list on the bottle. Urea and mineral oil are also beneficial ingredients.

* Glycerol or glycerin as a minor ingredient (later in the list of ingredients), since glycerol-related products may clog pores.

Creams are thicker than lotions and are generally used with more severe skin problems. Good moisturizers, such as Eucerin, Cetaphil, and Lubriderm, are available at grocery, drug, and retail stores.

If the patient has a history of sensitivity or allergic reactions to shin care products, test any new product on healthy skin before using it on an area with lymphedema.

Skin Soap

Moisturizing soap, such as Ivory, Dove, or Softsoap, is highly recommended for skin areas that are particularly dry or require more frequent daily washings since these soaps help the skin stay lubricated. A moisturizing soap is particularly beneficial during the winter when the skin tends to dry out more easily. Antibacterial soap (such as Dial) is suggested when the patient has been in an environment with greater exposure to infectious materials; for example after handling raw meat or garbage, house cleaning, yard work, pet or animal care. Deodorant or scented soaps should be avoided as these are harsher and tend to dry out the skin.

Tape for Bandages

Masking tape or cloth tape is used to secure bandages by taping to other bandages, not the patient's skin. Cloth tape is primarily used when wrapping the trunk and masking tape is used for other areas. Masking tape is widely available. Cloth medical tape—also known as silk tape, silk-like tape, or surgical tape—is available from medical supply companies and some drug stores.

Kinesio Tape

Kinesio tape is an elastic therapeutic tape that is sometimes used for lymphedema treatment (see "Kinesio Taping" on page 242). This tape is available from lymphedema supply companies. Kinesio tape comes in different widths and colors. Use the width recommended by the patient's therapist. Color is a matter of personal preference; all colors of Kinesio tape have the same properties,[1]

Notes

1   Per www.kinesiotaping.com/faq.php accessed in January 2009.

Chapter **18:**

Managing Bandages

The goal of this process is to make sure you have the bandaging materials that are needed, to care for bandages, and to monitor bandage condition. Skip this chapter if your patient is not using bandages.

The patient's therapist decides if a patient should use compression bandages and what bandaging materials are needed. A patient may need two or more sets of bandages to allow for washing bandages.

This chapter covers:

- Record keeping for managing bandages including getting started and changing bandaging requirements.

- Bandage care and inspection. Bandages are reused and replaced as they wear out.

- Bandaging materials including types and sizes of bandages, padding, stockinette, and other materials used with bandages.

If you are not familiar with these terms, you may want to start with "Bandaging Materials" on page 294, and then read the rest of this chapter.

Bandages and foam pads can be reused many times and are tracked using Equipment Forms. Multiple bandages of the same type and size can be tracked on one form.

Padding materials used for bandaging and gauze bandages are tracked as supplies using Supply Forms. These 'consumable' supplies come in rolls or sheets, are cut to fit, and are either used once or reused only a few times.

Getting Started

The Care Activity Forms for compression bandaging (see page 338) should list the bandages and supplies that are required for each affected area. If these forms have not been completed, the patient's therapist, or the patient (if they have been doing self care), should be able to tell you what bandages and supplies are required. It may be easier to fill in the Care Activity Forms, the Equipment Forms for bandages and reusable compression pads, and the Supply Forms for bandaging supplies at the same time.

Depending on how often bandages are used, the patient may need more than one set of bandages to allow for washing.

Determine the number of bandages needed in each type and size by counting up the number used in one set of bandages (including all affected areas) and multiplying by the desired number of sets of bandages. For example, a patient with lymphedema in both legs who uses three 10 cm bandages for each leg, needs six of these bandages for one set, or twelve for two sets of bandages.

For each bandage type and size and each reusable pad:

- Create one Equipment Form (see page 431) with the description and the number of bandages or pads required.

- Check how many reusable bandages or pads are on hand.

- Fill out an Item Needed Form, if additional bandages or pads have to be ordered.

- Update the Care Activity Forms to show where the bandage is used, if applicable.

Compression bandaging also requires consumable supplies, such as stockinette, cotton-like rolls, padding, etc. For each consumable supply item:

- Create a Supply Form.

- Check how much of the supply is available (if any).

- If the supply has to be ordered, add it to an Item Needed Form.

- Update the Care Activity Forms to show when and how the supply is used, if applicable.

Bandaging supplies can be managed and reordered with the other supplies, see page 281.

Perform the Review Needs and Place Orders process (see page 278) after you have completed the Getting Started process for all supplies, equipment, and medications.

Changing Bandage Requirements

Bandage usage in the care routine can change in several ways:

- Bandaging may be suspended due to an infection or other condition. A temporary suspension does not require any change in bandage management; the Weekly Care Plan should be updated to reflect the change.

- A patient who was not using bandages may start using bandages. This is the same as Getting Started (above) and involves Adding Bandages (page 290) or Adding Bandaging Supplies (page 290) for each item.

- A patient may discontinue the use of compression bandages. This is the same as Discontinuing Bandages (page 291) for each type and size of bandage used and Discontinuing Bandaging Supplies (page 291) for each supply item.

- The number of bandages of a given type or size that are used may change. This can be handled by updating the Equipment Form with the new number of bandages required; if more bandages are needed, add them to the Item Needed form.

- The type or size of bandages used may change. Handle this by Adding Bandages for the new type and size and Discontinuing Bandages for the type and size that is no longer being used.

- Supply usage may change. If a supply is added, see Adding Bandaging Supplies; if a supply is dropped, see Discontinuing Bandaging Supplies.

The subsections that follow explain the process for adding or discontinuing bandages or supplies.

Adding Bandages

Bandages that are added to the care routine may be new or may be a bandage size and type that had been used previously and discontinued.

If a completely new bandage type and size is added:

- Create a new Equipment Form with information about the bandage.

- Fill out an Item Needed Form if the item has to be ordered.

- Update the Care Activity Form to show when and how the bandage is used.

If a bandage size and type that had been used before and discontinued is added to the care routine:

- Look for an Equipment Form with the information about the bandage in the Inactive Equipment folder. Create a new form if you do not find one.

- Check to see how many reusable bandages are available.

- If new bandages have to be ordered, add them to an Item Needed Form.

- Update the Care Activity Form to show when and how the bandage is used.

Adding Bandaging Supplies

Supplies that are added to the bandaging routine may be completely new or they may be a type of supply that was used previously and discontinued.

If a new supply is added:

- Create a new Supply Form with the information about the item.

- Fill out an Item Needed Form if the item has to be ordered.

- Update the Care Activity Forms to show where the supply is used, if applicable.

If a supply is added that had been used before:

- Look for a Supply Form with the information about the item in the Inactive Supplies folder. Create a new form if you do not find one.

- Check if any usable supplies are available.

- If the supply has to be ordered, add it to an Item Needed Form.

- Update the Care Activity Forms to show when and how the supply is used.

Discontinuing Bandages

If the lymphedema care routine changes and a particular bandage type or size is no longer being used:

- Locate all remaining bandages of the specified type and size. Some of the bandages may be with the laundry.

- If you think this bandage type and size might be used again in the future, store any bandage(s) that are in good condition separately from current bandages and dispose of any bandages that are not usable. Mark the Equipment Form inactive and file it in the Inactive Equipment folder.

- If you think this bandage type and size will not be used again, dispose of the bandage(s) and the Equipment Form..

- Update the Care Activity Forms to remove any reference to this bandage.

Discontinuing Bandaging Supplies

If the use of a bandaging supply item is discontinued:

- Locate any remaining supplies. If you think this item might be used again in the future, then store the item separately from other supplies; otherwise dispose of it properly.

- Remove the Supply Form and mark it as discontinued. If you think the item may be used again, put the form in the Inactive Supplies folder.

- Update the Care Activity Forms to remove any reference to the supply.

Bandage Care

There are two parts to bandage care: washing bandages and inspecting bandages to see if they should be replaced. Inspection should be done once a week and is easiest to do after bandages have been washed and before they are rolled up.

Washing Bandages

Bandages that are worn all day and night should be washed every day for best results; this requires at least two sets of bandages. When bandages are only used at night, they may still need to be washed daily or several times a week for optimal effectiveness and to prolong the life of the bandages.

Washing allows the knitted bandage material to spring back to its original shape and makes the bandage easier to apply. Bandages that are not washed frequently tend to cause more skin irritation.

Stockinette should be washed with bandages. Foam rolls and chip bags can be washed with the bandages and air-dried. Padding is usually not washed unless it becomes soiled. Wash cotton padding by hand. Cotton rolls soiled by wound drainage should be replaced.

Prepare bandages for washing by unrolling them and placing them in a mesh garment bag along with the stockinette. Mesh laundry bags are available at most drugstores and help keep bandages from tangling. Each mesh bag should hold 5-10 bandages (depending on the size of the bag and the bandages). Wash in warm (104° F or 40° C) water on a gentle cycle with a mild liquid detergent that does not contain perfume, bleach, or fabric softener. Woolite liquid soap is not recommended for bandages.

Bandages can be air-dried or placed in the dryer on a medium setting; several drying cycles may be necessary. If time permits, take the bandages out of the dryer when they are still slightly damp and allow them to air-dry for the rest of the day. If the stockinette is frayed at the edges, the frayed areas may be trimmed off.

Once fully dried, the bandages should be rolled loosely (without pulling) so that the bandage does not become stretched out. A stretched-out bandage is more difficult to apply and is more likely to cause skin irritation. Bandages should not be ironed or cut. A mechanical or electrical bandage winder makes bandage rolling easier and faster. Bandage winders are available from lymphedema supply companies (see Appendix B, page 418).

Inspecting Bandages

Bandages are replaced based on wear and changes in condition, not a set schedule. Bandages should be inspected once a week to see if any bandages need to be replaced using the procedure provided here. Unless the patient has extra bandages, continue to use the old bandages until the replacements are available.

If a caregiver notices bandages that are worn, or otherwise in need replacing, while applying or washing bandages, they should mark the bandage for replacement at the next inspection.

Bandages that are used daily should last about 3-6 months depending on duration of use, general wear, and loss of elasticity. If the patient has two sets of bandages, the bandages will last longer and it will be easier to wash the bandages between uses.

Padding and gauze bandages will require more frequent replacement. Stockinette, cotton-like rolls and cotton will last approximately 2-4 weeks. Gauze finger/toe bandages may need to be replaced every 2-3 days. These materials are managed as supplies.

Inspect bandages after washing and before rolling. To inspect bandages:

- Locate all of the Equipment Forms that describe bandages.

- For each type and size of bandage:

  - Count all the bandages of this type and size, including those that are being worn. If there are fewer bandages available than required, determine how many additional bandages are needed.

  - Inspect the bandages that are not being worn for fraying, runs, loss of elasticity, or other signs of wear. Determine which bandages need to be replaced and mark the bandages.

  - Check the Equipment Form to see if replacement bandages have been requested, and how many. If additional replacements are needed (in addition to any previous request), add the information to the Item Needed Form and update the Equipment Form.

Receiving New Bandages

When new bandages are received:

- Remove and discard any metal clips provided with the bandages. These clips are usually not used for lymphedema care.

- Update the Equipment Form with the new bandage information. Save the receipt and physician's prescription, if needed for reimbursement.

- Mark each bandage with its size (if not marked) and the date received.

- Locate and discard any old bandages that are being replaced by these new bandages.

Bandaging Materials

This subsection explains different types of bandages, bandage sizes, and padding materials used in bandaging. Understanding these materials will help with both ordering and applying bandages properly.

There are several types of bandages available, and the therapist may recommend a combination of types to address specific needs. These include short-, medium-, and long-stretch, adhesive, and non-stretch bandages in different sizes as explained below. Short-stretch bandages are the main bandages used in lymphedema treatment.

Short-Stretch Bandages

A short-stretch bandage is made of 100% cotton knit material and extends by 40-90% of its original length when stretched. If applied correctly, the short-stretch bandage delivers a low resting pressure while the patient is sitting or sleeping and a high working pressure during movement.[1]

The low resting pressure makes the wrapped limb more comfortable during rest and the high working pressure (minimal stretch) improves the effectiveness of the muscle pump during movement, as described in the section on decongestive exercises. This provides the most effective swelling reduction for an affected limb.[2] The short-stretch bandages are comfortable enough to wear for long periods of time, making it possible to use bandages day and night. Available brands include: Comprilan,[3] Durelast, Idealbinde, Isoband, KomprimED, LoPress, Rosidal K. Finger and toe bandage examples include: Elastomull, KT Medical FingerBAND and ToeBAND, Mollelast, and Transelast.

Medium-Stretch Bandages

Medium-stretch bandages extend by approximately 60-140% of the original length when stretched. A medium-stretch bandage may be used for breast, chest wall, abdominal or genital swelling that requires compression with a lower working pressure, but enough elasticity to allow freedom of movement with minimal bandage slippage. Brands include: Lenkelast.

Long-Stretch Bandages

Long-stretch bandages, also known as Ace Bandages, extend by more than 140% of their original length when stretched.[4] Long-stretch bandages are often used in treating sports injuries (such as sprains) and to secure gauze dressings over wounds. These bandages are highly elastic and stretch easily as the person moves, allowing for relatively unrestricted mobility during various activities.

The bandage elasticity gives a low working pressure and reduces the effectiveness of the muscle pump compared to short-stretch bandages. The high resting pressure of the long-stretch bandage may make the wrap tight or uncomfortable when the patient is inactive or sleeping. Long-stretch bandages are occasionally used in lymphedema care for specific swelling conditions. Brands include: Ace Brand Elastic Bandage, Dauerbinde K.

Self-Adhering or Cohesive Bandages

Self-adhering or cohesive bandages apply a moderate stretch and have the advantage of adhering to another part of the bandage, eliminating the need for tape. Cohesive bandages can be used over short-stretch bandages to provide better foot or hand grip when the patient is walking with a cane or walker as explained in "Wheelchair-Bound Patients" on page 236.

Cohesive bandages also work effectively in areas where swelling diminishes quickly with compression, such as the scrotum in male genital edema. Self-adhering bandages must be applied very carefully with sufficient padding under the bandage to prevent skin issues and without overstretching the bandage, which can cause excess pressure on the wrapped body part. Brands include: Coban, Colastic.

Non-Stretch Bandages

Non-stretch bandages have little to no extension when stretched providing the highest working pressure and the lowest resting pressure. Non-stretch bandages help to minimize swelling, but restrict mobility and are not easy to use over joints. A non-stretch bandage may be applied to open wounds of the mid-arm or leg, or in the trunk area. Examples include non-elastic gauze and Gelocast Unna's Boot medicated gauze dressing.

Bandage Sizes

Bandages come in a variety of widths ranging from 2.5 centimeters (1 inch) to 20 centimeters (8 inches). Most bandages are 5 meters (16 feet) in length. Double length bandages (10 meters or 33 feet) are available in 10 and 12 cm widths for use on larger limbs.

Most patients use short-stretch bandages which are 6, 8, 10, or 12 centimeters in width. Smaller bandages (6 and 8 cm) are used for small body parts, such as the hand or foot, and larger bandages (10 and 12 cm or 15 and 20 cm) are used for large areas such as the upper arm or leg and the trunk. Four centimeter bandages are used on young children.

Gauze bandages 2.5 to 5 centimeters wide are used for finger and toe swelling and for very young children. These come in rolls that are 375 cm (150 inches) long.

Padding

Padding is used under short-stretch bandages to provide protection to the skin and to evenly distribute bandage pressure. This is especially important in bony areas and places with deep skin folds. Specialized pads may be used to further protect sensitive areas, such as the wrist or the ankle, and to increase pressure on problem areas with fibrotic (hardened) tissue. Some of the available padding items are described below. Prolonged exposure to sunlight or heat may degrade foam padding.

Stockinette and Gauze

Stockinette is a seamless tubular knit material available in a variety of types ranging from thin, light weight, open weave to thicker, close-mesh, jersey material. Gauze is sometimes used as padding or to keep other pads in place.

Both stockinette and gauze are available in widths ranging from less than one inch (2 cm) to about eight inches (20 cm), may be made of cotton, synthetic or blended materials, and come in rolls that can be cut to length as needed.

Cotton-like Rolls

Rolls of cotton-like material can be applied from the hand to the armpit and from the foot to the groin to provide basic skin protection and smooth out the limb to a more conical shape. Cotton-like rolls may be cotton or, more commonly, blends of polyester, polypropylene, and polyethylene. Examples: Artiflex, Cellona, Hartmann-Conco non-woven padding. Patients with very sensitive skin may be allergic to the synthetic blend.

Foam Rolls

Foam rolls are similar to cotton-like rolls and can be applied from the hand to the armpit or from the foot to the knee or thigh. The benefits of foam rolls are extra protection and the ability to wash the material as needed between uses. Examples: Rosidal Soft, Velfoam.

Foam Padding

Foam padding may be used to protect sensitive skin or to soften areas where the skin has hardened (fibrotic tissues). Foam padding comes in sheets that can be cut to fit a specific area. Pre-cut shapes are also available. The patient's therapist should specify the foam thickness and density for each application.

Soft or low-density foam is used to protect sensitive skin in areas such as the front of the ankle, the elbow, the back of the knee, and the hand. This foam may also be used on the trunk under a bra, girdle, or compression biker shorts. The most common colors are white and gray.

Firm or high-density Komprex foam can be used to apply pressure on fibrotic skin areas and can also be used in concave areas such as the palm of the hand or behind the ankle bones to even out bandage pressures. The padding is cut to fit over involved areas, including the calf and behind the ankle bones. The most common Komprex color is orange.

Komprex II is ribbed, fabric-coated foam with a special surface designed to provide directional compression for guiding lymph flow.

Specialized Pads

Special padding under short-stretch bandages can provide extra protection for sensitive skin, evenly distribute pressure over unusually shaped areas, or apply pressure on fibrotic areas. Specialized pads can also help channel lymph flow in certain directions. Chip bags, muffs, or Schneider packs are pieces of foam wrapped in stockinette (or other soft material) or between sticky cloth-tape (Hypofix, Cover-roll). Pads can be made by therapists in the clinic or purchased from lymphedema suppliers. Brands include JoViPak Multi-Purpose Pads, Peninsula Medical ReidSleeve Optiflow Packs, and Solaris Swell Spots.

Notes

1   **Textbook of Lymphology for Physicians and Lymphedema Therapists** by M. Földi, E. Földi, and S. Kubik (eds.), Urban & Fischer, p. 563, Germany, 2003.

2   **Textbook of Lymphology for Physicians and Lymphedema Therapists** by M. Földi, E. Földi, and S. Kubik (eds.), Urban & Fischer, p. 563, Germany, 2003.

3   BSN-Jobst Comprilan packing insert indicates that Comprilan is a short stretch bandage with a longitudinal elasticity of approximately 90%. BSN-Jobst, Inc., Rutherford College, NC.

4   **Lymphedema Management, The Comprehensive Guide for Practitioners** by J. E. Zuther. Thieme Medical Publishers, Inc. 2005. p. 113.

Chapter 19

Managing
Compression Garments and Aids

The goal of this process is to make sure the patient has the compression garments or aids they need, and to care for the compression garments and aids. If your patient uses garments or aids but not both, read only the appropriate parts of this chapter. Skip this chapter if your patient is not using either compression garments or aids.

The patient's therapist decides if a patient should use compression garments or aids and what garments or aids are needed. A patient may have two or more sets of compression garments to allow for care.

This chapter covers:

- Record keeping for managing compression garments and aids, including getting started and changing requirements. This process is the same for compression garments and aids.

- Care and inspection of compression garments and aids. Compression garments and aids are reused, and replaced as they wear out or the patient's needs change.

- Compression garment options, including the donning and doffing aids used to help get a garment on or off.

- Compression aid options.

If you are not familiar with compression garments or compression aids, you may want to read the last part of this chapter (starting on page 308) first, and then read the rest of the chapter.

Compression garments and aids are tracked using Equipment Forms. Multiple garments or aids of the same type and size can be tracked on one form.

Getting Started

The Care Activity Forms for putting on compression garments or aids (see page 338) should list the garments or aids that are required. If these forms have not been completed, the patient's therapist or the patient (if they have been doing self care), may be able to tell you what compression garments or aids are required for the patient's care routine. It may be easier to fill out the Care Activity Forms, the Equipment Forms for garments and aids, and the Supply Forms for any supplies that are required at the same time.

Depending on how often compression garments are worn, the patient may need more than one set to allow for washing. Most patients do not need multiple compression aids since compression aids are not washed frequently.

For each compression garment type and size or compression aid used:

• Create one Equipment Form (see page 431) with the description of each item and the number required.

• Check to see if the required garments or aids are available, if they are in usable condition, and how many there are.

• Fill out an Item Needed Form, if garments or aids have to be ordered.

• Update the Weekly Care Plan and Care Activity Forms to show when and how the garment or aid is used, if applicable.

• Add supporting activities to the Weekly Care plan: for compression garments, add "Washing Compression Garments" on page 305 each day and "Inspecting Compression Garments" on page 306 once week; for compression aids, add "Compression Aid Care" on page 307 once a week.

Compression garments may require special equipment, called a donning or doffing aid, or a lubricant to make it easier to put the garment on, see page 312.

If equipment, such as a donning aid, is required:

- Fill out an Equipment Form for each item.

- Check to see if the equipment is available and usable.

- If equipment has to be ordered, add it to an Item Needed Form.

- Update the Care Activity Forms to show when the equipment is used.

If a consumable supply item, such as lubricant, is required:

- Fill out a Supply Form for each item.

- Check to see how much usable supply is available.

- If the supply has to be ordered, add it to an Item Needed Form.

- Update the Care Activity Forms to show when the supply is used.

These supplies can be managed and reordered with the other supplies, see page 281.

Perform the Review Needs and Place Orders process (see page 278) after completing the Getting Started process for all supplies, equipment, and medications.

Changing Garment or Aid Requirements

Use of compression garments or aids in the care routine can change in several ways:

- Compression garment or aid use may be suspended due to an infection or other condition. A temporary suspension does not require any change in compression garment or aid management; the Weekly Care Plan should be updated to reflect the change.

- A patient who has not been using compression garments or aids may have one or both added to their care routine. This is the same as Getting Started (above) and involves Adding Compression Garments or Aids and possibly Adding Supplies and Adding Equipment for any donning aids required.

- Use of a compression garment or aid may be dropped from the patient's care routine. This is the same as Discontinuing Compression Garments or Aids for the item that was used, and possibly Discontinuing Supplies and Discontinuing Equipment for any associated donning aids.

- There may be a change in the type, or size, of compression garments or aids used. This can be handled by Adding a Compression Garment or Aid for the new type and size and Discontinuing a Compression Garment or Aid for the item that is no longer used.

- Donning and doffing aid usage may change. If equipment is added, see Adding Equipment; if equipment is no longer used, see Discontinuing Equipment; if a supply is added, see Adding Supplies; if a supply is dropped, see Discontinuing Supplies.

The subsections that follow explain the process for adding or discontinuing compression garments or aids and associated donning aid equipment or supplies.

Adding a Compression Garment or Aid

A compression garment or aid that is added to the care routine may be new or may have been used previously and usage was discontinued.

If a completely new compression garment or aid is added:

- Create a new Equipment Form with the information about the garment or aid.

- Fill out an Item Needed Form, if the item has to be ordered.

- Update the Weekly Care Plan and Care Activity Forms to show when and how the garment or aid is used.

If the compression garment or aid added to the routine had been used previously:

- Look for an Equipment Form with the information about the garment or aid in the Inactive Compression Garment and Aid folder. Create a new form if you do not find one.

- Check and see if there are any of the desired garments or aids still available and in usable condition, and how many there are.

- If the garments or aids have to be ordered, add them to an Item Needed Form.

- Update the Care Activity Forms to show when and how the garment or aid is used.

If this compression garment requires a new donning aid or lubricant, add the equipment or supplies as explained below.

Adding Equipment

A donning or doffing aid, or other equipment, added to the care routine may be new or used previously and usage was discontinued.

If a completely new equipment item is added:

- Create a new Equipment Form with the information about the donning or doffing aid.

- Fill out an Item Needed Form, if the item has to be ordered.

- Update the Care Activity Forms to show where the aid is used, if applicable.

If a donning or doffing aid added to the routine had been used previously and discontinued:

- Look for an Equipment Form with the information about the donning or doffing aid in the Inactive Equipment folder. Create a new form if you do not find one.

- Check to see if the donning or doffing aid is available and in usable condition.

- If the donning or doffing aid has to be ordered, add it to an Item Needed Form.

- Update the Care Activity Forms to show when and how the aid is used.

Adding Supplies

Supplies that are added to the compression garment routine may be completely new or they may be supplies that were used previously and usage was discontinued.

If a new supply is added:

- Create a new Supply Form with the information about the item.

- Fill out an Item Needed Form if the item has to be ordered.

- Update the Care Activity Forms to show when and how the supply is used.

If a supply is added that has been used before:

- Find the Supply Form with the information about the item in the Inactive Supplies folder. Create a new form, if necessary.

- Check to see how much usable supply is still available.

- If the supply has to be ordered, add it to an Item Needed Form.

- Update the Care Activity Forms to show when and how the supply is used.

Discontinuing a Compression Garment or Aid

If the lymphedema care routine changes and a particular type or size compression garment or aid is no longer being used:

- Locate all compression garments or aids of the specified type and size. Some compression garments may be with the laundry.

- If you think this compression garment or aid might be used again in the future, store any item(s) that are in good condition separately from current garments or aids; dispose of any garments or aids that are not reusable. Mark the Equipment Form as inactive and file it in the Inactive Compression Garments and Aids folder.

- If you think this compression garment or aid will not be used again, dispose of the equipment. Update the Equipment Form and file it under Inactive Compression Garments and Aids.

- Update the Care Activity Forms to remove any reference to this garment or aid.

If this garment or aid was the last garment or aid that required the use of a particular donning or doffing aid or lubricant, discontinue the equipment or supply as explained below.

Discontinuing Equipment

If the use of donning or doffing aid equipment is discontinued:

- Locate the equipment. If you think this item might be used again, then store it separately from current equipment; otherwise dispose of it properly.

- Update the Equipment Form and mark it as discontinued. Store the form in the Inactive Equipment folder.

- Update the Care Activity Forms to remove any reference to the aid.

Discontinuing Supplies

If the use of a supply item is discontinued:

- Locate any remaining supplies. If you think this item might be used again in the future, then store the supplies separately from other supplies; otherwise dispose of it properly.

- Remove the Supply Form and mark it as discontinued. If you think the item may be used again, file the form in the Inactive Supplies folder.

- Update the Care Activity Forms to remove any reference to the supply.

Compression Garment Care

Compression garment care includes washing garments daily and inspecting garments once a week as explained below.

Washing Compression Garments

Compression garments that are worn daily should be washed each day according to the manufacturer's instructions to remove skin oils and to allow the garment to return to its original shape. Garments that are not regularly washed become stretched and are less effective in controlling swelling. The patient may need two or more sets of garments to make washing and drying easier.

Prior to washing, turn the garment inside out. Hand wash garments or machine wash in a mesh garment bag (available at most drugstores) in warm water (up to 104°F or 40°C) on a gentle cycle. Use mild liquid detergent that does not contain perfume, bleach, or fabric softener. Juzo Detergent,

MediCare Wash, and Variance are examples of mild soaps for garments. Woolite is *not recommended* because it contains fabric softeners that may decrease the effectiveness of the garment.[1]

If garments are hand washed, roll them in a dry towel to remove any excess water (do not wring garments). Garments should be air dried, usually over a towel rack, or by laying them flat and away from direct sunlight or heat. Garments that do not have silicone bands or rubber threads may be dried in a dryer on a delicate setting, if necessary. Do not cut, iron, or dry clean compression garments.

Inspecting Compression Garments

With proper care, most garments will retain their compression for 3-6 months of daily use.[2] Lower extremity compression garments should be replaced every 3-4 months for patients who are ambulatory.[3]

As garments wear out, they lose their effectiveness in controlling swelling, slip down more frequently, and may become uncomfortable. See also "How can I tell if a garment doesn't fit?" on page 140.

Inspect compression garments for signs of wear and check their age. This can be done once a week, after washing garments. To inspect compression garments:

- Locate all the Equipment Forms that describe the compression garments.

- For each type and size of garment:

    - Count all the garments of this type and size, including those that are being worn. If there are fewer garments available than required, determine how many additional garments are needed.

    - Inspect the garments that are not being worn for fraying, runs in the fabric, loss of elasticity, or other signs of wear. Determine which garments need to be replaced and mark the garments.

    - Check the Equipment Form to see if replacement garments have already been requested, and how many. If additional replacements are needed (in addition to what was requested previously), add the information to the Item Order Request Form and update the Equipment Form.

Compression Aid Care

Compression aids should be inspected once a week and washed as needed.

To inspect compression aids:

- Locate all of the Equipment Forms that describe compression aids.

- Inspect each compression aid for fraying, deteriorating foam, loss of elasticity, or other signs of wear. Determine which aids need to be replaced and mark the aids.

- Check the Equipment Form to see if replacement aids have already been requested. If replacements are needed (in addition to what was requested previously), add the information to the Item Order Request Form and update the Equipment Form.

Compression aids that need cleaning should be washed and dried according to the manufacturer's recommendations. Each device may have slightly different instructions due to changes in the materials used. Check with the company that made the compression aid, or the fitter, if you do not have the care instructions for the compression aid.

Some compression aid manufacturers recommend that aids be re-checked periodically by a therapist or fitter to adjust the amount of pressure the garment provides.

Ordering Compression Garments or Aids

When the patient needs replacement compression garments or aids, contact the therapist for a follow-up appointment and have the patient's size re-checked. This is especially important when the patient is in the first two years of treatment or if there has been a recent change in the patient's swelling or body weight. If the patient has long-standing lymphedema and their limb size is stable, you may be able to order over-the-counter garments through a local or online garment distributor. Custom garments or aids generally require updated measurements by a therapist or certified fitter to reorder.

A physician's prescription, or letter of medical necessity, may be required for any garment or aid that will be reimbursed by the patient's insurance provider. Typically a physician's prescription is required to order or re-order compression garments that provide more than 20 mm Hg pressure.

Receiving New Garments or Aids

When a new compression garment or aid is received:

- Create or update the Equipment Form. Save the receipt and physician's prescription, if needed for reimbursement.

- Save the box or other identifying information so you have the specifications.

- Save the use and care instructions in the Product Information file.

- Mark each item with the date received.

- If this item replaces an existing garment or aid, dispose of the old item and cross out its entry on the Equipment Form.

For a new compression aid, it may be beneficial to have the therapist or fitter assess the garment for proper fit. If this is the first compression aid of its type, or if the design has changed, the therapist or fitter should show the patient or caregiver how to use the aid.

Compression Garment Options

Compression garments come in an assortment of styles, sizes, degrees of compression, and materials as described below. Some garments are available with other options including silicone bands to hold the garment in place, or zippers or Velcro to make the garment easier to put on and remove.

Compression garment style refers to the body area to be covered, and should not be confused with fashion. Available styles include arm sleeves, gloves, gauntlets or fingerless gloves, vests, knee high, thigh high, and waist high stockings, anklets, and foot or toe caps. For more detail and specific vendors, see "Garment Styles" on page 310.

Sizes

Pre-measured or over-the-counter compression garments come in sizes described as extra small to extra-extra-large or sizes 1-6. The patient's therapist or a certified fitter determines the compression garment size based on the patient's measurements and the manufacturer's size chart. Custom-made garments are specific to the patient's measurements.

Garment Pressure

Compression garment pressure ranges from relatively mild, or support garments, that provide less than 20 millimeters of mercury (mm Hg) pressure to very firm medical garments that provide more than 50 mm Hg pressure.

In the US, compression is graded from Class I 20-30 mm Hg, Class II 30-40 mm Hg, Class III 40-50 mm Hg, and Class IV over 50 mm Hg. Products from Germany use slightly different standards: Class I 18-21 mm Hg, Class II 23-32 mm Hg, Class III 34-46 mm Hg, and Class IV over 49 mm Hg.[4]

Custom garments in class I, II, and III generally provide less pressure but similar, if not more effective, swelling control than their over-the-counter counterparts. Class IV garments that provide more than 50 mm Hg pressure are custom-made only.

Garment Materials

Garments are made using a variety of materials and assembly techniques including circular knit (without seams), flat knit (with seams), and cut and sew (with seams) as described below.

Some patients may be allergic to garments because of latex, dyes, or other garment components. There are hypoallergenic garments available that are latex-free or the latex is shielded from the skin by wrapping it with cotton or lining the garment with silk.

Garments made with silver-impregnated fibers may contribute to fewer infections, enhance healing, keep limbs cooler, and reduce static.

Circular knit materials typically have elastic threads knit in a tubular shape to avoid a garment seam. Circular knit garments are available in standard sizes or custom-made to the patient's measurements. Circular knit garments apply an inward force against the patient's skin to prevent swelling. Circular knit material ranges from thin and sheer to very thick and opaque; the thicker the material, the better control of swelling. Sheer fabric garments may provide less control over severe swelling; however, they are more cosmetically appealing and are available in different skin tones, fashionable colors, and patterns. Circular knit garment companies include BSN-Jobst, Juzo, LympheDIVAs, Medi, and Sigvaris.

Flat knit materials are usually custom-made according to the patient's measurements and are constructed similar to the way yarn is knitted with needles; then, the fabric is brought into a cylindrical shape and sewn together. Flat knit garments are thicker than circular knit garments, lay flat against the patient's skin, and prevent fluid from pushing out. These garments offer the most effective control over severe swelling and are usually easier to put on than circular knit garments. Flat knit garment companies include BSN-Jobst, Juzo, and Medi.

Cut and sew garments are made from a woven material that is cut to the patient's measurements and sewn into the garment shape. Cut and sew garments are commonly used for burn-scar management and less frequently for mild cases of lymphedema. Cut and sew garments are custom-made and several companies offer a variety of colors, which is a particularly nice option. Manufacturers include Barton-Carey, Design Veronique, and Gottfried Medical.

Garment Styles

Garment styles for different affected areas are described below.

Head and Neck

Compression garments for head and neck swelling resemble hoods or ski masks. Most head and neck garments are custom-made, although some over-the-counter garments are available from Jobst Epstein and Facioplasty Supports.

Trunk, Breast and Genital

Compression garments for trunk, breast, and genital lymphedema may be off-the-shelf garments, specialized medical garments or pads, or a combination of these. Some medical garments include pockets for use with foam pads.

Support (light compression) bras, tops, and shorts are available at many sporting goods and department stores, and also online. When purchasing a support top or shorts for a patient, the caregiver should look for these key features:

- Nylon blends with Lycra/Spandex material. Cotton blends are available but generally stretch too much to provide effective compression.

- Clingy, tight fit to the patient's skin, but still comfortable to wear.

When purchasing support tops, specifically look for:

- T-shirt or tank top back, not a racer or T-back style.

- Scoop or V-neck styles that hide the garment under other clothing.

- Armholes that fit close to the armpit to minimize swelling of the chest wall over the edge of the shirt. If the patient has upper arm and shoulder edema, short sleeves are preferred over tank tops.

Common brands include Barely There, Danskin, Design Veronique, Hanes (for men), Marika, Sassybax, and Under Armour. Colors are usually white, black, and beige.

Medical compression tops and shorts are available through Durable Medical Equipment (DME) providers. Over the counter garments include the Bellisse Bra, Juzo Bra, and Jobst surgical vest designed for lumpectomy and post-mastectomy patients and Design Veronique compression bras for post-surgical swelling.

Custom-made shirts, vests, and shorts with a prescribed degree of pressure can be ordered from Barton-Carey, Gottfried Medical, Jobst, Juzo, and Medi.

Arm

Garments for arm swelling include sleeves, which extend from the wrist to the armpit or over the shoulder, gloves, and gauntlets (with only the thumb covered). Silicone bands are available to help keep garments from slipping down at the upper arm. Most patients with arm lymphedema will be placed in compression Class I or II garments.

Leg

Leg swelling garments include knee high, thigh high, and waist-high (pantyhose or men's leotard) stockings. Stockings may be open or closed-toe and come with or without silicone bands. Most patients with leg lymphedema will be placed in compression Class II or III garments. Figure 19-1 on page 312 shows pantyhose with suspenders on a child with primary lymphedema.

Note: Many leg garments are unisex; however, experience has shown that men's garments usually fit men better than unisex garments, especially at the foot. Since most men's feet are larger than women's feet, male patients may have problems with open-toed garments sliding into their foot arches.

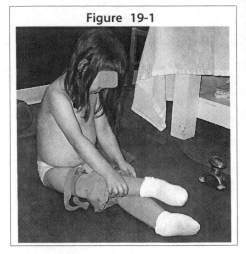

Figure 19-1

Donning and Doffing Aids

Donning and doffing aids are devices or lubricants that make it easier to get compression garments on or off. These aids can be obtained from the companies that sell garments (or may be included with garments), medical supply companies, or online vendors. Rubber gloves and non-slip rubber mats are household items that are readily available.

Rubber gloves: household rubber gloves (not medical gloves) with a textured (extra grip) surface will make it easier to don and doff garments, and help protect garments from fingernails or jewelry.

Metal Frame Donning Aids: Jobst Stocking Donner or Mediven Butler. The garment can be placed over the metal frame and the patient places their foot (or arm) into the garment and pulls the frame handles up for easier application.

Foot Slip: Arion Easy Slide, Jobst Foot Slip, Juzo Slippie Gator, Mediven Easy-On Slipper, or Sigvaris Silk. Many foot slips come with open-toed garments and make the stocking easier to put on; the foot slip also reduces the risk of the patient's toenails snagging the garment. Similar slips for closed toe stockings and for arm sleeves are also available.

Rubber mat: Dycem non-slip pad, Juzo Easy Pad, or other non-slip mat. Rubber mats are used by pressing the patient's heel against the mat to help move the garment on or off the foot. A similar technique can be used for an arm sleeve to inch it up the patient's arm, although this may not be necessary when the caregiver is assisting the patient.

Fitting Lotion or Silicone Lotion: Alps Silicone Fitting Lotion. Lotion makes the limb more slippery, so that the garment slides easily onto the limb. An added benefit is that the lotion moisturizes the limb.

Mediven Butler Off: The Butler Off is shaped like a long-handled shoe horn with an easy push handle and a hook at the back of the horn to catch the edge of the garment as it is pushed down the leg. The Butler Off is particularly helpful when a patient has trouble bending forward far enough to reach their foot.

Most donning and doffing aids are equipment and can be managed using an Equipment Form. Fitting lotion is a supply (since it is used up) and should be tracked using a Supply Form.

Compression Aid Options

A compression aid may be recommended by a lymphedema therapist as an alternative to compression bandaging for edema control and to simplify home care. The therapist should specify which aid(s) will best control the patient's swelling. Some compression aids have features for treating specific swelling issues.

All compression aids help control swelling but there are a variety of different options and issues to consider, as explained below. Finances and insurance reimbursement policies often influence the decision to purchase a compression aid. Other issues also arise, such as comfort and the ease of getting the aid on and off the patient. The caregiver or care arranger may be part of the decision making process and may want to research compression aid companies (see Appendix B on page 418). Discuss any patient-related concerns with the therapist or fitter before a final decision is made.

There are several options to consider when selecting a compression aid, including the type of foam, adjustability and durability.

Foam Types

There are several types of foam used in compression aids:

- Flat foam: provides uniform pressure throughout the garment in order to minimize pressure points, which may be a concern for patients with fragile skin or open wounds.

- Egg-crate foam: has bumps similar to an egg carton and may be used to soften fibrotic tissues.

- Channeled Foam Pieces: small chips or pieces of foam are sewn into a special fabric with a quilted pattern designed to help channel fluid out of affected areas.

- No foam: aids designed without foam are used to provide additional compression in a particular area, such as the lower leg. These aids are typically worn during the day and are sometimes used over a compression garment.

Adjustability

Certain foam compression aids are closed with a seam; these aids are pulled onto the patient's limb and then a Lycra "power sleeve" is applied over the aid to increase the overall amount of compression. In contrast, other compression aids wrap around the limb and close with Velcro straps or other closures. Aids with closures are easier to put on and may be adjusted (larger or smaller for lighter or firmer pressure) to accommodate swelling fluctuations. This may be an important consideration when swelling is relatively severe. Generally, compression aids with Velcro straps are stiff and bulky, restricting the patient's ability to move while wearing the aid.

Durability

Most compression aids have a 6-12 month guarantee against manufacturing defects but durability issues may arise depending on the patient's lifestyle and garment care. Consideration should be given to how gentle the patient will be with the aid and if the compression aid will be used day and night or only at night.

Notes

1   Care of Your Bandages and Garments patient handout, Bandages Plus, 2008.

2   Jobst Medical Leg Wear patient insert, BSN-Jobst, Inc., 2005.

3   "The Garments We Wear" by Paula Stewart. *Lymph Link* April-June 2007.

4   "The Garments We Wear" by Paula Stewart. *Lymph Link* April-June 2007.

Chapter 20

Managing Equipment

This chapter describes the process for managing equipment in terms of getting started, changing and replacing equipment. Lists of recommended equipment for care activities are included.

Equipment is tracked using Equipment Forms (see page 431).

Getting Started

The steps in getting started managing equipment include:

- Identify what equipment is being used, or will be needed, by reviewing the list of recommended equipment (see page 317) with the patient (if they have been doing their own care), the patient's therapist, and optionally, the patient's healthcare provider. If Care Activity forms (see page 338) have been completed, check these forms for equipment used.

- For each type of equipment that will be used in home care, fill out an Equipment Form.

- For each Equipment Form, check to see if the equipment is available and take the appropriate action:

  - If the equipment is available, update the Equipment Form with the information on the quantity on hand.

  - If an equipment item is not available or more are needed, add it to an Item Needed Form so it can be ordered.

Plan to do the Review Need and Place Orders process (see page 278) after you complete the Getting Started process for all supplies, equipment, and medications.

Changing Equipment Requirements

As the patient's care routine changes, there may be a need for additional equipment or the use of certain equipment items may be discontinued.

Adding Equipment

If a type of equipment is added, it may be new or used previously and discontinued. Separate instructions are provided below.

If new equipment is added:

- Create a new Equipment Form with the information about the equipment.

- Fill out an Item Needed Form if the equipment has to be ordered.

- Update the Weekly Care Plan and Care Activity Forms to show when and how the equipment is used.

If an equipment item is added that has been used previously:

- Look for an Equipment Form with the information about the equipment in the Inactive Equipment folder. Create a new form if necessary.

- Check to see if there is equipment on hand, if it is still usable, and how many are available (if more than one are needed).

- If the equipment has to be ordered, fill out an Item Needed Form.

- Update the Care Activity Form to show when and how the equipment is used.

Discontinuing Equipment

If the use of a care equipment item is discontinued:

- Return the equipment if it was rented or leased. If you think the equipment may be used again then store it safely; otherwise, dispose of it properly. In some cases, unneeded home care equipment can be sold or donated to an agency for recycling.

- Remove the Equipment Form and mark it as discontinued. If you think the equipment may be used again, put the form in the Inactive Equipment folder.

- Update any Care Activity Forms to remove references to using the equipment.

Replacing Equipment

Equipment may need to be replaced if it breaks, is lost, wears out, or no longer meets the patient's needs. If something must be replaced, add it to the Item Needed form.

Recommended Care Equipment

The right equipment can help make lymphedema care more comfortable for the patient and the caregiver. Details of the equipment needed will vary with the care routine. Care Activity Forms should list specific equipment requirements.

This section describes basic equipment by care activity. The patient's therapist can recommend medical aids for special needs such as a caregiver with limited strength and mobility and lifting equipment for large patients or patients with mobility limitations.

Skin Care

- Wash basin and floor covering for washing outside of the bath or shower.

- Long handled brushes for patients that have trouble reaching their feet.

- Mirrors and long-handled mirrors, if the patient is doing self-inspection of the skin and feet.

- Digital camera for taking photographs to record changes in swelling or skin condition over time; ideally the camera should record the date and time with each picture.

Remember to take the camera, or prints, to the patient's medical appointments if you are planning to discuss the images. Add a reminder to the appointment information in the Patient Notebook.

Taking Measurements

- A cloth tape measure or a specialized tape measure sold by lymph-edema supply companies. Ask the patient's therapist if they use centimeters or inches and use the same units, if possible (the conversion factor is 2.54 cm per inch).

- A calculator for comparing past and present measurement values.

- Digital thermometer. Glass and mercury thermometers are not recommended for use with children.

- Scale for weighing the patient. If a patient is obese, wheelchair bound, or has trouble standing, a special scale may be required and it may not be practical to weigh the patient at home.

Simple Lymph Drainage

- Massage table or adjustable bed that is accessible from the sides.

- Extra pillows, blankets, or towels that can be used as supports.

- Sheets or blankets to keep the patient warm.

Bandaging

- Mesh bag(s) for washing bandages.

- Movable table or cabinet to hold bandages and supplies.

- Stools of different heights for the patient and caregiver.

- Scissors or specialized bandage scissors for cutting padding materials.

- Mechanical or electrical bandage winder (optional).

Compression Garments and Aids

- Donning and Doffing Aids, see page 312.

Decongestive Exercise

Exercise equipment varies based what the patient's therapist recommends. Commonly used equipment includes:

- Broomstick or dowel about 30 inches (0.75 m) long.

- Hand weights, typically 1-3 pounds (0.5-1.5 kg).

Other Care Equipment

Depending on the patient and the affected area, it may be helpful to have:

- Chairs that fit the patient comfortably. A chair without arms is easier to use when bandaging patients who are mobile and stable; arm rests may be required for patients with balance issues or patients with trouble getting in and out of a chair.

- Stools in various sizes including a small step-stool and a medium height stool.

- Hospital bed that can be raised and lowered for easy access or transfer and has movable supports on the sides. Ideally, the bed should be positioned so that the caregiver has access to both sides. Make sure the wheels on the bed are locked during patient use.

- Transfer belt—a wide padded belt with an anti-slip surface on the inside and hand grips on the outside—to help move and support patients with mobility issues. Available from medical supply companies.

Some patients may require specialized lifting equipment or other devices to ease the burden on the caregiver. An Occupational Therapist (OT) can visit the home to evaluate specific needs, recommend solutions, and train caregivers on proper use of this equipment. The patient's doctor may have to order the OT evaluation, especially if the patient's insurance is expected to pay for or provide the care equipment.

Managing Care

This equipment is optional but may make care easier:

- File cabinet or file box for care management records. Employee records for hired caregivers should be kept in a locked file.

- All-in-one combination printer, copier, and facsimile machine for paperwork.

- Three-hole punch will make it easier to add things to notebooks.

Chapter **21:**

Managing Medications

Most patients take several medications for lymphedema or other conditions. Patients with lymphedema may have standby antibiotics, preventative (prophylactic) antibiotics, or topical medications.

The goal of this process is to make sure the patient has the medicines they need without purchasing more often than necessary. This procedure covers pills and topical medications (creams, powder, or spray). It does not cover managing injected medications, liquids, skin patches (transdermal medications), or perishable medications.

Adapt this procedure based on the time required to obtain each medication to provide at least a ten day margin of safety. Medications that can be obtained within 2-3 days should be reordered when a two week supply remains. Medications that take longer to obtain should be ordered further in advance. The Medication Form provides the information needed to track usage rates and the lead time between placing and receiving orders.

The Patient Notebook (see page 372) should include a complete list of all the medications the patient is taking, including over-the-counter medications and supplements. If this list is not available, or is not up-to-date, the caregiver and the care arranger should gather the information to create an accurate list.

A list of recommended over-the-counter medications that lymphedema patients should have on hand, in case they are needed, is provided on page 327. Compare this list with the patient's medication list and see if there are any medications that should be added. Check the patient's medication allergies or ask the patient's doctor before introducing any new medication.

The Weekly Care Plan (see page 333) should include any medications that the caregiver reminds the patient to take or gives the patient, and any topical medications the caregiver applies. The care plan will not list medications that are taken only as needed or medications that the patient takes on their own.

A Medication Form (see page 432) will be used for each of the patient's medications. The information on the form should include:

- The type of medication (pill, capsule, cream, etc.) and a description of the appearance of the medication or package.

- The standard storage location for the medication and any special storage instructions.

- Who prescribed the medication and for what condition.

- How and where the medication can be ordered or purchased, if known.

There should be a form for each of the patient's medications. If the caregiver is not responsible for managing or ordering a medication, note this on the form.

Getting Started

The steps in getting started managing medications include:

- Identify medications by checking the medication list in the Patient Notebook and any standby medications. If the Weekly Care Plan and Care Activity Forms have been created, cross check the plan and the medication list for medications used.

- For each medication that will be used in home care, fill out a Medication Form.

- Decide if the caregiver is responsible for managing each medication and mark the form appropriately.

- For each Medication Form where the caregiver is responsible for management, check and to see if the medication is available and take the appropriate action:

    - If a medication is available, update the Medication Form with the information on the quantity on hand so usage can be tracked. Estimate how quickly the medication will be used (see "Adding a Medication" on page 324) and consider ordering more if there is less than a two week supply on hand.

    - If a medication is not available, add it to an Item Needed Form so it can be ordered.

Plan to do the Review Needs and Place Orders process (see page 278) after you complete the Getting Started process for all supplies, equipment, and medications.

Changing Medications

If there is a change in the patient's medications:

- If one medication is substituted for another, follow the procedure for discontinuing the old medication (page 324) and adding the new medication (page 323). This applies if there is a change in the pill size, medication form, or a switch from brand name to generic or vice versa.

- If the change is only in the dosage or medication schedule, update the Weekly Care Plan and Care Activity form with the new dosage and schedule.

- If a medication is added, follow the procedure in Adding a Medication.

- If use of medication is discontinued, follow the procedure in Discontinuing a Medication.

Adding a Medication

If a medication is added it may be new or one that had been used previously and discontinued. Separate instructions are provided below.

If a new medication is added:

- Create a new Medication Form with the information about the medication.

- Fill out an Item Needed Form if the medication has to be ordered.

- Update the Weekly Care Plan and the appropriate Care Activity Form with the medication dosage and schedule.

- Add the new medication to the medication list in the Patient Notebook.

If a medication is added that has been used previously:

- Look for a Medication Form with the information about the medication in the Inactive Medications folder. Create a new form if necessary.

- Check to see if there is any of the medication on hand, if it is still usable, and how much is there.

- If the medication has to be ordered, fill out an Item Needed Form.

- Update the Weekly Care Plan and the appropriate Care Activity Form with the medication dosage and schedule.

- Add the medication to the medication list in the Patient Notebook.

Discontinuing a Medication

If the use of a medication is discontinued:

- Locate any remaining medication. If you think it may be used again in the future, then store it safely and separately from other medications; otherwise dispose of it properly. Ask the patient's doctor how to dispose of the medication safely.

- Remove the Medication Form and mark it as discontinued. If you think the medication may be used again, put the form in the Inactive Medications folder.

- Update the Weekly Care Plan and the relevant Care Activity form to remove the medication. If this was the only medication on the Care Activity form, remove the activity from the weekly plan destroy the Care Activity form.

- Update the medication list in the Patient Notebook.

Reordering Medications

The procedure for reordering medications varies depending on how the medication is used. Instructions are provided for pills, standby antibiotics, and topical medications.

If the patient's medications are covered by Medicare Part D or other health insurance drug benefits, the insurance program or the pharmacy benefit manager that administers the program may have specific rules on when and where medications may be purchased in order to receive reimbursement.

Managing Pills

Prescriptions and usage for pills typically follow one of these patterns:

- *Episodic usage*, for example a medication that is given for a 10 days. Typically the recommended number of doses is provided and the medication does not have to be reordered. Standby antibiotics are a special case, see below.

- *Consistent usage*, for example a medication that is taken every day or every week. Estimate the number of pills used per week and re-order when the quantity on hand is less than a two week supply.

- *As needed*, for example something taken for an occasional headache. Estimate the maximum number that could be used in one week and re-order when the quantity on hand is less than a two week supply.

Standby Antibiotics

Standby antibiotics for lymphedema infections are a special situation. A patient may be given a prescription for standby antibiotics so that treatment can start at the first sign of an infection. The standby prescription may be for a full course of antibiotics (typically 10 days) or just a few days supply.

If standby antibiotics have been prescribed for the patient:

- Fill the prescription (order the pills) as soon as possible. Do not wait for signs of an infection to develop.

- If an infection is suspected and the patient starts taking the standby antibiotics, contact the patient's health care provider and:

  - Follow the health care provider's instructions for treating the current infection and obtain additional medication, if necessary.

  - Ask to have the standby prescription replaced, if it can't be refilled. Replace the standby antibiotics that have been used.

- Check the standby medication every six months to make sure the medication has not expired. Contact the patient's health care provider for a replacement prescription, if necessary.

Managing Topical Medications

There are two ways to track topical medications and decide when to reorder:

- Monitor usage and reorder when the medication is getting low.

- Keep a spare container of each medication; when the current container is used up, open the spare container and order more.

The first method works well for creams or powders where one container lasts several weeks and you can tell how much remains. The second method is better if containers are used up quickly and for spray medications where it is hard to tell how much remains. If several containers are used per week, re-order when there is less than a two week supply on hand.

Decide how you want to track each of these medications and fill in the Reorder information on the Medication Form. You can always change the reorder method if needed.

Recommended Medications

Prescribed medications are determined by the patient's health care providers according to the patient's specific condition. This section lists over-the-counter medications that you might want to have on hand, in case they are needed. Check the patient's list of medication allergies and ask the patient's doctor before introducing any new medication.

Topical medications:

- Athletes foot cream, powder, or spray.

- Jock itch or skin fungus cream or spray.

- Antibiotic cream.

- Anti-itch cream or spray.

Other medications:

- Anti-inflammatory drugs such as aspirin, ibuprofen (Advil, Motrin), naproxen (Aleve), or acetaminophen (Tylenol).

- Antihistamines such as Benadryl.

Arranging and Managing Care

Arranging care is a multi-step process, as explained in the chapters that follow:

- Evaluating Care Needs

- Finding and Paying for Care

- Preparing for Care

- Training Caregivers

We describe a complete process. Feel free to use as much, or as little of this process, as you think is needed, depending on your situation.

You may need to repeat part or all of this process at different times because of changes in the patient's care needs, to replace a caregiver, or for other reasons. Save your notes and information.

Chapter 22

Evaluating Care Needs

Evaluating care needs is an easily overlooked but very important step in arranging lymphedema care. The results of this evaluation will help you determine:

- What care is needed, when, and for how long.

- What caregiver skills and other abilities are needed.

- Caregiver goals and the nature of the care relationship.

This chapter describes the process for evaluating what care is required and making plans to provide the care. Depending on the patient's situation, a professional evaluation and plan may be required (page 349). Even if a formal evaluation is not required, we recommend documenting the care routine as described below.

This chapter outlines a complete process for coordinating team care; adopt as much or as little of this process as needed for your patient's situation. You can begin with just an outline weekly care plan and add more detailed instructions and records as needed.

The overall process includes:

- Weekly Care Plan and associated Care Activity instructions as explained in this chapter, starting on page 333.

- Patient Notebook with information on the patient and their medical condition, see page 372.

- Caregiver Handbook with specific information and instructions for the caregiver, see page 375.

- Managing supplies, equipment, and medication as explained in the previous section (page 269).

The Weekly Care Plan provides a template showing care activities in a typical week. This template is then copied and modified to plan and schedule specific care activities for each week. During the week, the form is used to document care provided and other activities.

The current and future Weekly Care Plan and the Care Activity forms should be stored in the Caregiver Handbook for easy reference and use. During the week, the Weekly Care Plan is updated to record the patient's condition and care provided; completed forms can be stored in the Patient Notebook.

Both the Patient Notebook and the Caregiver Handbook may contain health information, financial information, and personal information for the patient and others. These documents should be kept confidential in order to protect the privacy of all parties.

The Patient Notebook and Caregiver Handbook can be combined in one notebook, if desired. Using separate notebooks minimizes the amount of paper to be carried to medical appointments.

There are several online services offering tools to help coordinate caregivers, see the list in Appendix B (page 420). These tools are especially useful if everyone involved is comfortable using an online service and if caregivers or care coordinators are in different locations. If you use an online service, we suggest maintaining paper records as backup in case the online service is not available. You may be able to print pages from the online service for this purpose.

Weekly Care Plan

The weekly care plan serves three purposes:

1. Planning and coordinating what care is required, when, and who will provide it.

2. Providing instructions for care providers. Specific instructions can be recorded on Care Activity Forms (see page 425) or you can reference specific pages in this book.

3. Record keeping to show what care was provided, what medication the patient has taken, and to document changes in the patient's condition. See "Recording Care Activities" on page 340.

The care plan need only cover the aspects of the patient's day where assistance or instructions are required. This can include lymphedema care activities that the patient can do independently, lymphedema care activities that require caregiver assistance, and other care activities.

Planning may involve making trade-offs between the ideal level of care and what can be achieved with the resources available. The patient's therapist can help create a plan that balances keeping the patient's swelling controlled with the amount of time the patient and caregiver can spend on lymphedema care.

Weekly Care Plan Overview

The form for the Weekly Care Plan (see page 424) has several parts:

*   Weekly schedule showing:

    -   Time and Care Activity columns show what needs to be done at different times of the day. The columns for days of the week can be used to show variations in schedule if some days are different, such as weekends.

    -   Directions: mark this column to show if instructions are provided on a Care Activity Form or insert the page number to reference instructions in this book.

- Help/Who: use this column to show if assistance is required for an activity and optionally the type of assistance required (if special skills are required) and the number of people needed. This area can also be used to show who is scheduled to help with each activity.

- Days of the week: cross out days when an activity is not planned, check off each activity and day as it is completed.

• Notes: use this area to record any changes in the patient's condition including any changes in skin appearance, swelling, the patient's general activity level, emotions, or other unusual findings. Add additional pages if needed.

The amount of planning detail required varies based on the patient's situation. For example:

• A female breast cancer survivor with upper extremity lymphedema might only need two care routines:

- Morning self-care which she does independently. This can be shown on the Weekly Care Plan but a description is not needed.

- Evening lymphedema care that includes some activities where caregiver assistance is required, such as SLD and applying compression bandages. As a minimum, Care Activity Forms should be created to document the steps where caregiver assistance is required.

• A young child with primary lymphedema may need assistance with lymphedema care three times a day for SLD, all using the same Care Activity descriptions.

• An older man with lower extremity lymphedema, limited mobility, and other health issues may have his whole week planned out including:

- Weekday morning and evening lymphedema care with a hired caregiver who also prepares his meals and helps him with other activities. Care Activity forms should be used to document each step of the lymphedema care; this level of detail may not be needed for other activities.

- Senior Day Care where lunch is provided during the week.

- Assistance from his adult children on weekends.

Listing Care Activities

Make a list of care activities before creating a weekly plan. Once you have this list, it will be easier to set the sequence of activities and work out a schedule. Start with a list on a piece of scratch paper or a computer file; this information will be added to the weekly plan in the next step.

The patient's therapist, the patient (if they have been doing self care), or current caregivers should be able to help you identify care activities. It may be easiest to have the patient or caregiver describe a typical day, and what they do, in order to identify care activities.

First, list the major lymphedema care activities and any other health care activities or activities of daily living where the patient requires assistance every day. Depending on the patient's care needs, these activities can include:

- Skin care (see page 45) at least once a day, typically either morning or evening. If this includes applying topical medications, check to make sure the medications are on the patient's medication list.

- Simple lymph drainage (see page 67) one or more times per day. Frequently this will be done after skin care.

- Compression bandaging (see page 95) or compression garments and aids (see page 133), depending on when the patient wears compression and what type their therapist recommends. A common schedule is to put on compression garments in the morning and change to either compression bandaging or compression aids before bed.

- Decongestive exercises (see page 143), one or more times per day. The patient may need to put on additional compression before exercising and remove it afterwards.

- Medications: list the patient's medications and group them together by time of day to identify the related care activities. Add activities for medications the caregiver gives the patient that are not part of another care activity like Skin Care.

Second, add care activities that may not happen every day. For example:

- Taking Measurements (see page 339) is typically done once a week. It may be easiest to schedule this just before bathing or skin care to wash off the measurement marks.

- If a bath or shower is not a daily event and the patient requires assistance with bathing or related lymphedema care, add the appropriate care activity to the plan.

- Instrumental activities of daily living such as cooking, shopping, laundry, cleaning, transportation, etc.

Third, add supporting activities for taking care of equipment and supplies. For example:

- If the patient uses compression bandages, add an activity for Washing Bandages (see page 292) every day, or on a schedule recommended by the patient's therapist, and fill out a Care Activity Form with specific instructions, if needed. Also add a weekly activity for Inspecting Bandages (see page 293).

- If the patient uses compression garments, add an activity for Washing Garments (see page 305) every day, or on a schedule recommended by the patient's therapist, and fill out a Care Activity Form with instructions, if needed. Also add a weekly activity for Inspecting Garments (see page 306).

- If the patient uses a compression aid, add a weekly activity for Compression Aid Care (see page 307), and fill out a Care Activity Form with any necessary instructions, if needed. Compression Aid care includes inspection and washing as needed.

- If a caregiver is responsible for managing supplies, bandages, compression garments and aids, equipment, or medications (see page 269), add the appropriate weekly activities to the plan. If necessary, fill out a Care Activity Form with specific procedures for each activity.

Emotional care and support is part of every interaction between the patient and caregiver and does not appear on this list as a care activity.

Creating the Weekly Care Plan

Start with a blank Weekly Care Plan form (see page 424) and make a template that can be copied to create a specific plan for each week. Either print or copy a blank paper form and mark it up in pencil or edit the electronic version of the form in the computer and save it under a new document name.

To create a Weekly Care Plan template:

- Fill in the Patient name but leave the "Week of" area blank.

- Add the care activities to the form in sequence by time of day, for example morning and evening. For help identifying care activities, see "Listing Care Activities" on page 335.

- For each activity where caregiver assistance is required, fill in the column for "Help/Who." See "Caregiver Assistance Required" below.

- For each activity that requires instructions, you can either:

    - Fill out a Care Activity Form (see page 425) with specific instructions and mark the column to show that there are instructions.

    - Use instructions provided in this book and put the page number in the instructions column.

- Many patients have a different routine on weekends than they do during the week. Modify the plan to reflect these differences by day of the week, if appropriate.

- For medications, group the medications the patient should be given by time of day and fill out a Care Activity Form (see below) with the medications, dosage, and specific instructions for each group of medications. If there are medication that are not given every day, cross out the boxes for the days that do not apply.

Caregiver Assistance Required

For activities that require caregiver assistance:

- Mark the "Help/Who" column to distinguish care activities that require specific caregiver skills or qualifications. For example, lymphedema care requires a trained lymphedema caregiver; other care activities may require a nurse, physical therapist, occupational therapist, housekeeper, etc.

- Note the number of people needed in the "Help/Who" column for those activities (if any) that require multiple caregivers. For example, bandaging an obese patient may require the help of two or more people.

- Adjust the schedule and plan to accommodate caregiver scheduling constraints, if necessary. For example, caregivers may only be available at certain times of the day, or caregivers provided by an agency (see page 357) may have to be scheduled in fixed time blocks or require a minimum number of hours per visit.

Care Activity Instructions

General instructions for many care activities are included in this book. In some situations you will want to prepare specific instructions and document them on Care Activity Forms (see page 425). The patient's therapist, the patient (if they have been doing self care), or caregivers should be able to help you document instructions.

You may want to copy and markup instructions for:

- Specific SLD sequences for each affected area (see page 78).

- Exercise routine worksheets (see page 146) include an area for tracking a week of exercise. You can copy the relevant pages, or download the forms from the book Web site, and use these to track exercise.

Use the "Care Activity Checklist" on page 339 to make sure that your Care Activity Forms are complete.

Care Activity Checklist

Are supplies and equipment for each task in preparation?

☐ Skin care: moisturizing creams or lotions, topical medications, medical gloves, soap, washcloth, towels, etc.

☐ Taking Measurements: marker, tape measure, calculator, etc.

☐ Compression bandaging: padding, tape, scissors, etc. Does the list of bandages include the specific quantity, size, and type in the sequence in which they are used?

☐ Compression garments or aids: donning or doffing aids.

☐ Decongestive exercise: exercise equipment, towel, drinking water, etc.

Other things to check:

☐ Simple Lymph Drainage: sequences for each affected area?

☐ Is additional compression needed for exercise?

☐ Exercise routines for each affected area?

☐ Remove additional compression after cooling down?

☐ Reminder to record the activity after it is completed?

Planning Care for the Week

A specific weekly care plan based on the template created above is the major tool for coordinating care. The care arranger may want to prepare plans for several weeks in advance in order to schedule caregivers.

To prepare a weekly plan, make a copy of the Weekly Care Plan template and:

- Fill in the start date for the Week; dates for each day of the week are optional.

- Mark up the plan to reflect any changes to the normal routine such as holidays, medical appointments, or lab tests.

- Schedule caregiver(s) for each day and activity where assistance is required. If there are multiple caregivers, mark up the plan to show who works when.

Recording Care Activities

During the day, the Weekly Care Plan helps the caregiver know what they should be doing and can also be used to record the care provided:

- Care Activity: initial or check-off each activity after it is completed in the row for the activity and the column for the day.

- Use the Notes area to record any activity that is skipped or modified, changes in the patient's condition, etc. Record the date and time, and initial each note.

- If the patient is weighed or their temperature is taken, record these readings in the appropriate area.

- Medications: initial or check-off each medication given in the column for the day.

At the end of the week, move the completed Weekly Care Plan form to the Patient Notebook and switch to the plan prepared for the coming week.

If measurements are taken, record these on the Arm or Leg Measurement Form in the Patient Notebook.

Routine, Respite, and Backup Care

Most patients need three types of caregivers:

- Routine caregivers who help on a regularly scheduled basis.

- Respite caregivers who can substitute for a routine caregiver on a pre-arranged basis. For example, to allow a caregiver to go on vacation or have time away for other reasons.

- Backup caregivers who can be available on short notice in the event of an illness or other unexpected change in caregiver availability. Respite caregivers may not be available on short notice to provide backup care.

All too often, arrangements for respite and backup care are neglected until a primary caregiver becomes burned out, hurt, or ill. Adequate respite care is important to support the health of the routine caregivers (see "Caring for the Caregiver" on page 381). Knowing that they have respite and backup care options helps patients, their families, and caregivers feel more secure.

It may be difficult to recruit caregivers for respite and backup care only. Caregivers may be more willing to help, and easier to train, if they also provide some routine care on a scheduled basis.

Routine Care Needs

The Weekly Care Plan shows when routine caregivers, or additional routine caregivers, are needed in terms of care activities that do not have anyone—or the appropriate number of people for activities requiring more than one person—scheduled to help. By looking at the care plans for several weeks into the future you can determine what additional resources are required in terms of time-of-day and days-of-the-week. From this you can calculate the number of hours needed per day and per week.

Respite Care Needs

Respite care provides time off for routine caregivers. There are several approaches to providing caregivers with planned substitute care and temporary relief from the daily responsibilities of caring for the patient. Respite care can take place in an adult day center, in the home of the person being cared for, or in a residential setting such as an assisted living facility or nursing home.

The desired amount of respite varies from caregiver to caregiver. Family and other informal caregivers may need more or less time away depending upon the person providing the care, their health, and their other obligations.

Hired caregivers may have legal rights to vacation, holidays, and other time off under the terms of their employment agreement (see "Written Contracts" on page 364) and state labor laws. Check with your lawyer or the state department of labor or employment in the state where the caregiver is employed.

If a caregiver is hired through an agency, the agency may be responsible for managing respite care and backup care issues, and providing an alternate caregiver if needed. For more information, see "Working with an Agency" on page 357.

Backup Care Needs

Every lymphedema patient who needs caregiver assistance on a daily basis should have at least one designated and trained backup caregiver. Additional backup caregivers should be recruited when:

- Routine caregiver absences have become common or are expected to increase.

- Backup caregivers have limited availability and may not be able to help when needed.

Caregiver Job Description

A job description is a useful way to organize and document caregiver skill requirements and may be useful for recruiting caregivers or hiring through an employment agency. Employment agencies may provide templates for job descriptions.

Respite and backup caregivers may not need all the same skills as routine caregivers, and you may want to prepare two different job descriptions. Some aspects of the care routine can be skipped, simplified, or postponed if necessary.

Fill out the Job Description(s) as follows:

- Job title: either 'Routine Caregiver' or 'Respite/Backup Caregiver' and the patient's approximate age, gender, and condition. For example: 'Respite/Backup Caregiver for a four-year-old girl with lower extremity lymphedema.'

- Duties: select the applicable lymphedema care duties from the list in "Lymphedema Care Duties" on page 343 and add any duties that are required for other health conditions, or to support the patient's activities of daily living, or instrumental activities of daily living. Use the information from the Weekly Care Plan and Care Activity forms if they are available.

- Other requirements: list any specific requirements for doing the job or conditions of employment. For example, if the position requires a driver's license, car, the ability to move or transfer the patient, specific language skills, etc.

Lymphedema Care Duties

☐ Skin Care

☐ Taking Measurements

☐ Simple Lymphatic Drainage

☐ Compression Bandaging

☐ Compression Garments or Aids

☐ Decongestive Exercise

☐ Emotional Care and Support

☐ Record Keeping (general)

☐ Managing Supplies and Equipment including care supplies, compression bandages, compression garments and aids, other equipment, and medications.

- Work schedule: for routine care outline the days and hours needed in a typical week (based on the Weekly Care Plan, if you have one); for respite care, say 'for temporary assignments' and outline the hours and time period required; for backup care, say 'substitute caregiver available on short notice.'

- Work location: provide a general description of the care setting and neighborhood but you may not want to disclose the actual address in the job description or ads. For example, 'for in-home care in the University Heights area.'

Duration of Care

Lymphedema care is usually required throughout the patient's life but the type of caregiver assistance needed, the reasons that the patient needs assistance, and the amount of caregiver time required each week may change. For example:

- Young children with lymphedema will need less assistance with the physical aspects of self-care as they get older. The child's need for emotional support and encouragement may fluctuate over time.

- Patients with degenerative physical or mental conditions may need long-term care and increasing amounts of assistance over time.

- Severe lower extremity swelling can become easier to care for, and require far less caregiver assistance, as the swelling is reduced through treatment.

Care requirements can also change based on the phase of lymphedema treatment (see "Phases of Treatment" on page 36). During an intensive treatment phase, the patient may need less assistance with daily care at home, but they may need to have their bandages washed daily.

The patient's therapist and doctor should be able to estimate how long caregiver assistance will be needed and what to expect in terms of the amount of assistance required in the future. Adjust the work schedules in the job descriptions as necessary.

Other Considerations

There are several other factors to be considered when recruiting caregivers, managing the expectations of the patient, caregiver, and care arranger, and building effective relationships between the caregiver and patient. These factors include:

- The patient's overall situation and the goals of lymphedema care.

- Reasons why the patient needs assistance with care.

- Communications abilities or preferences.

- Patient attitude towards self-care and knowledge of the home care routine.

The care arranger should keep these factors in mind when recruiting and interviewing caregivers. In some cases, you may want to add this information to the caregiver job descriptions.

Patient Situation and Care Goals

What is the patient's overall health situation? What are the goals of lymphedema home care? Depending on the patient's age, medical condition, knowledge and attitude the goals of the caregiver and lymphedema care could include:

- Helping the patient learn self-care skills and become more independent.

- Improving the patient's motivation and compliance with daily care.

- Providing a terminally ill patient with palliative care and comfort.

Reasons for Assistance

Why does the patient need assistance? Does the patient have:

- Physical conditions that affect self-care such as limited joint range of motion, issues with grip strength and dexterity, or obesity. What changes in the patient's physical condition are anticipated?

- Mobility limitations? Does the patient need assistance transferring or walking? Is the patient homebound (unable to leave the place of residence without a supportive device, special transportation, or another person)?

- The ability to learn and organize self-care activities?

- Signs of depression or dementia that affect the patient's ability or willingness to care for themselves? See "Depression" on page 191 and "Alzheimer's Disease or Dementia" on page 232.

Communication Abilities

Evaluate the patient's communication skills:

- Does the patient have issues with hearing or speaking?

- Can the patient communicate effectively in English?

- What is the patient's preferred language?

Self-Care Attitude and Knowledge

Patient attitudes towards lymphedema and lymphedema care impact the patient's willingness to accept care and cooperate with a caregiver. Lymphedema evokes a number of emotional responses, and patient attitudes can range from anger or denial to acceptance and full cooperation. For more information on emotions and attitudes, see the chapter on "Emotional Care and Support" (page 189).

☐ Does the patient accept that they have lymphedema?

☐ Does the patient acknowledge the need for lymphedema care?

☐ Is the patient willing to cooperate with lymphedema care?

☐ How well does the patient know the lymphedema care routine?

☐ Does the patient have the ability to remember the care routine?

☐ Is the patient motivated to perform self-care activities?

Chapter 23:
Finding and Paying for Care

The process of finding care involves defining care requirements, researching available options, and selecting the best available alternative. This process may be repeated if there are changes in care needs, care provider availability and cost, or the patient's financial situation.

We suggest that you:

- Find a guide to help you navigate the care and reimbursement system.

- Create a comprehensive plan covering all care needs, including lymphedema treatment.

- Develop a budget if there are financial constraints.

- Explore options for financial support.

- Look at the most appropriate options: working with an agency, direct hiring, or recruiting informal caregivers.

Informal caregivers— including family members, friends of the patient, or volunteers—provide the bulk of the home care for lymphedema and other conditions. Hired caregivers play an important role in providing routine care for those who require, or prefer, paid care and in providing respite or backup care for informal caregivers. In future years, we expect that hired caregivers will become more common because the baby boomer generation has fewer children who can provide informal care.

Many patients end up with a patchwork of formal and informal caregivers to cover the range of services they need on the days when they routinely need care, plus respite or backup care when a regular caregiver is ill, injured, or on vacation.

Informal caregivers may have to be recruited and encouraged; we provide specific suggestions in "Recruiting Informal Caregivers" on page 366.

In most cases, hired and informal caregivers will need training on how to provide lymphedema care. In addition to the instructions in the Lymphedema Care Skills section (page 43), we provide some pointers in "Training Caregivers" on page 378.

Lymphedema home care is ongoing, but the patient's need for assistance, and the availability of specific resources, may change over time. Likewise, the patient's eligibility for insurance and other sources of payment may vary based on changes in the patient's condition, the type of care needed (short-term, long-term, or palliative care, see page 39), financial resources, and coverage. Plan to revisit this chapter as often as needed.

Find a Guide

A wide variety of home care services are available, but service eligibility and reimbursement rules can be very complicated. Fortunately, there are experts who can help with this process. Start by talking with the patient's doctors and lymphedema therapist about problems with home care activities and the types of assistance and equipment that are needed. They may be able to suggest resources and strategies for obtaining assistance.

To find a case manager who can guide you through the various care options, contact:

- National Association of Professional Geriatric Care Managers at 520-881-8008 or www.caremanager.org.

- US national Eldercare Locator at 1-800-677-1116 or www.eldercare.gov.

- The Area Agency on Aging for the county and state where the patient lives.

- City, county or state health departments or visiting nurse association.

- American Cancer Society at 1-800-227-2345 or www.cancer.org.

- Discharge planners or social workers at hospitals where the patient has been treated.

- In Canada, start with www.canada.gc.ca or call 1-800-755-7047.

Eldercare and cancer care programs can provide useful information on local resources, even if the patient is not elderly or a cancer survivor. Eldercare agencies may also be sources of help from senior volunteers or seniors seeking employment.

Evaluating care options is easier once you know the range and extent of services required and what resources are available in your area. In addition to providing resource information, a case manager can help identify sources of financial support.

Create a Comprehensive Care Plan

Lymphedema care should be arranged as part of a comprehensive care plan that covers the patient's requirements for lymphedema care, care for any complications of lymphedema (such as wounds), and care for other medical conditions. The patient may also need assistance with:

- Activities of daily living(ADL) and personal care such as eating, bathing, dressing, transferring, toileting, etc.

- Instrumental activities of daily living (IADL) that support independent living such as cooking, shopping, laundry, cleaning, transportation, etc.

- Companionship to provide a social outlet or for safety monitoring.

Hired caregivers provided by home care agencies are predominantly paraprofessionals:

- Certified Nursing Aide (CNA) provides basic patient care under the direction of nursing staff.

- Home Health Aide (HHA) provides personal health care and help with activities of daily living.

Home Health Care Services for adults living in the community provide mostly Home Health Aides, with some Nursing Aides. Residential facilities are primarily staffed with Home Health Aides while nursing facilities employ mostly Nursing Aides.

Depending on the situation, you may want to arrange a professional evaluation by a geriatric care manager, nurse, or social worker, and have them develop a comprehensive plan of care taking into account physical, cognitive, emotional, and social issues. Medicaid and other insurance programs may provide this assessment as part of their service.

The person doing the assessment may not be familiar with lymphedema care. If you have created a Weekly Care Plan (see page 333), make copies of the plan and associated Care Activity descriptions for them. It may also be helpful to arrange for them to speak with the patient's lymphedema therapist or doctor.

The plan should cover:

- Types of care required and the desired times of day and days of the week.

- Expected duration of the care need, if care is temporary.

- Requirements for specialized equipment or home medications, if any.

- Transportation needs for the patient, if appropriate.

Develop a Budget

Anyone with limited financial resources will need to budget for lymphedema care and other expenses in order to make informed decisions about what they can afford. The patient may need to provide a budget and financial information to qualify for needs-based financial support. A care manager can help you with this process.

An evaluation of personal financial resources involves looking at:

- Assets: including liquid assets like checking and savings accounts and other assets such as property or investments.

- Liabilities or debt: money owed on mortgages, credit cards, unpaid bills, etc.

- Income: including retirement benefits, Social Security, etc.

- Expenses: for living expenses, health care, insurance, etc. The cost of lymphedema care is discussed in more detail below.

- Insurance benefits for medical and home health care expenses.

- Tax status of expenses: medical expenses are tax deductible in certain circumstances. This helps reduce the effective cost of care for the patient or a person who can claim the patient as a dependent.

Budgeting is an ongoing process. Plan to update your budget any time there is an important change in the cost of care, other expenses, expense reimbursement, or income.

For more information on budgeting for healthcare expenses of all types, see the resources in Appendix B (page 420).

Costs of Lymphedema Care

Lymphedema home care can be expensive, and many home care costs are not covered by health insurance or other reimbursement programs. Although the need for caregiver assistance with home care may be temporary, other lymphedema home care costs will be ongoing.

This section outlines a budget for lymphedema home care. It does not include other medical expenses such as therapist sessions, doctor visits, or medications.

There are four types of expense associated with lymphedema home care:

1. People costs for providing care, if paid caregivers are used.

2. Supplies such as padding, lotions, tape, etc. that are used once or only reused a few times.

3. Bandages, compression garments and aids with a limited useful life.

4. Medical Equipment such as compression pumps or lifting devices.

Each type of expense is treated differently for reimbursement as explained below. The subsections that follow will help you budget for these costs and understand the reimbursement issues.

The types and quantities of supplies, bandages, and compression garments or aids required can change during the course of lymphedema treatment. For example, more bandages may be required during an Intensive Phase, or treatment series, than during the Maintenance Phase, see "Phases of Treatment" on page 36.

People Costs

There are several options for hiring caregivers:

- Reimbursed care is typically paid for, managed, and controlled by the insurance provider. Although this is not the most common source of care, it has its own set of issues and is usually provided through an agency that has been approved by the insurance provider, see "Working with an Agency" on page 357.

- Contracting with an agency to provide certain levels of care for certain time periods, typically in blocks of four hours. The agency is responsible for hiring, scheduling, and supervising the care provider(s).

- Employees hired by the patient or the person coordinating care. See "Direct Hiring" on page 360.

- Family reimbursement programs pay family members for providing home care, subject to restrictions on who may be paid and what services are covered. These programs are offered by some state and federal government programs for the elderly or disabled, by other local agencies in some areas, and by some long term care insurance programs.

A care manager can help you locate resources and estimate the cost of these options in your area. In general, contracting with an agency will be more expensive than hiring employees directly, but it will also require less time on the part of the person arranging care.

Supply Costs

Supplies for lymphedema home care are discussed in "Managing Supplies" (page 281) and include items that are used once, or only reused a few times.

If the patient is just starting lymphedema care, ask the patient's therapist to help you estimate what supplies will be required, the purchase price for each item, and how frequently each supply will need to be purchased. They can also explain how supply requirements are likely to change over time.

If you are managing supplies using the process provided in this book, the Supply Forms will provide the information you need to track supply usage and estimate future supply costs.

Purchase price can be converted to a monthly budget cost based on the useful life of the item:

- Disposable supplies or supplies that require replacement each month: estimate the quantity that will be used up in a month and multiply by the cost of each supply.

- Supplies that last longer: divide the cost by the useful life in months. For example, if an $18 bottle of donning lubricant lasts for 6 months, the cost is about $3/month.

Unfortunately, very few insurance programs provide realistic payment (or any payment) for lymphedema care supplies.

Bandages, Compression Garments and Aids

Bandages, compression garments, and compression aids can be reused repeatedly until the item wears out, or the item is no longer suitable for the patient. See "Managing Bandages" (page 287) and "Managing Compression Garments and Aids" (page 299) for more information.

If a patient is just starting lymphedema care, ask the patient's therapist to help you estimate what bandages, compression garments, or aids will be required, the purchase price for each item, and how long each is likely to last. The therapist can also explain how requirements are likely to change over time. For example, a compression garment may wear out or may need to be replaced by a different size garment as the patient's limb size changes.

If you are managing bandages, compression garments, and aids using the process provided in this book, the Equipment Forms will provide the information you need to track and estimate costs.

Efforts are underway to convince Medicare and other insurance providers that compression bandages are not "personal comfort items." Until these rules are changed, this is an expense the patient and their family must absorb.

Coverage of compression garments and aids by Medicare, Medicaid, and other insurance programs varies between states and companies. Some programs consider these to be durable medical equipment and pay part or all of the cost based on the rules for Medical Equipment described below.

In recent Medicare appeals cases it has been determined that compression garments and compression aids are covered services under the Social Security

Act because they meet the statutory definition of prosthetic devices. This is good news but it will take time for this coverage ruling to be adopted by all Medicare regions and other programs. For more information see the chapter on Reimbursement Policy Issues in **Voices of Lymphedema**[1] or contact Bob Weiss, NLN Patient Advocate at LymphActivist@aol.com.

Medical Equipment Costs

Several types of equipment may be required for home care, as described in "Managing Equipment" (page 315). Certain items of equipment that are medically necessary may be covered by Medicare or other insurance reimbursement programs. Typically, this includes treatment devices like sequential compression pumps, lifting equipment, hospital beds, etc. These items are considered to be "durable medical equipment" (DME) with a long useful life.

Many health plans will pay some or all of the cost of durable medical equipment based on a doctor's order and a formal approval process. Medicare, for example, will pay 80% of the cost to rent, purchase, or service approved medical equipment and expects the patient to pay the other 20%, this can be a considerable amount of money for some equipment.

In order to receive reimbursement for medical equipment, the patient's therapist or medical doctor may have to place the order. Many health care plans will only pay for equipment that is purchased from an approved supplier. Physicians can appeal a denial by providing a letter of medical necessity.

Paying for Care

Every organization that pays for medical care has its own rules about the types of care they will cover (short-term, long-term or hospice care, see page 39), what home care services are covered (if any), who may provide these services, and coverage limits. Rules for federal programs, like Medicare, often vary from state to state. Although we cannot explain all of these rules, we provide suggestions for finding out what services are covered.

In general, organizations that pay for care will require:

- Doctor's order or prescription explaining the medical necessity for the care.

- Care provided by an agency that is accredited or accepted.

- Written care plans and periodic progress reports from the agency.

Health care agencies may require written authorization before they will discuss care with anyone other than the patient.

If you think the patient may be eligible for paid care:

- Look for a care manager or other specialists who can help you with this process.

- Make a list of all the organizations that may provide coverage for the patient (see below) and apply to each of them.

- If the patient currently needs short-term or long-term care, ask about coverage for other types of care so you know what options may become available in the future.

US resources include:

- Medicare covers health care for people age 65 and up, and for younger people with certain disabilities. See www.medicare.gov or call 1-800-633-4227 for more information.

- Medicaid pays medical costs for people with limited income and resources; this is a federal program administered by each state. See www.cms.hhs.gov or call 1-800-633-4227 for more information.

- Veterans Affairs (VA) care for eligible veterans and surviving spouses. See www.va.gov or call 1-800-827-1000.

- Other government programs such as state or county Indigent Care Programs, Civilian Health and Medical Program of the Uniformed Services, Indian Health Services, and Workers' Compensation Programs.

- Health Savings Accounts (HSA) and other tax-favored health plans may be used to pay for qualified medical expenses for yourself, your spouse or a dependent. Qualified medical expenses can include over-the-counter medications and expenses not covered by other plans; see IRS Publication 969 for details.

- Long-term care insurance may cover some caregiver services.

Canada offers a variety of caregiver resources and benefits. For more information, see www.canada.gc.ca or call 1-800-755-7047.

The federal Family Medical Leave Act (FMLA) provides certain employees with up to 12 weeks of leave to care for a child, spouse, or parent or because the employee is unable to work due to a medical condition. Although this leave is unpaid, health benefits are maintained during the leave and the employee's job is protected. Some states have family leave programs for caregivers.

Specific Resources

There are some specific resources available to help support the cost of lymphedema care and/or supplies, especially if the lymphedema is cancer-related. These options include:

- NLN Garment Fund, founded by the Marilyn Westbrook family, provides compression stockings and sleeves to qualifying National Lymphedema Network members. For more information, call the NLN at 1-800-541-3259/510-208-3200 or see www.lymphnet.org.

- Lance Armstrong Foundation offers some resources and can help connect patients with other sources of support. See www.livestrong.org or call 1-866-467-7205.

- Lymphedema support groups may be able to connect members with local resources or may offer support programs. See the support group listing on www.LymphNotes.com.

- Susan G. Komen for the Cure offers grants through their local affiliates that can include lymphedema care. To find your local affiliate, see www.komen.org or call 1-877-465-6636.

Tax Deductions and Credits

Favorable tax treatment of care expenses may help reduce the financial burden of care. If the patient is not paying for their own care, the person who is paying may have to claim the patient as a dependent in order to take tax deductions or credits. Contact your tax advisor or the IRS for more information.

Medical expenses may also be tax deductible. These expenses may include medical care, medications, supplies, equipment, medical care insurance premiums, transportation for medical care, amounts paid for qualified long-term care services and limited amounts for qualified long-term care insurance contracts. There are a number of conditions that apply, see IRS Publication 502 for more information.

You may be able to claim a Child and Dependent Care Credit if you pay for someone else to provide care for a person who is your dependent (which may be a child, parent, or other financial dependent) so that you may work. There are a number of conditions that apply, see IRS Publication 503 for more information.

Working with an Agency

Many types of agencies offer home care services. The types of care services offered, the role of the agency, and their prices may vary considerably. For example:

- Home health care agencies assign and supervise teams of caregivers including nurses and therapists. Medicare certified agencies meet federal standards and provide services that may be reimbursed by Medicare and Medicaid.

- Home care agencies provide care aides or attendants. These agencies are licensed in some states.

- Registries or staffing agencies match clients with care personnel. They may or may not screen care personnel or handle employment taxes.

When evaluating an agency you will want to know:

- Type of organization and ownership: government, for profit, nonprofit? Are fees fixed or on a sliding scale?

- Is the agency licensed or regulated? By whom?

- How does the agency screen their personnel? Do they conduct a background check and a criminal record check?

- Are agency personnel bonded or insured for liability? Are they covered by workers compensation insurance? Will the care arranger be responsible for providing any insurance?

- Who is responsible for screening, supervising, paying caregivers, and paying employment taxes (see page 362)?

- If a caregiver is sick or on vacation, who arranges for a substitute caregiver?

- Will the agency provide a written plan that identifies specific tasks and services to be provided? Will the family be notified of any changes in this plan?

- What is the charge for care, what is included and what extra charges or minimum charges apply? Will there be charges for travel, overtime hours worked, specific procedures, or services that are not performed?

- What forms of payment are accepted? Will the agency bill the patient's insurance provider directly? How often will you be billed and what are the payment terms?

- Types of services provided and rates. What are the rules about what care activities agency staff may provide?

Quality information for Medicare approved home health providers is available online at www.medicare.gov.

Caution: In-home health care has become a very popular franchise business. By early 2008, there were more than 3,400 franchising companies in this market.[2] With such rapid growth, you can expect wide variability in the quality and experience level of managers and caregivers.

Agency Interview Questions

Here are some questions you can use when interviewing an agency:

- How long has the agency been in business (in your area)? Ask for, and check references from doctors, patients, and other care arrangers.

- How large is your staff in this area? How many of these are supervisors?

- Does your agency have experience caring for other patients with lymphedema?

- How are care needs assessed and documented? How does the agency coordinate care with the doctors and other people who are important to the patient's care?

- How are emergencies handled?

- How are problems resolved? What are the policies and the process for resolving disputes?

Consumer Rights

A patient and their care arranger have consumer rights that are guaranteed under state and federal licensing laws that set standards for home health agencies. Most agencies require clients to sign a contract that lists these rights and defines their relationship with the agency before any care begins. Review the rights and responsibilities listed in the contract and consider filing a complaint if these rights are violated.[3]

Individuals receiving home health care retain the rights to:

- Information about the plans for their care, costs, and changes in care or agency policies.

- Quality care including care planning, safe and adequate care, and referrals to more suitable care if desired.

- Privacy and dignity while receiving care and in protecting medical information.

- Timely and adequate response to any complaints about treatment or services, including a prompt hearing to address any complaints.

The patient or care arranger also has responsibilities, including the duties to:

- Notify the agency of changes in condition, schedule, or preference for care.

- Follow prescribed care—including asking questions about treatment and accepting consequences for not following the care routine.

- Report problems with services that are inadequate.

- Be financially responsible and pay for services as agreed.

- Treat agency personnel respectfully, provide a safe environment, and respect home health care personnel and their property.

Direct Hiring

Direct hiring, where the patient or the person coordinating care is the employer, may be less expensive than using an agency but the process is more complicated and can be time consuming. The employer will be responsible for finding and screening help, employment taxes (see page 362), insurance (see page 364), etc.

Unfortunately, there is currently no directory or mechanism for locating trained lymphedema caregivers. Hopefully, something like this will be created in the future; check www.LymphNotes.com for the latest information.

We can suggest two paths for locating caregivers:

- Networking through lymphedema therapists and support groups to locate people with experience as lymphedema caregivers who may be able to assist.

- Locating caregivers and arranging for them to learn lymphedema care skills.

Care coordinators, volunteer and employment agencies, other patients or care coordinators, caregivers, and other networks can help you locate caregivers.

The Caregiver Information Form (see page 427) can be used to organize information about hired or volunteer caregivers.

Lymphedema Networking

You may be able to locate people with experience as lymphedema caregivers by networking through lymphedema therapists and treatment centers, lymphedema or cancer support groups, etc. Referrals to caregivers may also be available from other patients, care arrangers, or care providers.

Medical professionals are prohibited by law from disclosing patient names or other information without permission. However, you can network through them by providing cards or flyers that they can pass on to people who may be able to help you. These cards or flyers should contain contact information for the person who is coordinating care, not the patient.

Individual Interview Questions

Interviewing a lymphedema caregiver is not that different from interviewing any other personal care provider. You want to cover the basics in order to make sure this is someone that you will be comfortable with and can rely upon. In addition to the interview, you should check references, verify credentials (if the caregiver has a healthcare credential), check for a criminal record, and you may want to have a service conduct a background check. Criminal record checks for home care providers are available from government agencies in many states.

If you find someone with experience providing lymphedema care, ask about:

- Daily care routine for other patients and what they did, as caregiver.

- How they view the role of the caregiver and what they like and dislike about their work.

- Experience recognizing infections or other lymphedema emergencies.

If you are screening someone without lymphedema experience, you may need to explain what lymphedema is and what causes it, and assure them that lymphedema is not contagious. At the same time, you want to be sure that they understand (or are willing to learn) basic precautions for infection control.

If you are hiring someone who will need training in lymphedema care, look for:

- Willingness to learn and an ability to retain new information.

- Patience and commitment to stick with something, despite obstacles.

- Organized and systematic approach to activities.

Consider asking these questions when interviewing potential caregivers:

- How long have you been doing this type of work? What do you like about it?

- What is your experience and where did you work previously?

- What specific skills and training do you have? Do you have CPR certification or other emergency first aid training?

- Do you drink or take drugs?

- How would you handle a medical emergency?

- What are the basic sanitary precautions for infection prevention?

- Are there any tasks in the job description that you are not comfortable with?

Before hiring a caregiver, be sure that he or she is:

- Capable of communicating clearly with you and the patient.

- Someone that you and the patient are comfortable with.

- Physically able to perform the duties of the job safely and in good health overall.

- Able to provide valid identification (driver's license or state id), a Social Security card, and documentation for employment (see below).

- Cleared by a reference check (see "Reference Check Questions" on page 363) and a background check or criminal record check.

- Able to get to the work location on schedule, if applicable.

Employment Taxes

If you pay people to provide care, you may be required to pay federal or state employment taxes. These taxes do not apply if your payments go to a person who is in business as an independent contractor with multiple clients, a company, a nonprofit organization, or a government agency.

If you hire a caregiver as an independent contractor and you pay more than $600 per year for services, you may be required to give the contractor a 1099 form and file a copy with the IRS. See the Instructions for Form 1099-MISC for more information.

Federal payroll taxes include income tax, Social Security, Medicare, and unemployment tax. The rules on who must pay taxes and tax rates are subject to change. See the current version of IRS Publication 926 Household Employer's Tax Guide for details. The following summary of the 2008 rules is provided as an example:

- You are not required to withhold federal income tax from your household employee's wages. But if your employee asks you to withhold tax, you can.

> ### *Reference Check Questions*
>
> ☐ How long have you known the applicant? In what context?
>
> ☐ Was the applicant reliable? Dependable? Courteous? Trustworthy?
>
> ☐ What were your impressions of the quality of their care or work?
>
> ☐ Why is the applicant no longer working for you?

- You must withhold and pay Social Security and Medicare taxes if during the year you pay wages of $1,600 or more to any one household employee who is not your spouse, your child under the age of 21, your parent (subject to certain conditions), or an employee under the age of 18 (subject to certain conditions).

- You must also pay federal unemployment tax if you pay wages of $1,000 or more in any calendar quarter to employees who are not your spouse, your child under the age of 21 or your parent.

If you are required to pay federal employment taxes you will need to:

- Obtain an employer identification number (EIN) before you file employer tax forms. See IRS Form SS-4 for instructions on obtaining an EIN by phone, online, or by mail.

- Decide how you will make tax payments and keep records; see IRS Publication 926 for details.

- When you hire an employee, you must obtain documentation that the person can legally work in the United States and complete US Citizenship and Immigration Services (USCIS) Form I-9, Employment Eligibility Verification.

- Have each employee show you their Social Security card and complete a Form W-4, so you know how much tax to withhold (if any).

- When you pay your employee, withhold federal income tax (optional), Social Security and Medicare taxes, and make advance payments of the earned income credit (if applicable). See Publication 926 for rates and procedures.

- In January, give each employee Form W-2, Wage and Tax Statement copies B, C, and 2.

- In February, send Form W-2 copy A to the Social Security Administration.

- In April, file Schedule H (Form 1040), Household Employment Taxes, with your federal income tax return (Form 1040). If you do not have to file an income tax return, use the option to file Schedule H by itself.

Each state has different rules for payroll taxes. Contact your state tax agency to find out if you need to pay state unemployment tax; state taxes may apply even if you are not required to pay Federal Unemployment Tax. You should also determine if you need to pay or collect other state taxes or carry workers' compensation insurance.

Payroll processing services can help you with accounting and tax filings. There are a number of firms that specialize in household payroll.

Insurance

Make sure employees are covered by insurance in the event of an accident at the care location. Some homeowner's or renter's insurance policies automatically cover household employees. Check with the insurance agent to see if existing policies include employee coverage and cover employees working at the care location, especially if the caregiver's employer does not live at the location where the care is provided.

Written Contracts

A written employment agreement or contract is prudent any time you are hiring an employee or contractor. See "Contract Checklist" on page 365 for a list of points you may want to include in the contract. Check with your lawyer to see what is appropriate for your situation. In some situations, a contract may help the patient and caregiver feel more comfortable as discussed in "Roles, Goals, and Relationships (page 389).

Contract Checklist

Employer: name, address, contact information.

Other people and their responsibilities: patient (if not the employer), others who may provide direction.

Employee: name, address, contact information, Social Security number.

Duties and responsibilities: describe what is expected of the caregiver.

Work schedule: including work hours, break times, days off, holidays, etc.

Work location(s): where care will be provided.

Pay: including wages, benefits (if any), paid sick leave (if any), paid vacation (if any).

Pay policy: what is the policy on paying the caregiver if the patient is hospitalized, traveling, or does not need care temporarily for other reasons?

Pay procedure: time cards or other records required, how and when payments are made.

Expenses: mileage, meals that are paid or provided, etc.

Other rules or requirements:

- Prohibited behaviors: smoking, consuming alcohol or other substances, etc.

- Bringing guests or other persons to the care location.

- Personal use of the telephone, television, computer, etc.

- Requirements for providing a car, driver's license, insurance, etc.

- Reasons for termination without advance notice.

- Requirement for giving advanced notice before quitting.

Signatures: employer, employee, date signed, effective date.

Written agreements are especially important if:

- A hired caregiver will be living with the patient. The agreement should explicitly state that the caregiver may only stay in the home while they are employed.

- Family members are hired as paid caregivers with funding from a government program or long-term care insurance.

- An individual is being paid as an independent contractor rather than an employee.

- A patient is arranging their own care or care is being arranged at a distance.

- The agreement involves things that will happen if the patient is hospitalized, no longer competent to manage their own affairs, or dies.

Recruiting Informal Caregivers

Informal caregivers may volunteer, but more commonly you will have to be proactive in recruiting people and letting them know what specific help is needed. For practical advice on how to do this, see the resources in Appendix B (page 420), especially:

- **Share the Care** book and www.sharethecare.org website.

- **Lotsa Helping Hands** at www.lotsahelpinghands.com.

Screen volunteers that you don't know before accepting them as a caregiver to make sure you and the patient will be comfortable working with them. You may want to adapt the interview questions provided on page 361. You may also want to check references and get a criminal background check.

Supervising Caregivers

All caregivers deserve encouragement, support, and monitoring. Appropriate supervision varies depending on the type of relationship between the caregiver and the care arranger or patient and the scope of the caregiver's responsibilities. Hired caregivers should have regular supervision, especially if they are employed by the patient or care arranger.

Informal caregivers also need guidance, oversight, clear instructions, and emotional support in appreciation of their efforts.

Supervising a lymphedema caregiver involves looking at several things:

- Is the caregiver competently performing their duties for lymphedema care, record keeping, and assisting with the activities of daily living (if applicable)?

- Does the caregiver provide appropriate emotional care and support to the patient?

- Are there signs of problems with the caregiver's behavior or the relationship between the caregiver and the patient? Specific signs are given below.

Note that the first item is competent performance of care duties and not swelling reduction or improvement in the patient's lymphedema.

If the person arranging care is not the patient, the care arranger should establish a regular routine for checking in with each caregiver. If practical, the care arranger should check daily duties twice a month and weekly duties once a month.

Other ways to check on the performance of the caregiver include:

- Speaking with the patient without the caregiver present.

- Visiting unannounced or on short notice.

- Using a Web cam or "nanny cam" device to communicate with, or monitor, the patient and caregiver. Video or audio recording systems can be used for surveillance as well.

When a caregiver is doing a good job, the care arranger should provide frequent, positive feedback and should encourage the patient to do the same (assuming the patient is not the care arranger). Give praise immediately, as deserved, so the caregiver feels recognized and valued.

Discuss any problems as they arise. Don't bottle them up. Problems should be discussed objectively and calmly. When offering corrections, first comment on a part of the task that has been done correctly. Then let the care provider know pleasantly and firmly how you want the task to be performed.

Give clear instructions and training when needed. If things are not done ideally, remember that being flexible and picking your battles will save you stress and aggravation. Encourage the caregiver to let you know if he/she does not understand you. Be respectful of your caregiver, this encourages them to be respectful of you.

If a caregiver is expected to pay care expenses and be reimbursed, there should be clear written guidelines about the types of expenses that will be reimbursed and an appropriate budget. All expenses should be documented by receipts, and the receipts should be checked before the caregiver is reimbursed.

A caregiver who is not the patient's spouse or a close family member should not be added to the patient's financial accounts such as checking, savings, credit card, Social Security, etc. Protect the financial information of the patient and other household members from caregivers without a legitimate need for this information.

If you hire caregivers directly, keep in mind that you are their employer. Plan to provide periodic performance reviews. Establish a performance review schedule at the time of hiring so a performance review does not seem like punishment or criticism. Keep written records of your employee reviews and any disciplinary issues.

Tell-tale signs of possible patient abuse include:[4]

- Bruises, pressure marks, broken bones, abrasions, and burns may indicate physical abuse, neglect, or mistreatment.

- Unexplained withdrawal from normal activities, a sudden change in alertness, and unusual depression may be indicators of emotional abuse.

- Sudden changes in financial situations that may be the result of exploitation.

- Bedsores, unattended medical needs, poor hygiene, and unusual weight loss are indicators of possible neglect.

- Belittling, threats, and other uses of power and control are indicators of verbal or emotional abuse.

- Strained, tense relationships or frequent arguments between the caregiver and patient are also signs.

If a caregiver is hitting, screaming, endangering the patient's health, or making you or the patient feel afraid, that is abuse. Tell the patient's family or friends immediately and call the police. Make a report to Adult Protective Services if the patient is over 18 or Child Protective Services if the patient is a minor.

If you suspect theft, confront the caregiver and ask for his/her explanation. If you are certain that something of value is missing, call the police.

You will need to fire a caregiver if:

- You, or the patient, do not feel comfortable with the person or they are not cooperative.

- The caregiver becomes unreliable and frequently arrives late or misses work without advance notice.

- They violate the conditions of their employment agreement (see page 364).

- You suspect abuse, theft, or any illegal or improper behavior.

If you decide to fire a caregiver, document the date and your reasons for termination.

Notes

1   **Voices of Lymphedema** edited by Ann Ehrlich and Elizabeth McMahon. Lymph Notes, 2007.

2   "Taking Care of Business: why in-home health care is one of the hottest concepts in franchising today" by Simona Covel. *The Wall Street Journal*. March 17, 2008.

3   "Rights and Responsibilities in Home Health Care" by the California Health Care Foundation. Available at www.calnhs.org/homehealth/index.cfm?itemID=107139&sectionID=106337.

4   Adapted from "Warning Signs of Elder Abuse" by the National Center on Elder Abuse, www.ncea.aoa.gov.

Chapter **24:**

Preparing for Care

There are a number of things that may need to be done in preparation for having someone help with care initially. This information may need to be revised periodically based on changes in the caregiver relationship or setting.

These include:

- Documenting the care routine, as discussed in "Evaluating Care Needs" (page 331), if this has not been done.

- Assembling a Patient Notebook, if you don't have something similar. The Patient Notebook is discussed on page 372.

- Ensuring that the caregiver has appropriate access to the patient's health information under federal privacy laws, as explained on (page 374).

- Putting together a Caregiver Handbook with information a caregiver may need to understand and carry out their duties, as explained on page 375. This Handbook is an important tool for training caregivers as discussed below.

- Preparing the home to make things easier for the caregiver and patient, including obtaining special equipment, if needed, and setting up standard locations for things. See page 377.

- Training caregivers, see page 378.

Patient Notebook

The Patient Notebook is an essential tool for coordinating caregivers and the patient's medical team. This is especially important in the event of an emergency, or if the patient is unable to provide medical information.

The Patient Notebook should include:

- Patient information including contact information, basic medical information, allergies, and insurance information. Use the Patient Information Form (see page 426) or equivalent.

- Additional medical information and patient medical history, if appropriate. See the "Medical Information Checklist" on page 373 for a list of topics to be included.

- Medication List covering all current medications including the medication name, form and dosage, instructions for taking the medication, who prescribed the medication, and for what condition(s). This should also include any injected medications, patches (transdermal medication), topical creams or ointments, over-the-counter medications, vitamins or herbal supplements, and complementary or alternative medications taken on a routine or as needed basis.

- Weekly Care Plan forms that have been completed and show the patient's condition and care provided during past weeks. The Weekly Care Plan for the current week should be in the Caregiver Handbook.

- Arm or Leg Measurement Forms, if applicable, for each affected area (see page 60 for instructions, page 428 and page 429 for forms). The patient's therapist may supply baseline or best day measurements.

- Exercise tracking worksheets as explained in the "Decongestive Exercise chapter (page 143). This would include a master worksheet for each of the patient's exercise routines, worksheets for the current week, completed worksheets for past weeks, and blank worksheets.

- Release of Medical Information forms, if appropriate. Health care providers may require written authorization before discussing a patient's condition with the caregiver if the patient is not present, or is incapacitated, as explained in "Privacy Laws and Caregiver Access" on page 374.

Medical Information Checklist

Medical information should include:[1]

☐ Patient identification: including name, address, telephone number, date of birth, and health plan identification numbers.

☐ Emergency contacts: name, telephone numbers, and relationship.

☐ Medical team: name, specialty, telephone number, group or affiliation, office address. Be sure to include the patient's lymphedema therapist, dentist, and other specialists.

☐ Health insurance or Medicare coverage information.

☐ Diagnoses or medical conditions currently affecting the patient. For a lymphedema patient, this would include the areas affected by lymphedema and the condition of each area.

☐ History of illnesses, surgeries, and major medical procedures with dates; include any implanted medical devices such as pacemakers.

☐ Allergies or other sensitivities to medications, latex, food, or environmental factors.

☐ Considerations for medical and diagnostic procedures. For example, no blood pressure, IV placement, or blood draws from an arm that is affected by lymphedema or at risk for lymphedema.

☐ Religious beliefs that may impact medical care, such as transfusions.

• Living Will, Advanced Care Directive, Do Not Resuscitate Instructions, Medical Power Of Attorney, or Organ Donor Authorization, if appropriate.

A brightly colored three ring binder works well for this purpose. Label the notebook with the patient's name and decorate it with a picture of the patient to make it easier to select the right notebook. Select a standard location to store the notebook so that everyone knows where to find it.

The caregiver or the patient should:

- Take the notebook to medical appointments and record any changes in medications, future appointments, etc. Take both the Patient Notebook and the Caregiver Handbook to therapist appointments.

- Record any changes in condition, medications, etc. If there are changes to the home care routine or medications, the Weekly Care Plan should be updated to reflect these changes.

- Keep a list of questions to be asked at the next medical appointment in the Patient Notebook. It may easiest to keep a separate list for each health care provider.

Privacy Laws and Caregiver Access

Federal privacy regulations requiring health care providers to protect the privacy of patient health information can block caregiver access in certain situations. This section explains these rules and actions that you may need to take in advance to facilitate caregiver access to the patient's medical team and information.

Providers may share information with family members, friends, or others involved in providing care or paying for care subject to these rules:

- Patient is present and has the capacity to make health care decisions: information may be disclosed if the patient agrees to disclosure, is given an opportunity to object and does not object, or if the provider decides from the circumstances that the patient does not object.

- Patient is not present or is incapacitated: provider may disclose information if the provider is reasonably sure the person is involved in the patient's care and the provider believes the disclosure to be in the patient's best interest.

- Persons with legal authority to make health care decisions on behalf of the patient have the same information rights as the patient. Examples include a person granted a health care power of attorney or a general power of attorney by an adult; a court appointed legal guardian of an incompetent adult; and a parent, guardian or other person acting in the role of parent (*in loco parentis*) for a minor child.

If you anticipate a situation where a caregiver without legal authority—especially a caregiver who is not related to the patient—may need to communicate with the patient's health care providers by phone, without the patient present, or while the patient is incapacitated, you should make arrangements in advance. Identify the health care provider(s) where agreements are needed, contact each one to find out what documentation they require, if any, and ask them to document the agreement with a note in the patient's file. Update this information if there is a change in caregiver or health care providers.

For HIPAA information, contact the US Department of Health and Human Services Office for Civil Rights (www.hhs.gov/ocr/hipaa/). Psychotherapy notes are subject to different rules.

Caregiver Handbook

A Caregiver Handbook is an important tool for training and coordinating caregivers, and contains the Weekly Care Plans, Activity Forms, and other information as described below.

We suggest keeping the Caregiver Handbook separate from the Patient Notebook so there is less paper to be carried to medical appointments. If you decide to use one notebook for both, use tabs to show different subjects. Both notebooks contain confidential information and should be protected.

Suggested Caregiver Handbook contents include:

- Weekly Care Plan form for the current week used to document patient condition and care activities; you may want to clip this form to the front of the notebook. At the end of the week, move the completed form to the Patient Notebook and replace it with the form for the new week.

- Care Activity Forms that provide caregiver instructions.

- Weekly Care Plan forms for the upcoming weeks. These should show caregiver work schedules for the coming weeks.

- Weekly Care Plan template used to create plans for specific weeks.

- People: names, photos, contact information for patient, family, friends, neighbors, other caregivers, and other people a caregiver is likely to encounter. It may be helpful to provide some information about each person.

- Emergency Contacts: 911 or equivalent medical emergency services number; patient's primary care provider emergency number; the nearest urgent care facility with address and directions; care coordinator; family and friends to contact in the event of an emergency. This could be a duplicated copy of the Patient Information Form (page 426).

- Standard Locations for things within the home; see page 377.

- Local Information, covering places where the caregiver and patient may go on a routine basis including addresses, maps, and directions if needed. This might include locations for medical appointments, hospital, shopping, social activities, etc.

- Sick Day Procedure: outline what the caregiver is expected to do if they are ill or otherwise not able to work as scheduled. This should cover who should be notified, who is responsible for arranging a substitute caregiver, etc.

- Hospitalization Procedure: outline what the caregiver should do if the patient is hospitalized. This should cover who should be notified, what should be packed for lymphedema care, what is expected of the caregiver while the patient is in the hospital, etc.

- Emergency Relocation Procedure: outline in general terms what the caregiver is expected to do if the patient must be moved temporarily due to an emergency such as a fire or extreme weather.

Depending on the situation, you may also want to include this information:

- Procedures for documenting hours worked by paid caregivers.

- Process for documenting expenses that are paid by the caregiver and reimbursed.

- A way for the caregiver to keep the care arranger informed of their availability for scheduled work hours and as backup.

- Caregiver contact information (see page 427) if a caregiver is expected to contact other caregivers for assistance or backup care.

Preparing the Home

If care is going to be provided in the home, it may be necessary to prepare for care activities and the presence of caregivers. This may include obtaining care equipment and establishing standard locations for things, as explained below.

You may also need to:

- Make sure the home is accessible and safe for the patient and caregiver.

- Remove or protect valuables. Store jewelry, cash, checkbooks, credit cards, and financial information where they are secure and not visible.

- Eliminate temptations for the patient and caregiver. Food, drinks, toys, etc. that are off limits should be kept out of sight or locked up.

Standard Locations

Lymphedema care requires an amazing amount of stuff. Make coordination easier by establishing standard storage locations for things. For example:

- Patient Notebook and the patient's identification and healthcare cards.

- Caregiver Handbook, messages for caregivers, and a copy of this book (if it is referenced in the care plan).

- Files for the forms and information used to manage supplies, equipment, and medications as described in "Managing Orders" (page 271).

- Bandages, compression garments, and other lymphedema care supplies.

- Medications should be stored in a location that is safe and accessible. Avoid exposing medications to moisture and handling medications over a sink.

- Keys, cordless phones, mobile phones, etc.

- Emergency supplies: flashlights, radio, extra batteries, bottled water, stored food, etc.

It may be easier for caregivers to find things, and put things away in the assigned location, if cabinets and other storage areas are labeled to show their contents.

Training Caregivers

Identify what caregivers need to know and create a checklist for orienting new caregivers, see "Training Checklist" on page 379 . You may need to adapt the level of detail in the training materials depending on how much the caregiver knows about lymphedema and home care.

Update the orientation checklist as the care routine changes or new orientation items are identified. This may seem like overkill at first, but it can prevent a lot of grief if a caregiver, or the patient, has to orient a new caregiver unexpectedly.

Currently your options for training caregivers include this book and, hopefully, a cooperative lymphedema therapist. We hope this book will help spur the development of additional training materials and programs; check www.LymphNotes.com for the latest information.

Training tips:

- Lymphedema care is a hands-on skill and there is no substitute for actually doing the care, seeing what happens, and getting feedback and support. Arrange time for the caregiver and patient to meet with the therapist and go over the care routine.

- Encourage questions, even seemingly dumb questions, and get answers if you don't know.

- Training can be tiring for the caregiver and the patient. Watch for signs of fatigue and take a break or stop before either becomes stressed.

Training Checklist

☐ Roles and responsibilities: who is the care coordinator, who is the patient, who are any other people that the caregiver will be dealing with and what are their roles?

☐ Best ways to communicate with the care coordinator and any family members.

☐ Lymphedema basics: lymphatic system function, causes of lymphedema, effects of lymphedema, treatment methods.

☐ Weekly and daily care routine for this patient as described in the Weekly Care Plan and Care Activity forms, see page 333.

☐ Patient Notebook contents, usage, and maintenance, see page 372.

☐ Caregiver Handbook contents and usage, see page 375.

☐ Standard locations for information, things, and supplies, see page 377.

☐ Procedures and logistics for other activities, if appropriate.

☐ Special needs or procedures in the event of an emergency.

Notes

1   "Health-Record Checklist" in *AARP*, January 2008.

Caring for the Caregiver

Caregivers need care and support to reduce the risk of injury or burnout. This section provides practical tips on:

- Body mechanics and techniques for working safely and avoiding injury.

- Roles and goals of lymphedema care and different types of caregiver relationships

- Emotional demands of being a caregiver, and protecting yourself from burnout.

Chapter 25

Body Mechanics

Being a caregiver can be physically demanding and stressful. In order to protect yourself from injury it is important that you:

- Learn and practice proper body mechanics, as explained below.

- Know your limitations and get help from other people, or mechanical devices, for tasks that you cannot manage safely by yourself.

- Get enough rest, exercise, and eat right. Most of the suggestions for Diet and Nutrition (page 265) apply to caregivers as well as patients.

Body mechanics describe the way we stand and move to make the best use of our strength, prevent injuries, and minimize fatigue. These are simple skills that will help you control and balance your body so that you may safely assist another person.

You may want to teach some of these skills to your patient to help them become more aware of how they move and to help them move more safely. Together, you can work out ways in which the patient can move and position themselves based on their abilities.

The patient's lymphedema therapist may provide specific suggestions to help you move the patient as part of the care routine. Don't be afraid to ask questions or ask for help solving problems.

The basic principles of good body mechanics are:

- Keep your spine in an optimal position—straight with a slight inward curve in the lower back—during activities, while resting, and while sleeping.

- Use large muscles, especially your legs, to do the heavy work instead of straining smaller muscles in the arms or lower back. See Figure 25-1.

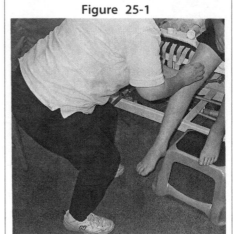

Figure 25-1

General Guidelines

Follow these rules:[1]

- Warm-up and stretch before heavy lifting or other demanding activities.

- Never lift more than you can handle comfortably and safely. Get help if you are not sure you can lift something safely.

- Create a firm base by planting your feet about shoulder width apart, with one foot a half step behind the other.

- Use your leg muscles to do the lifting and keep your back straight.

- When lifting objects from the floor or a low starting point, use a basic squat lift. Squat down keeping the back straight, hold the object close to your body and tighten your stomach muscles as you stand, letting your leg muscles do the work.

- Inhale just prior to lifting, 'set' or tighten your abdominal muscles, and breathe out through pursed lips as you lift.

- Stay close to your work or anything you are lifting.

- Communicate with the person you are moving or anyone who is helping you. For example, "1, 2, 3, Go!" or "Ready, Set, Lift!"

- When moving things, push rather than pulling to protect your back and neck.

- Balance rest and activity to conserve your energy and avoid fatigue.

Situations to Avoid

Replace these high risk movements with the suggested alternatives.

Try to avoid	Instead
Twisting your trunk while reaching or lifting	Bend your knees, move your feet, and turn your whole body
Squatting for prolonged periods of time	Use a stool or support
Carrying or lifting weight unevenly on one side of your body	Carry weight evenly with both arms. See Figure 25-2 on page 386.
Leaning forward from the waist during standing activities or when lifting	Try bending your hips and knees or sitting on a stool
Craning your neck forward during activities	Adjust your position to remain comfortable. If vision is a problem, you may need 'middle vision' glasses or trifocals for detailed tasks like bandaging or working on a computer.
Sitting on the floor with your knees turned in and feet splayed out to the sides, this compresses the knee joints and strains the ligaments	Sit straight or with feet crossed in front of the body
Extended reaching	Use a long handled tool or change your position

Specific Techniques

According to the American Academy of Orthopedic Surgeons, home caregivers are at greatest risk for back pain when:[2]

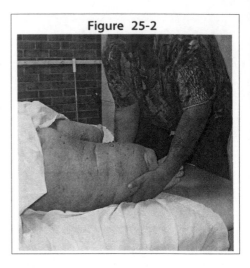

Figure 25-2

- Pulling a person who is reclining in bed into a sitting position. Instead of pulling, have the patient bend their knees and roll to the side, then bring the feet over the edge of the bed while pivoting the body so the person rises up to a position sitting at the edge of the bed.

- Transferring a person from a bed to a chair. Help the patient sit up (see above) and then help them stand by placing your arms around the person's back and clasping your hands together or holding a transfer belt securely wrapped around their waist. Keeping the person close to you, shift your weight back allowing the patient to rise up off the bed, and then pivot, turning the patient toward the chair. Slowly lower the person into the chair by bending your knees. Encourage the patient to assist in the transfer as much as they are able.

- Leaning over a person for long periods of time. Use a stool or other support to minimize leaning, or place one knee on the bed for better body leverage (in Figure 25-2 the caregiver has his right knee on the bed). Periodically take a break, stand up straight, and stretch your back before resuming the activity.

First Aid for Back Pain

If you are in severe pain or have crushing chest pain, call 911 or your local emergency telephone number and get help. Seek emergency treatment if you experience pain or pressure in your neck or head; tingling or loss of sensation in your arms, legs, or genitals; partial or complete loss of movement in any body part; or loss of bowel or bladder control.[3]

The following may be used for mild to moderate back pain:[4]

- Apply a cold pack (if available), or a homemade ice pack using a plastic bag, to the injured area for about 10 minutes of every hour. If the area is affected by lymphedema, wrap the cold pack as described on page 264.

- Rest for short periods in a comfortable position.

- Stand with your feet about shoulder width apart, place your hands on your hips, and gently bend backwards 5-10 times within your pain tolerance. Repeat this exercise throughout the day.

- Walk frequently for short distances on a level surface.

- When sitting, use a small pillow at the lower back for support. Avoid sitting for long periods of time.

If your pain does not go away within a few days, contact your doctor for medical advice.

Dress for Success

Proper clothing is important:

- Wear supportive shoes that give adequate traction and support.

- Use knee pads or a cushion if you are kneeling or working on your knees.

- Clothing should be comfortable, fit properly, and not be restrictive. Avoid long belts or scarves that can catch on things or trip you.

Some people find that a 'back belt' is helpful when lifting; ask your doctor or physical therapist if this is appropriate for you.

Notes

1   **The American Physical Therapy Association Book of Body Maintenance and Repair** by Marilyn Moffat and Steve Vickery, Holt Paperbacks, 1999.

2   "Lifting Techniques for Home Caregivers" by the American Academy of Orthopaedic Surgeons, http://orthoinfo.aaos.org/topic.cfm?topic=A00096 accessed on April 25, 2008.

3   **Emergency Response** by American Red Cross, Staywell, 2001, pg 317.

4   **The Comfort of Home** 3rd edition by Maria Meyer and Paula Derr. Care Trust Publications, 2007, page 312

Chapter 26

Roles, Goals, and Relationships

Caregivers must work with each patient in a way that is appropriate to the patient's situation. What is appropriate depends on the patient's age, health, state of mind, and prior relationship with the caregiver (if any).

Understanding care goals and the patient's needs, shapes the caregiver's role and relationship as explained below. The care relationship will be more comfortable and emotionally supportive for everyone when there is agreement on the goals of care and the role of the caregivers. If there is friction or tension between the caregiver and patient, check for disagreement over goals and roles (see "Emotional Care and Support" on page 189).

Get help if your relationship is not working or is upsetting you. There are many organizations that can help, see the Caregiver Resources in Appendix B (page 420). Respite care may also be helpful, see page 398 and also page 341.

Care Goals

As discussed earlier, care may be short-term, long-term, or palliative (see page 39) and there may be different care goals (see page 39).

Care goals are also influenced by the specific reasons why the patient needs caregiver assistance, as discussed in "Evaluating Care Needs" (page 331).

Caregiver Roles

In addition to helping with care, caregivers can take additional roles with their patients and these roles will shape the caregiver-patient relationship. These roles can include a mix of:

- Teacher, to help the patient learn the home care routine.

- Cheerleader, or coach, to motivate and encourage a patient who knows, or is learning, the care routine to follow it carefully and regularly.

- Supervisor, to monitor and manage the home care routine.

In some cases these roles are obvious. For example:

- Children need physical assistance but also need instruction and encouragement.

- Adolescents are expected to learn the care routine and be able to provide at least some aspect of home care for themselves; the caregiver's role will involve more motivation and supervision. Instruction will be needed for adolescents who are newly diagnosed or when the care routine changes.

- Younger adults that have recently been diagnosed with lymphedema will need instruction and possibly physical assistance initially. Once they have learned the routine, a caregiver would expect to provide more encouragement than supervision.

In other cases, especially with older adults, the appropriate roles may not be obvious and may change over time as the patient's physical condition or mood changes. Listening carefully and communicating effectively will help prevent misunderstandings over these roles. For more information and an example, see the chapter on "Communicating Effectively" (page 205).

Caregiver Relationships

Having a preexisting relationship with the person receiving care can make care giving more rewarding or more complicated.

Are you physically close and personally involved in physical care giving, or are you arranging care giving from a distance? Do you know the patient only because you are a hired employee, or did you have a personal relationship before becoming their caregiver?

Having a formal contract can be important and appropriate even if you are a relative or friend. A contract clarifies expectations and can protect your personal relationship from problems that may arise in the course of care giving. Contracts are discussed below and on page 364.

Specific tips on establishing a successful caregiver relationship are provided below for parents, children, spouse or partner, and friends; we also provide some suggestions on dealing with family that can be used by anyone. For more information on these topics, see **Overcoming the Emotional Challenges of Lymphedema**, specifically Chapter 22 for friends and family members and Chapter 23 for parents of children with lymphedema.

Parent as Caregiver

When a child has lymphedema, it is commonly the parents who provide care. As a parent, you bring special strengths to care giving. You care about your child and have a strong emotional commitment to your child's welfare. You know your child's personality and can adapt your approach to suit the child. These are tremendous strengths.

At the same time, because you care so deeply, you may have more negative emotional reactions to your child's condition than a hired caregiver. When your child has lymphedema, it is easy to focus on the negative. You may be angry about the unfairness of such an illness. You may worry too much about the future. You may be on the lookout for problems more than is needed.

Your goal is for your child to become as independent as possible and to successfully take over self-care for themselves. As children go through different developmental stages, they vary in their eagerness to be independent, and their willingness to accept guidance and advice from parents.

Deliberately emphasize the child's strengths and positives when thinking about or talking to your child. Be a kind of crystal ball showing your child the most positive view of themselves and the future.

Focus on the progress that has been made, or that is possible. Look ahead and plan. Over time you should move from directly providing care, to providing guidance, and eventually to just providing praise.

Child as Caregiver

Sometimes the role described above is reversed and a child becomes a caregiver for a parent (or grandparent).

If you are an adolescent or adult child and will be providing care to a parent, or other relative, discuss in advance what to expect from each other. Problem-solve together. Make plans that are realistic for the short-term and the long-term. If you are in high school and providing care, what will happen when you go to college, get a job, or marry?

If you are an adult child providing care, what financial arrangements will be made? What will be the roles of siblings or other relatives?

Expect old family patterns to arise. If you have areas of conflict, try to talk about them beforehand and find ways to resolve them or keep them from interfering with care giving.

Spouse or Partner as Caregiver

Frequently, the spouse or partner is the caregiver. This is an increasingly common situation as the population ages and as people live longer, develop chronic conditions, and remain in their homes.

If your partner develops lymphedema and needs care giving from you, this can either strain your relationship or strengthen it. As both caregiver and partner, you are taking on a new role. Find ways to adapt care giving so it fits into the normal pattern of your relationship as much as possible.

If you have usually been the nurturer in the relationship, care giving may feel natural and acceptable to both of you. On the other hand, if your spouse has usually been responsible for taking care of you, find ways for your spouse to continue to nurture you.

Let your partner do as much as possible independently. This is especially important if he or she has been very independent in the past. Protect your partner's self-respect. Keep the relationship as normal as possible.

Protect yourself physically and emotionally. You cannot help your partner if you become physically unable to provide care giving, nor if you burn out emotionally. Ask for help. Arrange respite care. Communicate with your partner about how both of you are feeling. Work to solve potential problems when they are small—before they become major difficulties.

Friend as Caregiver

In some cases, a friend steps in as caregiver. A friend may provide occasional help or regular, ongoing care. The suggestions for the partner-caregiver (above) also apply to the friend-caregiver.

Clarify in advance what will be expected. Discuss tasks and expectations. How long and how often will you provide care? What exactly will you do? Who will train you? Who is available to answer questions or to help in unexpected situations? If you are being paid, have a formal contract that spells out the job requirements, hours, payment, vacations, and other issues. Contracts are discussed on page 364.

If you are a friend who is providing care, the key message is: protect your friendship. Continue to share the interests or activities that made you friends in the first place.

Let your friend take care of you in some way in return. Keep a mutual give and take. A balanced relationship feels better to both caregiver and care recipient.

Dealing with Family

As a caregiver, you are likely to have at least occasional contact with the patient's family members or you may be part of the family (as discussed above). Family can be a source of conflict as well as support.

Family members may know little about lymphedema or they may be misinformed. They may offer food that is not healthy for the lymphedema patient. They may want to continue activities that are unhealthy or unsafe for their family member with lymphedema.

Family members may live far away from the patient. Even family members who live nearby, if they do not see the care you are providing, may not understand the day-to-day demands of care giving.

Sometimes family only get involved during a crisis or during brief visits. Family members who are not involved in daily care giving may feel guilty. Guilt is not a pleasant feeling and when people feel guilty, they can react in several ways:

- Withdrawing and having no contact. This may be happening if family members don't return phone calls or e-mail messages.

- Blaming themselves. This may be occurring if family members seem to be oversensitive or feel easily criticized or attacked.

- Getting angry. This shows up in ways like criticizing the caregiver, criticizing the care giving arrangements, not listening to what you say, demanding that their ideas be followed, arguing over money, and so on. Anger may stem from worries about their relative's health, financial stress, fear of being criticized for not doing more, guilt, uncertainty, sadness, or other uncomfortable feelings.

Remember that however difficult they are to deal with, these family members are probably feeling bad themselves. Use the effective listening and communication skills described in the chapter on "Communicating Effectively" (page 205) to defuse problem situations.

Chapter **27:**
Emotional Demands

Care giving is emotionally satisfying. It can also be emotionally demanding. As a caregiver, you may be a target for anger from the patient or from their family members. You may feel discouraged or blame yourself when things go wrong or the patient's condition does not improve. You may feel stressed. Planning for respite care (see page 398) is important to prevent caregiver burnout.

When the Patient Becomes Angry

Patients with lymphedema have lots of reasons to be angry. They can't do things they used to do. Both lymphedema swelling and compression can make their body feel heavy, uncomfortable, and hot. Swelling or other medical problems can cause pain.

If medical treatment caused lymphedema or if lymphedema wasn't diagnosed or treated early, the patient may be angry at all health care professionals, including caregivers. They may be angry because self-care and compression can be time-consuming, boring, repetitive, and remind them that they have a chronic condition.

The patient can get angry with you about things that are not your fault. Anger about other issues can get directed at the caregiver. You are there; other people aren't. You can become the target for anger about lymphedema in general. Of course, you should not have to put up with verbal or physical abuse, but sometimes letting the patient express angry feelings may be helpful.

Here are some tips for dealing with angry outbursts:

- Stay calm, sympathetic, and matter-of-fact.

- Think of anger as a brief summer storm that passes and is gone, clearing the air.

- Be curious. Listen for the feelings or concerns that may lie behind the anger.

- When the person is calmer, ask them how the two of you can work together to make things better.

- Some patients calm down quickly if they are distracted. Others respond to comforting words said in a soothing voice, to a familiar calming song, or when given a favorite stuffed animal or comforting object.

When Lymphedema Doesn't Improve

Being a caregiver is harder when things don't go well. Lymphedema swelling may increase and infections can occur. The patient may not follow self-care recommendations despite your best efforts to motivate them.

When problems persist, it is disheartening. You can feel guilty and begin to blame or criticize yourself. Here are some thoughts to remember.

Sometimes, there is nothing more to be done. Some problems are caused by factors that are out of your control. Remember, lymphedema is a chronic condition and swelling will fluctuate.

Sometimes, a patient's lack of improvement is a sign that you have something to learn. This is a chance to become a more effective caregiver. If you made mistakes, or need to change what you are doing, don't waste time on self-blame. Spend your energy instead on correcting the mistakes, learning what to do instead, and improving your care giving.

Just like Maria in the story on page 397, you or the patient, may get discouraged if lymphedema does not continue to improve, or if flare-ups occur. When you feel this way, talk to someone who will tell you what is reasonable to expect and whether you need to change what you are doing. Use this as an opportunity to learn.

Story: Maria and Anna

Maria was caring for Anna. She did SLD in the areas Anna couldn't reach. She used lotion on the skin and tried to use compression the way the lymphedema therapist had demonstrated. She and Anna walked every day.

And still Anna's lymphedema didn't improve. In fact, she even had a sudden worsening of her swelling and got an infection from an insect bite. Maria felt terrible, *"What am I doing wrong?"* She thought, *"I'm no good as a caregiver. I ought to just quit because I'm not helping."*

Luckily, Maria talked to Anna about these feelings and together they called Anna's lymphedema therapist. The therapist reminded Maria that Anna's swelling used to be much worse before it was treated and that with Maria's help, Anna was more mobile and had maintained the gains of treatment. The therapist praised Maria for seeing the early signs of infection.

Anna, Maria, and the therapist agreed to have Maria come with Anna to the next therapy appointment so the therapist could check what Maria was doing and answer any more questions.

Maria felt much better. Anna was very relieved because she liked Maria and enjoyed having her as a caregiver.

When You Feel Stressed

Care giving can be demanding and stressful, especially if you feel like you do not have the resources to meet the demands that are being made.

Here are some things that you can do when you are feeling stressed:

- Use stress reduction techniques, such as exercise, relaxation (page 177), and deep breathing (page 162). This breathing relaxes the body and reduces stress chemicals in the body as well as moving lymph.

- Face and resolve problems. Un-addressed problems cause stress.

- Reach out for emotional, spiritual, and practical support. Find someone supportive to talk to about the pressures and demands of care giving. Talk about your feelings. Talk about what you do and what you expect of yourself and the patient.

- Take care of your physical health. Are you getting enough sleep and exercise? What are you eating and drinking (see page 265)? Keep your doctors' appointments and follow recommendations for any health conditions you have.

- Take care of your emotional health. Spend some time each day doing things that you enjoy and that give you pleasure. Focus on what is going right, the good things that happen each day, the blessings in your life, and everything for which you are grateful day-to-day. Positive emotions counteract the effects of stress.

- Listen to your body. Muscle tension or pain can be the body's way of telling you that you are overburdened. Are you clenching your jaw or grinding your teeth? Are you getting headaches, neck aches, shoulder pain, or upset stomach? Know your body's stress signals and listen to them.

- Pay attention to your emotions. Are you feeling stressed, overwhelmed, irritable, or impatient? These can be signs that you are getting burned out and need a break.

Respite Care

Because care giving is demanding, every caregiver needs a respite now and again. You will be a better caregiver if you take care of yourself physically and emotionally.

- Arrange for someone to take over so you can have regular vacations.

- Plan respite care in advance—before you get to a crisis (see page 340). Do not wait until you feel overwhelmed or are at the end of your rope.

- Have a plan for back-up care in case you become ill or incapacitated. Who will take over care giving? Who will care for you if you need it?

- Be realistic in your expectations of yourself. Enlist other people to help with care giving when possible and appropriate. Accept help that is offered. Ask for help if you need it.

Caregiving calls for balance. Care for yourself, so you can continue to care for the patient. A caregiving team can't exist without a functioning caregiver.

Understanding the Lymphatic System

This appendix provides additional detail on the lymphatic system:[1]

- Lymphatic system structure and lymph node locations

- Lymph transport with a functional lymphatic system from the leg, through the trunk, and from the arm.

- Dysfunctions of the lymphatic system that result in lymphedema.

Lymphatic System Structure and Function

Lymph makes a one-way journey from the spaces between cells throughout the body to the lymphatic ducts that empty into the subclavian veins (or venous angle) located just under the collarbone at the terminus. At this endpoint, the lymph returns to the venous circulation and once again becomes blood plasma.

The *terminus* is below the triangular indentation on either side of the base of the neck that is formed in front by the collarbone (clavicle), on the side by the neck, and in the back by the top of the shoulder muscle; see Figure A-4 on page 407.

Excess fluid is removed from the tissues by tiny lymphatic capillaries that connect to progressively larger collectors and trunks or ducts. This fluid is called tissue fluid while it is in the tissues and lymphatic fluid, or lymph, while it is in the lymphatic system. As the lymph is transported, it passes through lymph nodes where it is filtered and processed.

Lymphatic Capillaries

Fluid in the spaces between tissue cells (interstitial spaces) can flow into a *lymphatic capillary*. These *lymphatic capillaries* begin as open-ended tubes with walls that are only one cell in thickness. Each of these individual cells is fastened to nearby tissues by an *anchoring filament*. As the nearby tissues move, the filament pulls the tube walls apart and allows fluid to enter the lymphatic capillary.[2] Millions of these tiny capillaries are grouped together in mesh-like formations throughout the body.

Approximately 70 percent of these are *superficial capillaries* that are located near, or just under, the skin. The remaining 30 percent, known as *deep lymphatic capillaries,* surround most of the body's organs.[3]

Lymphatic Pre-Collectors and Collectors

Lymph flows from the capillaries into slightly larger *pre-collectors* that have walls that are about three cells thick. The pre-collectors merge into thicker vessels known as *collectors* and these eventually connect to larger vessels known as lymphatic trunks or ducts.

Lymphatic Trunks

The *lymphatic trunks*, which are the largest lymphatic vessels, are located deep within the body near blood vessels. These lymphatic collectors and trunks contain valves that are similar in structure to those found in veins. The purpose of these valves is to permit lymph to flow in only one direction (see Figure A-1 on page 401).

The segment of the vessel between two valves is known an *angion* or *lymphangion.* The smooth muscles in the walls of the lymph vessels contract in a wave-like motion at a rate of one contraction every eight to twelve seconds. This rate of motion, which equals five-to-seven contractions per minute, pushes the lymph forward and helps to draw more lymph into the capillaries.[4]

As the lymph flows through the body, it receives more help from the action of deep breathing, the pulsing motion of nearby blood vessels and the movement of muscles (muscle pumps) and joints (joint pumps).

Figure A-1: Vein and Lymphatic Vessel Compared

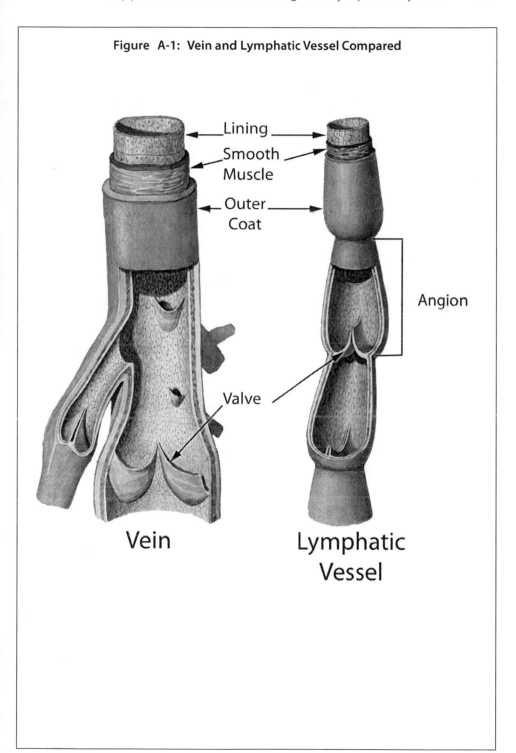

Lining

Smooth Muscle

Outer Coat

Angion

Valve

Vein

Lymphatic Vessel

Lymph Nodes

Lymph nodes are bean-shaped structures ranging in size from as small as a pinhead to as large as an olive. The primary function of the lymph nodes is to act as defensive barriers against infections and malignant disorders by filtering lymph and destroying pathogens.[5] Lymph nodes concentrate the lymphatic fluid by removing most of the water and returning the water to the bloodstream through blood vessels connected to the nodes. In a healthy lymphatic system, this greatly reduces the volume of fluid to be transported by the lymphatic system.

Lymphocytes, specialized white blood cells that defend against non-self or altered cells, are concentrated in the lymph nodes. Some lymphocytes produce antibodies that circulate through the blood and bind to non-self substances. Lymph nodes contain a mesh of tissue tightly packed with lymphocytes and macrophages. As lymph is filtered through this mesh, harmful microorganisms are attacked and destroyed.

Each part of the lymph node has a specific role (see Figure A-2 on page 403):

- A *protective capsule* surrounds and protects each lymph node.[6]

- The *afferent lymphatic vessels* around the outer surface of the node carry lymph into the node. *Afferent* means toward.

- The lymph flows into the *cortex* or outer portion of the node. Here the lymphocytes engulf and destroy damaged cells, cancer cells and foreign particles such as bacteria and viruses. These lymphocytes block or slow the spread of cancer until the lymph node is overwhelmed by the disease.

- Next, the lymph flows into the *medulla*, which is the central portion of the node. Here the lymph is filtered to remove waste products and about 40 percent of its liquid content is removed.

- The *efferent lymphatic vessels* carry the filtered lymph out of the node. These vessels connect to other lymphatic vessels or nodes and carry the lymph toward the trunks that drain the filtered lymph into the subclavian veins where it becomes plasma again.

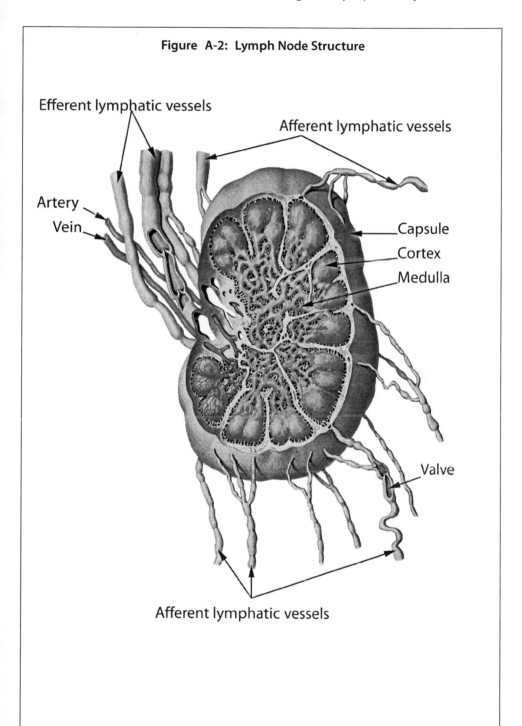

Figure A-2: Lymph Node Structure

Efferent lymphatic vessels

Afferent lymphatic vessels

Artery

Vein

Capsule

Cortex

Medulla

Valve

Afferent lymphatic vessels

Unequal Drainage Areas

A unique feature of the lymphatic system is that it divides the body into unequal drainage areas or territories. A simplified view of these territories is shown in Figure A-3 on page 405. The upper right quadrant drains on the right side and the other three quadrants drain on the left side. Lymphedema therapists use the term 'watershed' to describe a boundary between territories, not a drainage area.[7]

The *right lymphatic duct* is much smaller than the left thoracic duct and removes lymph from the right hand and arm, upper right quadrant of the trunk, and the right half of the head and neck to the terminus on the right side of the neck. At the terminus, it connects into the right subclavian vein (see Figure A-7 on page 411 and Figure A-4 on page 407).

Three quarters of the body—including both lower extremities and the upper left quadrant—drain on the left side through the *thoracic duct* which empties into the left subclavian vein at the terminus (see Figure A-9 on page 413).

Lymph Node Locations

Lymph is filtered and processed as it passes through lymph nodes located along the lymphatic vessels. There are between 600 and 700 lymph nodes located throughout the body. A person is born with a set number of lymph nodes and lymph nodes do not regenerate or vanish.[8] Lymph nodes can change size, and enlarged lymph nodes may indicate that the body is fighting an infection.

Most lymph nodes are located where pathogens are likely to enter the body, such as around the intestines in the abdomen (see Figure A-8 on page 412) and in the head-neck area (see Figure A-4 on page 407).

About half of the lymph nodes are in the abdomen, the rest are clustered in the major groups listed below, located around major joints, or located singly along the lymphatic vessels.

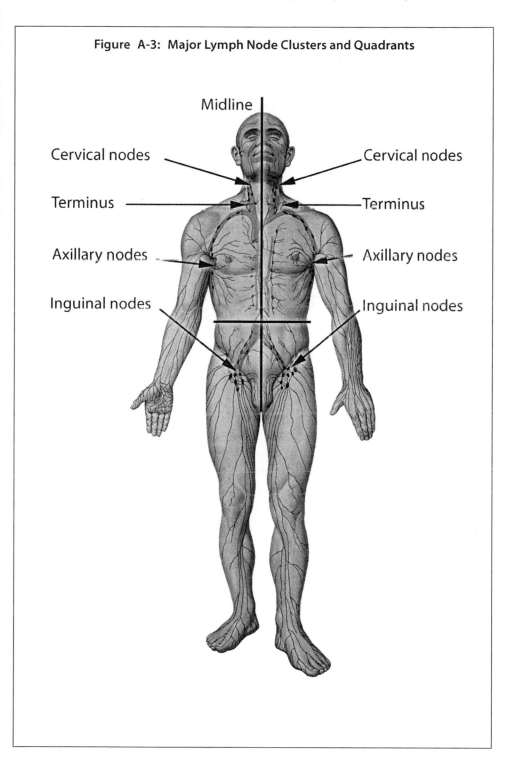

Figure A-3: Major Lymph Node Clusters and Quadrants

Midline

Cervical nodes

Cervical nodes

Terminus

Terminus

Axillary nodes

Axillary nodes

Inguinal nodes

Inguinal nodes

The major clusters of lymph nodes are:

- **Supraclavicular lymph nodes** above the collarbone near the terminus (see Figure A-4 on page 407).

- **Cervical lymph nodes** along the sides of the neck (see Figure A-4 on page 407).

- **Occipital lymph nodes** at the back of the head (see Figure A-4 on page 407).

- **Auricular lymph nodes** around the ears (see Figure A-4 on page 407).

- **Axillary lymph nodes** in the armpits (see Figure A-7 on page 411).

- **Antecubital lymph nodes** in the elbow (see Figure A-7 on page 411).

- **Inguinal lymph nodes** located at the upper thigh near the groin (see Figure A-5 on page 408).

- **Popliteal lymph nodes** located at the back of the knee (see Figure A-6 on page 409).

Lymph Transport from the Leg

The upward flow of lymph from the feet to the trunk depends largely on motion of muscles and joints in the legs during exercise and other activities. This motion stimulates both the superficial and deep lymph flow to the inguinal lymph nodes and the trunk (see Figure A-5 on page 408 and Figure A-6 on page 409).

Muscle Pumps

The muscles that are most helpful in stimulating this upward flow of lymph are known as *major muscle pumps*. The major muscle pumps of the legs are the plantar muscles on the bottoms of the feet, the calf muscles in the lower leg, and the thigh muscles in the upper leg.[9]

Joint Pumps

The bending and straightening of the larger joints also stimulate the upward flow of lymph and these joints are known as *major joint pumps*. The major joint pumps of the lower body are the ankles, the knees and the popliteal lymph nodes behind each knee, and the hips and inguinal lymph nodes.[10]

Figure A-4: Head and Neck Lymphatic Structures

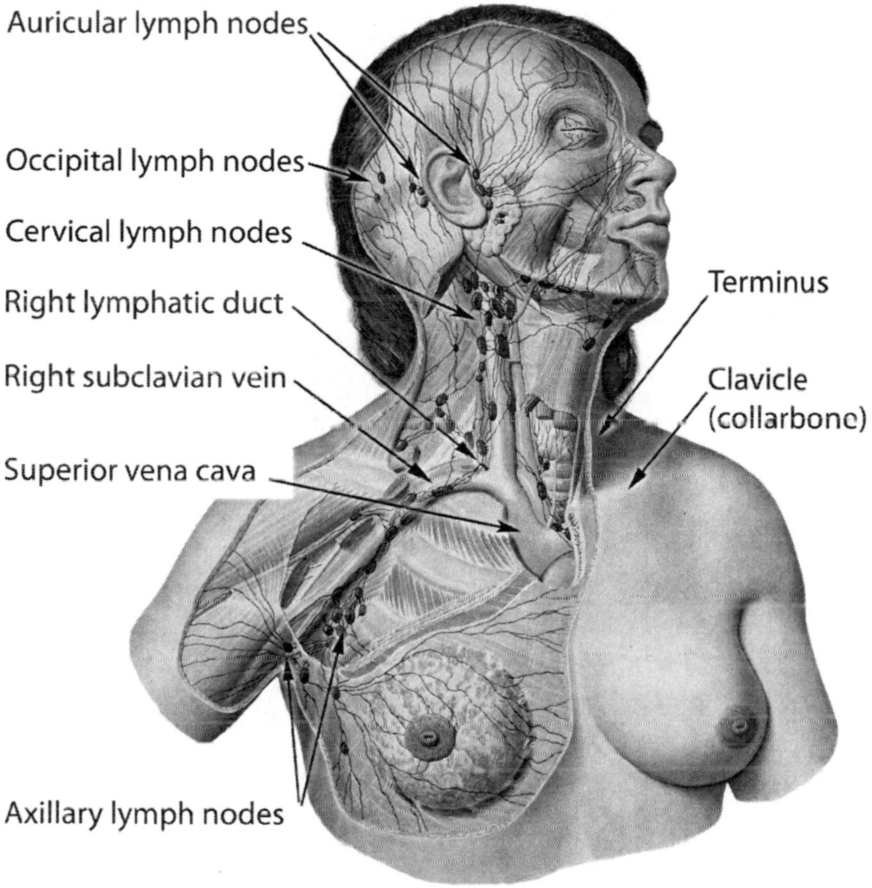

Auricular lymph nodes

Occipital lymph nodes

Cervical lymph nodes

Right lymphatic duct

Right subclavian vein

Superior vena cava

Terminus

Clavicle
(collarbone)

Axillary lymph nodes

Figure A-5: Leg front view, superficial Lymphatic Structures

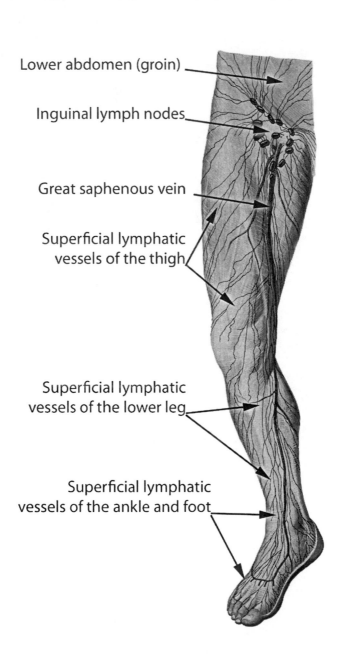

Lower abdomen (groin)

Inguinal lymph nodes

Great saphenous vein

Superficial lymphatic vessels of the thigh

Superficial lymphatic vessels of the lower leg

Superficial lymphatic vessels of the ankle and foot

Figure A-6: Leg rear view, deep Lymphatic Structures

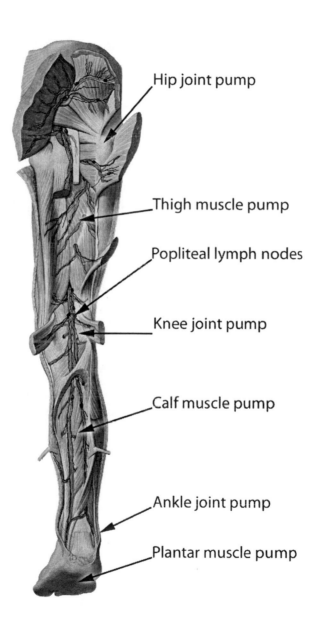

Hip joint pump

Thigh muscle pump

Popliteal lymph nodes

Knee joint pump

Calf muscle pump

Ankle joint pump

Plantar muscle pump

Lymph Transport through the Trunk

Major lymphatic vessels carry lymph upward from each leg into the trunk. Here, these vessels merge to form the *cisterna chyli*, which is a small pouch located below the diaphragm that temporarily stores lymph as it travels upward from the legs and lower trunk (see Figure A-9 on page 413). Lymph vessels from the small intestine and other internal organs flow into the cisterna chyli.

From the cisterna chyli, the *thoracic duct* carries lymph upward through the chest to the terminus at the left side of the neck. The thoracic duct empties into the subclavian vein and returns the lymph to the venous circulation as plasma. The muscles of the diaphragm help pump lymph through the thoracic duct; deep breathing enhances this action.

Lymph Transport from the Arm

The flow of lymph from the hand and arm to the axillary lymph nodes in the armpit depends on the muscles and joints in the arms. Lymphatic collectors along the fingers and the back and front of the hand pass the wrist to join collectors in the forearm. The collectors from both sides of the forearm converge at the antecubital lymph node cluster and joint pump in the elbow. See Figure A-7 on page 411.

Collectors from the forearm and the inside of the upper arm connect to the axillary lymph nodes and the joint pump in the armpit. Collectors on the outside of the upper arm and shoulder connect to the supraclavicular lymph nodes near the terminus.

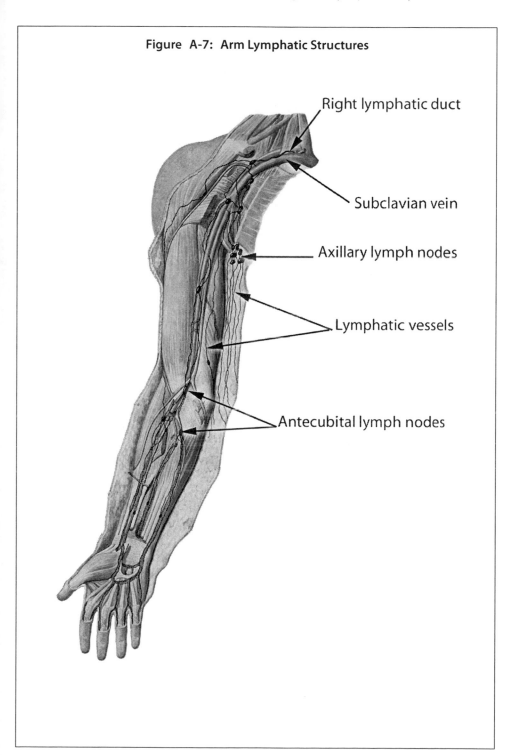

Figure A-7: Arm Lymphatic Structures

Right lymphatic duct

Subclavian vein

Axillary lymph nodes

Lymphatic vessels

Antecubital lymph nodes

Figure A-8: Lower Abdomen Lymphatic Structures

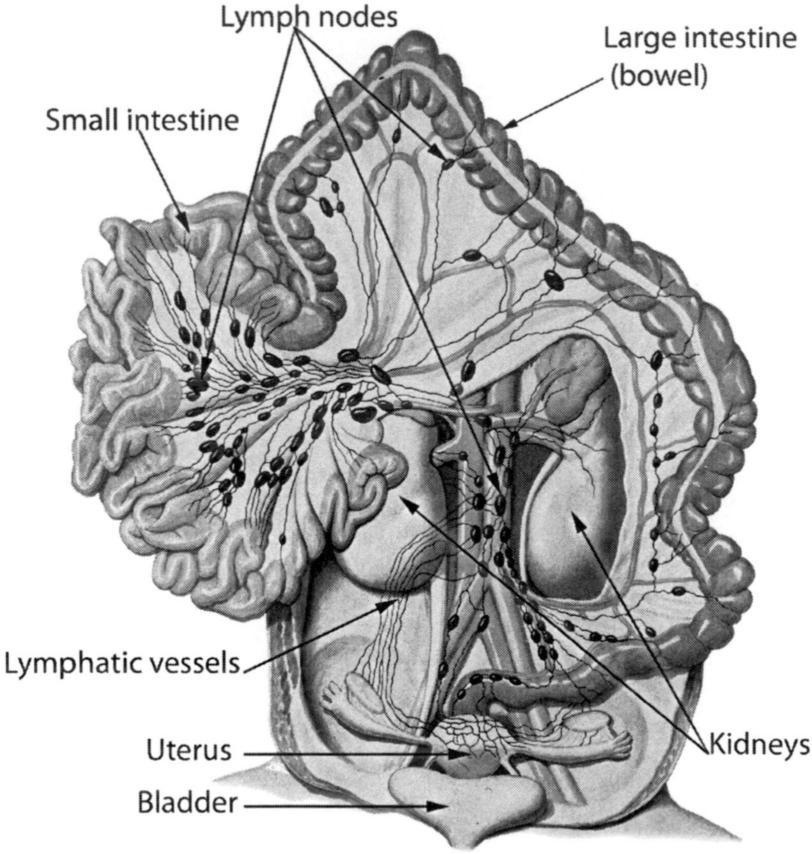

Figure A-9: Trunk with Deep Lymphatic Structures

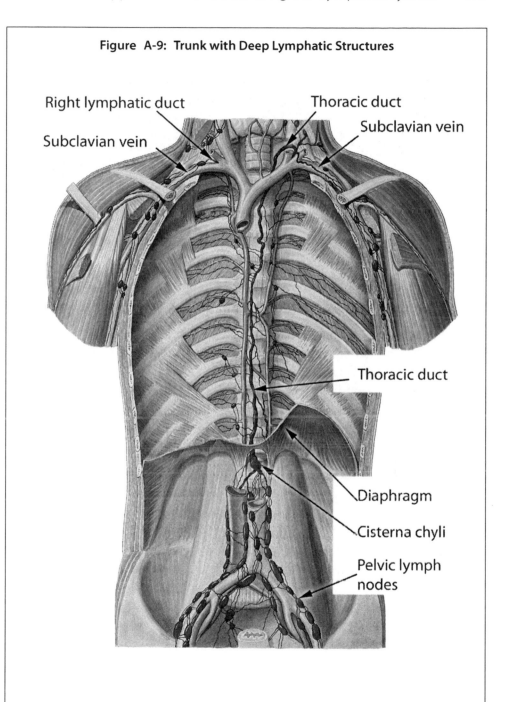

Right lymphatic duct

Thoracic duct

Subclavian vein

Subclavian vein

Thoracic duct

Diaphragm

Cisterna chyli

Pelvic lymph nodes

Lymphatic System Dysfunctions

Each cause of lymphedema interferes with the function of the lymphatic system in a different way. Lymphedema may result from a combination of these causes:

- Primary lymphedema is a congenital condition with several variations. A wide variety of lymphatic developmental abnormalities have been observed, including:

    - *Aplasia,* the absence of lymphatic vessels or nodes;

    - *Hyperplasia,* an excess number or enlargement of ineffective lymphatic vessels or nodes; or more commonly,

    - *Hypoplasia,* where there are fewer lymphatic structures than normal and those that are present are small and incomplete.[11]

- Trauma, large scars and burns (including radiation) often lead to tissue injuries which may destroy lymphatic vessels and impair normal lymphatic function in the skin. As wounds heal, lymphatic capillaries grow by sprouting from existing lymphatics. The ability to regenerate varies with the consistency of the connective tissue and the size of the injured area. Inflammation can destroy lymphatic vessels and infection interferes with lymphatic regeneration, possibly due to fibrosis.

- Lymph node dissection is a surgical procedure in which lymph nodes are removed; lymph node biopsy is a procedure where lymph node parts are removed surgically or with a sampling device. Both procedures damage lymph nodes and lymphatic vessels, resulting in more lymphatic fluid (since damaged nodes are not able to concentrate fluid) and less ability to remove fluid from the involved area. In cases of breast cancer, the axillary nodes are damaged and lymphatic drainage from the arm, breast, and trunk is disrupted; for prostate and other pelvic cancers, the inguinal or pelvic nodes are damaged, impairing lymphatic drainage from one or both legs.

- Obesity and lipedema increase the amount of fat in the body. Lymphatic vessels in the skin drain through the layer of fat located just under the skin (subcutaneous fat). As this fat layer becomes thicker and denser, it becomes harder for the lymph to pass through the fat. Subcutaneous fat separates the skin from the large muscles and may interfere with the natural pumping action of the muscles.

- Inactivity, paralysis, or muscle damage decreases the pumping action of the large muscles and joints that normally stimulates the drainage of lymph.

- Filariasis is caused by parasitic worms (filariae) that live in the lymphatic vessels and cause lymphatic vessel dilation and blockage. Filariasis is a tropical disease spread by mosquitoes. Treatment includes medication to kill the parasites and prevent infections due to breaks in the skin, combined with other lymphedema treatments.

Notes

1   **Living Well With Lymphedema** by Ann Ehrlich, Alma Vinjé-Harrewijn, and Elizabeth McMahon. Lymph Notes, 2005.

2   "Lymphedema Strategies for Management" by S. R. Cohen, ,D. K. Payne, et al. in Cancer Rehabilitation in the New Millennium, Supplement to *Cancer* 2001, 980-987.

3   **Modern Treatment for Lymphoedema, 5-E** by Judith R. Casley-Smith and J. R. Casley-Smith. The Lymphoedema Association of Australia, Inc., 1997, p. 25.

4   **Compendium of Dr. Vodder's Manual Lymph Drainage** by R. Kasseroller, Haug, 1998.

5   "The Lymphatic System in Pathology" by B. Lasinski in C. C. Goodman, et al. **Pathology Implications for the Physical Therapist 2-E**. Saunders, 2003, p. 484.

6   **Modern Treatment for Lymphoedema, 5-E** by Judith R. Casley-Smith and J. R. Casley-Smith. The Lymphoedema Association of Australia, Inc., 1997, p. 20.

7   **Lymphedema Management The Comprehensive Guide for Practitioners** by J. E. Zuther. Thieme 2005, p. 13.

8   **Lymphedema Management The Comprehensive Guide for Practitioners** by J. E. Zuther. Thieme 2005, p. 12.

9   **Textbook of Lymphology for Physicians and Lymphedema Therapists,** M. Földi, E. Földi, and S. Kubik eds. Urban & Fischer, 2003, p 514-516.

10 **Textbook of Lymphology for Physicians and Lymphedema Therapists,** M. Földi, E. Földi, and S. Kubik eds. Urban & Fischer, 2003, p. 514.

11 **A Primer on Lymphedema** by D. G. Kelly. Prentice Hall, 2002, p. 30.

Resources

Lymphedema Resources

Books

Living Well With Lymphedema by Ann Ehrlich, Alma Vinjé-Harrewijn, and Elizabeth McMahon. Lymph Notes, 2005.

Overcoming the Emotional Challenges of Lymphedema by Elizabeth McMahon. Lymph Notes, 2005.

Voices of Lymphedema edited by Ann Ehrlich and Elizabeth McMahon. Lymph Notes, 2007.

Lymphedema by the American Cancer Society. American Cancer Society; 2006.

Lymphedema: A Breast Cancer Patient's Guide to Prevention and Healing by Jeannie Burt and Gwen White. Hunter House, 2005.

Websites

Lymph Notes www.LymphNotes.com offers:

- Informative articles about lymphedema and related topics, and stories about people with lymphedema.

- Resources for treatment, supplies, support groups, etc.

- Support via the online forums.

National Lymphedema Network (NLN) www.lymphnet.org.

Lymphovenous Canada www.lymphovenous-canada.ca

Lymphedema Organizations

Organizations for patients and professionals (see **Voices of Lymphedema** for more information on these organizations and other resources):

- NLN: National Lymphedema Network, serving patients and professionals. www.lymphnet.org.

- LANA: Lymphology Association of North America, therapist certification, www.clt-lana.org.

- PLAN: Parents' Lymphedema Action Network, for parents of children with lymphedema, contact via NLN.

- LRF: Lymphatic Research Foundation, promoting and supporting lymphatic research, www.lymphaticresearch.org.

- ASL: American Society of Lymphology, establishing lymphology as a medical specialty in the US, www.lymphology.org.

- ISL: International Society of Lymphology, professional organization, www.u.arizona.edu/~witte.

- LAO: Lymphovenous Association of Ontario, patient group, www.lymphontario.org.

Lymphedema Bandages and Supplies

- ACOLS Store: www.acols.com or 1-800-863-5935.

- Bandages Plus: www.bandagesplus.com or 1-800-770-1032.

- Lymphedema Products: www.lymphedemaproducts.com or 1-866-445-9674.

See also the lymphedema resource directory on www.LymphNotes.com.

Compression Garment and Aid Companies

Most compression garment or aid manufacturers sell through medical supply companies, specially trained fitters, or therapists; some companies have their own sales departments. This list also includes makers of related clothing and donning or doffing aids. See "Managing Compression Garment and Aids" starting on page 299 for more information.

- Barely There: www.barelythere.com
- Barton-Carey: www.bartoncarey.com
- Bellisse: www.bellisse.com
- Circaid: www.circaid.com
- Comprefit: www.comprefit.com
- Compression Design: www.compressiondesign.com
- Danskin: www.danskin.com
- Design Veronique: www.DesignVeronique.com
- Dycem: www.dycem.com
- Farrow Medical/Farrow Wrap: www.farrowmedical.com
- Gottfried Medical: www.gottfriedmedical.com
- Hanes: www.Hanes.com
- Jobst: www.jobst-usa.com
- JoViPak: www.jovipak.com
- Juzo: www.juzo.com
- LympheDIVAs: www.lymphedivas.com
- Marika: www.Marika.com
- Medi: www.mediusa.com
- Peninsula Medical/ReidSleeve: www.reidsleeve.com
- Sassybax: www.sassybax.com
- Sigvaris: www.sigvaris.com

- Solaris: www.solaris-tribute.com

- Telesto Medtech: www.telesto-medtech.com

- Under Armour: www.UnderArmour.com

Caregiver Resources

Books on Caregiving

- **American Medical Association Guide to Home Caregiving** edited by Angela Perry. Wiley 2001.

- **The Comfort of Home** by Maria Meyer and Paula Derr. CareTrust Publications 2007.

- **The Complete Legal Guide to Senior Care** by Brette McWhoter Sember. Sphinx Publishing 2003.

- **Elder Care 911** by Susan Beerman and Judith Rappaport-Musson. Prometheus Books 2002.

- **The Eldercare Handbook** by Stella Mora Henry. Collins 2006.

- **How Can I Help?** By Monique Doyle Spencer. Adams Media, 2008.

- **How to Care for Your Parent's Money While Caring for Your Parents** by Sharon Burns and Raymond Forgue. McGraw Hill 2003.

- **Share the Care** by Cappy Caposssela and Sheila Warnock. Fireside 2004.

Budgeting and Direct Hiring Information

- Intuit (www.intuit.com) offers Quicken software for managing bills, payments and other information for multiple insurance plans including Medicare and supplemental plans.

- Family Health Budget (www.familyhealthbudget.com) offers tools for building a healthcare budget.

- Internal Revenue Service (IRS) www.irs.gov or 1-800-829-1040.

- US Citizenship and Immigration Services (USCIS), www.uscis.gov or 1-800-870-3676.

- Tax Counseling for the Elderly (TCE), call 1-800-829-1040.
- Volunteer Income Tax Assistance Program (VITA), call 1-800-829-1040.

Online Care Coordination and Information

- Care Central: www.carecentral.com
- Care Pages: www.carepages.com
- Caregiver Helper: www.caregiverhelper.com
- Caring Bridge: www.caringbridge.org
- Lotsa Helping Hands: www.lotsahelpinghands.com

Online Caregiver Resources

- AARP: www.aarp.org
- American Association for Homecare: www.aahomecare.org
- ARCH National Respite Network: www.archrespite.org
- Care.com: www.care.com
- Caregiver Alliance www.caregiver.org
- Caring Connections (www.caringinfo.org) a service of the National Hospice and Palliative Care Organization.
- Caring.com: www.caring.com
- Eldercare Locator/National Association of Area Agencies on Aging: www.eldercare.gov
- Empowering Caregivers: www.care-givers.com
- Family Caregiver Alliance: www.caregiver.org
- Family Caregiving 101: www.familycaregiving101.org
- Lance Armstrong Foundation: www.livestrong.org
- National Alliance for Caregiving: www.caregiving.org

- National Association of Professional Geriatric Care Managers (www.caremanager.org).

- National Clearinghouse for Long-Term Care Information: www.longtermcare.gov

- National Family Caregivers Association (www.nfcacares.org or www.thefamilycaregiver.org)

- Rosalynn Carter Institute: www.rosalynncarter.org

- Strength for Caregiving: www.strengthforcaring.com

- Well Spouse Association: www.wellspouse.org

Care Management Forms

Forms for planning and managing care, supplies, equipment, etc. are provided below. Letter sized versions of these forms can be downloaded from the book website (www.Lymphedema-Caregiver.com).

Form	Form Page	Instructions
Weekly Care Plan Form	424	333
Care Activity Form	425	338
Patient Information Form	426	372
Caregiver Information Form	427	375
Arm Measurement Form	428	63
Leg Measurement Form	429	64
Supply Form	430	281
Equipment Form	431	287, 299, 315
Medication Form	432	321
Item Needed Form	434	277
Order Form	435	277
Vendor Form	433	278

Forms for planning and tracking exercise routines start on page 149.

Weekly Care Plan

Patient: _____   Week of: _____

Time	Care Activity	Directions	Help/Who	M	T	W	T	F	S	S

Form to accompany Lymphedema Caregiver's Guide by Mary Kathleen Kearse, et. al. © 2009 by Lymph Notes, all rights reserved.

Care Activity Form

Patient:	

Care Activity:	Affected Area:

Preparation (supplies):

Instructions:

After (clean up, put away, record):

Form to accompany Lymphedema Caregiver's Guide by Mary Kathleen Kearse, et. al. © 2009 by Lymph Notes, all rights reserved.

Patient Information Form

Patient:						
Address: Telephone: Date of birth:	Health insurance plan(s): Identification numbers:					
Medical conditions/diagnoses:		Lymphedema affected areas:				
Emergency services number (911 equivalent): Urgent care facility:			Care coordinator:			
Primary medical care provider:				Lymphedema therapist:		
Other medical specialists:					Dentist:	
Emergency Contacts:						Allergies and other information:

Form to accompany Lymphedema Caregiver's Guide by Mary Kathleen Kearse, et. al. © 2009 by Lymph Notes, all rights reserved.

Caregiver Information Form

Caregiver:	
Address: Telephone: E-mail:	Schedule/Availability:
Emergency Contacts:	Other information:
Agency Information (if applicable):	Employee Information (if applicable):
Start date:	End date:
Notes:	

Form to accompany Lymphedema Caregiver's Guide by Mary Kathleen Kearse, et. al. © 2009 by Lymph Notes, all rights reserved.

Arm Measurement Form

Patient:

Affected Arm left/right/both (circle one)

Units: cm/inches (circle one)

Date/Time	Hand	Wrist	Mid-Forearm	Upper Arm
GOAL (uninvolved arm)				
BEST DAY				
Measurement				
Difference from Best Day				
Measurement				
Difference from Best Day				
Measurement				
Difference from Best Day				
Measurement				
Difference from Best Day				
Measurement				
Difference from Best Day				

Notes

Form to accompany Lymphedema Caregiver's Guide by Mary Kathleen Kearse, et. al. © 2009 by Lymph Notes, all rights reserved.

Leg Measurement Form

Patient: _____

Affected Leg left/right/both (circle one)

Units: cm/inches (circle one)

Date/Time		Arch of Foot	Ankle	Mid-Calf	Mid-Thigh
	GOAL (uninvolved leg)				
	BEST DAY				
	Measurement				
	Difference from Best Day				
	Measurement				
	Difference from Best Day				
	Measurement				
	Difference from Best Day				
	Measurement				
	Difference from Best Day				
	Measurement				
	Difference from Best Day				

Notes

Form to accompany *Lymphedema Caregiver's Guide* by Mary Kathleen Kearse, et. al. © 2009 by Lymph Notes, all rights reserved.

Supply Form

Patient:

Item: | **Reorder when:**

Order History

Order Date	Received On	Quantity/Size	Vendor	Cost/Reimbursement	Notes

Form to accompany Lymphedema Caregiver's Guide by Mary Kathleen Kearse, et. al. © 2009 by Lymph Notes, all rights reserved.

Equipment Form

Patient:

Item: **Quantity required:**

Order History

Order Date	Received On	Quantity/Size	Vendor	Cost/Reimbursement	Notes

Form to accompany Lymphedema Caregiver's Guide by Mary Kathleen Kearse, et. al. © 2009 by Lymph Notes, all rights reserved.

Medication Form

Patient:

Item: _____   Reorder when:

Storage location:

Order History

Order Date	Received On	Quantity/Size	Vendor	Cost/Reimbursement	Notes

Form to accompany Lymphedema Caregiver's Guide by Mary Kathleen Kearse, et. al. © 2009 by Lymph Notes, all rights reserved.

Vendor Form

Patient:

Company:
Address:

Telephone:
Web Site:
Contacts:

Products:

Ordering information:

Notes:

Form to accompany **Lymphedema Caregiver's Guide** by Mary Kathleen Kearse, et. al. © 2009 by Lymph Notes, all rights reserved.

Item Needed Form

Patient:

Item	Quantity/ Size	Date Added	Date Ordered	Vendor	Notes

Form to accompany Lymphedema Caregiver's Guide by Mary Kathleen Kearse, et. al. © 2009 by Lymph Notes, all rights reserved.

Order Form

Patient:

Vendor:

Order Date:
Order Number:

Received Date:

Item	Quantity/Size	Ordered	Received	Notes

Form to accompany Lymphedema Caregiver's Guide by Mary Kathleen Kearse, et. al. © 2009 by Lymph Notes, all rights reserved.

Index

About the Authors

Mary Kathleen (Kathy) Kearse, PT, CLT-LANA, has practiced physical therapy for 24 years in a variety of clinical settings and has worked full time with lymphedema patients for the past eight years. Her primary goal is to provide the best possible care for her patients in all aspects of their treatment and she has put her creative energy into developing solutions for problems faced by clients with special needs. She is an advocate for lymphedema patients and their caregivers, encouraging better quality of life through swelling management.

Kathy is a LANA certified lymphedema therapist and an active lymphedema educator making presentations on lymphedema, risk reduction techniques, and the treatment of pediatric and adolescent patients at local, regional, and international meetings. Her prior publications include "Case Study: Treatment of Two Siblings With Congenital Primary Lymphedema" in *NLN Lymph Link*.

Elizabeth McMahon, PhD is a clinical psychologist who brings to this book over 25 years of experience in helping patients, many of whom have chronic medical conditions. Elizabeth shares her expertise in helping these individuals learn the skills necessary to manage the anxiety, depression, and other emotional issues that may be part of living well with a chronic condition like lymphedema.

She is the coauthor of **Living Well with Lymphedema** (Lymph Notes 2005), the author of **Overcoming the Emotional Challenges of Lymphedema**

(Lymph Notes 2006), and the co-editor of **Voices of Lymphedema** (Lymph Notes 2007). Elizabeth has done multiple presentations on lymphedema-related topics for therapists and patients. In 2008, she presented a seminar on "Responding to Non-Compliance and Preventing Personal Burn Out" at the NLN International Conference.

Ann Ehrlich, MA is a professional medical writer with secondary lymphedema following breast cancer treatment. She is active on the Lymph Notes web site (www.lymphnotes.com), coauthor of **Living Well with Lymphedema** (Lymph Notes 2005), and co-editor of **Voices of Lymphedema** (Lymph Notes 2007).

Got Lymphedema? At risk for Lymphedema?

Get your free Lymphedema Wallet Card from LymphNotes.com. Carry this card with your insurance and ID cards to let emergency personnel know about your condition.

To receive your free wallet card, please send an e-mail to cards@lymphnotes.com. Be sure to include your postal address with your request.

Do you have a lymphedema support group?

No To find a support group, check the Lymphedema Resources directory on LymphNotes.com
and/or
Join our online support group in the Lymph Notes Forums: LymphNotes.com/bb/

Yes Be sure that your group is listed on Lymph Notes. To add your group, e-mail the information to groups@lymphnotes.com

Printed in the United States
213075BV00002B/6/P

9 780976 480679